Clinical Approaches in Endodontic Regeneration

Clinical Approaches in Endodontic Regeneration

Current and Emerging Therapeutic Perspectives

Henry F. Duncan • Paul Roy Cooper

Editors

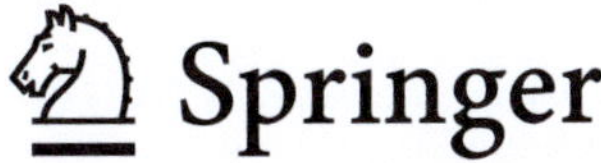 Springer

Editors
Henry F. Duncan
Dublin Dental University Hospital
Trinity College Dublin
University of Dublin
Dublin, Ireland

Paul Roy Cooper
School of Dentistry
University of Birmingham
Birmingham, United Kingdom

ISBN 978-3-030-07262-9   ISBN 978-3-319-96848-3   (eBook)
https://doi.org/10.1007/978-3-319-96848-3

This Springer imprint is published by the registered company Springer Nature Switzerland AG
The registered company address is: Gewerbestrasse 11, 6330 Cham, Switzerland

Foreword

Reflecting on the last 40+ years, we have experienced a golden age of pulp biology research with immense advances in our understanding of the structure and behaviour of the dental pulp both in health and after injury. While much of this research has focused more on the basic science aspects, it has provided a strong and robust platform from which we can now start to see clinical application of this knowledge and the emergence of regenerative endodontics in its broadest context as a clinical reality. New therapeutic strategies and approaches are always exciting for any clinical speciality, and this is especially true for endodontics where more traditional surgical protocols have centred mainly on effectively sealing the root canal(s) of the tooth. Exploitation of the bioactive properties of the dentine-pulp complex, its natural wound healing capacity and application of the principles of tissue engineering are all helping to underpin future clinical endodontic strategies. It is thus a great pleasure for me to offer this foreword to introduce a text, which fills a significant gap in the published literature. This text offers the reader an exciting and unique vision of where endodontics is going in the future. Few recent texts have offered more than a snapshot of clinical direction in endodontics, but the editors of the current work have brought together a strong group of experts to specifically provide focus on clinical direction based on recent advances in our understanding of pulp biology.

Paul Roy Cooper and Henry F. Duncan have strong reputations globally for their contributions and expertise in pulp biology and endodontics. The partnership of these researchers epitomises the characteristics of a first-class scientific-clinical partnership. Their research spans pulp stem cell biology, bioactive signalling molecules, inflammatory mediators and epigenetic mechanisms and has led to many novel and significant contributions. They are very well placed to provide the editorial leadership for the current text and have brought together a panel of distinguished authors for the various chapters who provide a wealth of experience and expertise on a range of key topics important to the future directions of clinical endodontics. The topics have been brought together in such a way that the overall scope of this text is much greater than the simple summation of the individual components. It will appeal to postgraduates, residents in training, researchers and practising clinicians, and I am sure it will help to inspire many people in the clinical endodontics areas. I am grateful to the editors and authors for providing us with this valuable insight and know that the text will become essential reading for those working in the area.

Anthony (Tony) J. Smith
Oral Biology, School of Dentistry
University of Birmingham
Birmingham, UK

Preface

At the inception of this project, we discussed with Tony Smith the need for another textbook in the pulp biology and regenerative endodontics field. We agreed that there was little point in investing effort in creating yet another encyclopaedic, largely scientific-based reference text, but in our view, there was room for a shorter and more focused clinical-translational book which would be the current 'go to' text in the field. The proposed volume should be 'cutting edge' and underpinned by current science but should discuss the implications on clinical therapy as well as the avenues for future research. As a result, we contacted an array of clinical and basic-scientist international friends, collaborators and colleagues working at the forefront of pulp biology, regenerative endodontics and vital pulp treatment research/practice to enlist their help with this project.

This resulting international book combines the clinical practice and the scientific base underpinning vital pulp treatment, by journeying through modern views on pulp disease, deep caries and pulp exposure management, before leading to an analysis of the biological aspects of regenerative techniques such as angiogenesis, neurogenesis, inflammation and epigenetics. In the latter chapters, practical considerations relating to bioengineering, biomaterial choice, revitalisation and cell homing-/stem cell-based procedures are discussed and their likely therapeutic impact being considered. Aimed at inspiring dental students, postgraduates and research-minded dental practitioners, this translational book summarises state-of-the-art scientific knowledge on dentine-pulp interactions and regenerative endodontics while highlighting to readers the opportunities for recent developments to be incorporated into their everyday practice. Included in each chapter is a discussion of the potential developments in each aspect of this exciting rapidly developing field.

Fundamentally, why should students and practitioners learn about current and emerging therapeutic strategies in endodontic regeneration? Perhaps the best answer is that over the last 10 years there has been a complete shift in dental treatment provision from the destructive 'drill and fill' doctrines of the past to novel methodologies promoting minimally invasive, biologically based dental restorative solutions. For patients with pulpal damage, this has resulted in a move away from invasive root canal treatment towards more conservative dental procedures aimed to protect the pulp and harness its natural regenerative capacity or replace the necrotic pulp with biological tissue. However, these new principles can be difficult to instil effectively in dentistry, as putting these regenerative endodontic strategies into practice requires a working understanding of the scientific processes of pulp/periapical disease and repair/regeneration. Therefore, an underlying theme of this book was to mix clinical chapters relating to disease and treatment with more basic science elements covering the processes of inflammation and regeneration.

That said, although the text is translational, readers will not find a pulp biology 'cookbook' indicating how to perform every regenerative endodontic procedure. Indeed biological procedures rarely lend themselves to this approach, and rather a scientific understanding of the importance and mechanisms behind the biological processes was deemed to be more important. Developing this book and working with our colleagues from around the world has been an enjoyable procedure, and as always it is the collaboration between us all as clinical and basic scientists which will continue to drive this field forward. We realise that at some point in the future, this book will pass its 'sell-by date', but in the meantime, hopefully, we have captured the 'here and now' of the field. We sincerely hope you enjoy the book and that it stimulates you the reader to foster a biological rather than technical outlook for the management and replacement of damaged pulp tissue in your everyday practice.

Dublin, Ireland   Henry F. Duncan
Birmingham, UK   Paul Roy Cooper

Contents

Current and Emerging Innovations in Minimally Invasive Caries and Endodontic Treatments

W. J. Wolters and L. W. M. van der Sluis

1.1   Introduction

Apical periodontitis (AP) is caused by an inflammatory reaction by the host immune system in response to the presence of bacteria (planktonic state or biofilm) and their products which are close to, in or outside the root canal system (i.e. periradicular around the root apex) (Haapasalo et al. 2011). Research indicates that the majority of both primary and resistant apical periodontitis cases have a radiographically visible apical periodontitis, which is associated with a periradicular biofilm (Wang et al. 2013). The goal of root canal treatment is to remove these bacteria and the associated biofilm in the root canal system to prevent or heal AP.

A biofilm develops when bacterial cells accumulate and aggregate at a liquid-solid interface. Biofilms are composed of bacteria encased in a matrix of highly hydrated extracellular polymeric substances (EPS) (Flemming and Wingender 2010). The matrix facilitates nutritional uptake and dispersal (Stewart and Franklin 2008) and gives the biofilm its viscoelastic properties. An established biofilm is very stubborn and difficult to remove due to these properties (Peterson et al. 2015), and the matrix also provides protection from chemical and mechanical disruption delivered via cleaning procedures and disinfectants (Stewart and Franklin 2008; Chavez de Paz 2007). Furthermore, if conditions become unfavourable, bacteria in the biofilm can enter a state of dormancy in which they can survive harsh conditions or chemical attacks, and examples of persistent bacterial cells have been identified which can survive almost many forms of disinfection regime (Flemming and Wingender 2010).

The complex root canal anatomy consists of isthmuses, oval extensions, and lateral canals, which often will not be reached by root canal instruments during root canal

W. J. Wolters (✉) · L. W. M. van der Sluis
Center of Dentistry and Oral Hygiene, University Medical Center Groningen, Groningen, The Netherlands
e-mail: w.j.wolters@umcg.nl; l.w.m.van.der.sluis@umcg.nl

© Springer Nature Switzerland AG 2019
H. F. Duncan, P. R. Cooper (eds.), *Clinical Approaches in Endodontic Regeneration*,
https://doi.org/10.1007/978-3-319-96848-3_1

preparation. In the areas where root canal files does reach the root canal walls during preparation, a smear layer with dentine debris is produced. This layer adheres to the root canal walls and is forced into the dentinal tubules (Pashley et al. 1988; Drake et al. 1994; Violich and Chandler 2010). Dentine is a porous material containing tubules with a diameter varying from 0.6 to 3.2 μm, with a length of up to 2 mm. These are accessible to microorganisms, and bacterial colonization of the root canal results in biofilm formation on the canal wall and in the dentinal tubules (Haapasalo et al. 2011). As a result of the persistence of the biofilm and the complexity of the root canal anatomy, it is not possible to totally eradicate the biofilm (Wang et al. 2012) and the smearlayer. As a result complete healing of AP is difficult to achieve (Wu et al. 2006).

The European Society of Endodontology (ESE) states that; 'Following successful root canal treatment the contours of the periodontal ligament space around the root should radiographically be normal' (European Society of Endodontology 2006). However, seemingly normal periapical radiographs lack sensitivity and underestimate the incidence of AP with histological cadaver studies showing that around 40% of cases remain undetected with this method (Wu et al. 2006). Research shows that the majority of root canal systems of endodontically treated teeth with radiographic signs of AP are infected. What they also show is that the majority of endodontically treated teeth *without* signs of AP are also infected or contaminated (Molander et al. 1998). These studies utilized paper point sampling and culturing of bacteria to arrive at their conclusion, which by modern microbiological standards is not a very sensitive methodology. If this research were to now be repeated using modern molecular techniques, all investigated teeth would likely be revealed as infected, harbouring many types of bacteria.

Since elimination of bacteria from a root canal system is near impossible, it becomes apparent that new approaches are required to prevent the development of AP. The bacterial colonization and infection of the root canal system should be prevented so that AP will not ensue. Vital pulpectomy (complete removal of the pulp) is a procedure that has been advocated to achieve this aim when irreversible pulpal damage is suspected and this procedure has been employed with good results (Sjogren et al. 1990; Marquis et al. 2006).

In many endodontic studies the absence of AP is radiographically assessed using the periapical index (PAI). This index links radiographic appearance to histological findings (Brynolf 1967). A higher score has been shown to be indicative of an increase in inflammatory tissue. In several publications low PAI scores of 1 and 2 are combined to represent the healing or success group (Wu et al. 2006, 2009). Here the success rate of endodontic treatments, of both AP and vital cases, is influenced by the decision of the researcher to include or exclude the PAI score of 2 in the healing or success group. If cases with the PAI score of 2 are not included in the success group and only PAI score 1 is used, representing absence of inflammation and normal radiographic appearance (European Society of Endodontology 2006), the success rate of conventional endodontic treatment reduces to only 70% and not 94% in vital pulpectomy cases (Ørstavik et al. 2004).

Cone beam computed tomography (CBCT) is a relatively new imaging modality used to evaluate root canal treatment and has shown that conventional endodontic treatment success rates drop even further, around another 10%, in comparison with standard evaluation of the treatment result using periapical radiographs (Abella et al. 2012; Al-Nuaimi et al. 2018). This, however, is not the only problem with conventional endodontic treatment of vital teeth. Conventional root canal treatment is time consuming and expensive. It weakens teeth and reduces the survival rate by causing apical cracks that possibly result in vertical root fractures (Shemesh et al. 2010; Liu et al. 2013).

1.2 Conclusion

Conventional endodontic treatment of teeth with vital pulps is less successful than expected. Bacteria and associated biofilms, present in the root canal system, are difficult to remove, and it is also possible that in time all root-filled teeth will become infected. This means that other treatment options must be considered. What are the alternative procedures to a full pulpectomy and root canal treatment?

1.3 Minimally Invasive Approaches

Recent research has suggested that pulp vitality can be preserved in more cases preventing the development of AP. Preservation of pulp vitality starts by following a conservative policy in the treatment of deep carious lesions and the inflamed/infected pulp. In the future, regenerative endodontic procedures (REPs) which have been defined as 'biologically based procedures designed to replace damaged structures, including dentine and root structures, as well as cells of the pulp-dentine complex' (Murray et al. 2007) may also offer opportunities in treating advanced cases of infected/necrotic pulps. If endodontic regeneration is to be successful, then infection control, biomaterials and stem cells must be integrated during treatment (Cao et al. 2015).

Research has shown that pulps, exhibiting symptoms of irreversible pulpitis, contain a stem cell/progenitor cell population. Further research and identification of the specific properties of these cells will help to establish if these cells could serve as a source of endogenous multipotent cells for dental tissue regeneration procedures in the future (Wang et al. 2010). Presently, there are no clinical protocols for undertaking this approach in the general practice, and dental tissue engineering remains an academic/research subject, which at present has offered mixed results, as the tissues generated cannot be designated as true pulp tissue (Cao et al. 2015; Saoud et al. 2016).

The principle objective of modern endodontics is the conservation and maintenance of pulp vitality, particularly when treating teeth with deep carious lesions. In the past thorough excavation has led to many pulp exposures, and application of a capping material was considered unpredictable. The most frequently used capping material was calcium hydroxide (CH), introduced to the dental field in 1921. It became the 'gold standard' of direct pulp capping materials for several decades, but direct capping was only advocated on vital pulps which had been accidentally injured and demonstrated no other symptoms (Baume and Holz 1981). This classically meant that conventional root canal treatment was indicated for teeth whose pulp was exposed during excavation of deep carious lesions, perhaps due to the limited success of calcium hydroxide capping in these cases (Dominguez et al. 2003; Li et al. 2015; Kundzina et al. 2017). Although calcium hydroxide was considered the gold standard, several disadvantages with its use have been reported: presence of tunnels in the dentine barrier, extensive dentine formation obliterating the pulp chamber, high solubility in oral fluids, the lack of adhesion and degradation after acid etching (Li et al. 2015). In recent years several new bioceramic materials have been developed; however, mineral trioxide aggregate (MTA), a tricalcium silicate-based material, seems to be the most promising as a direct pulp capping agent for use after carious pulp exposure (Bogen and Kuttler 2009; Torabinejad and Parirokh 2010) due to its excellent sealing properties and biocompatibility (Torabinejad and Parirokh 2010). Success rates of up to 85% have been reported in the cases where it has been used (Kundzina et al. 2017).

MTA demonstrates superior performance compared with calcium hydroxide: it reduces inflammation, hyperaemia and tissue necrosis. As well as creating thicker dentine bridges with minimal tunnel flaws, the apposition of dentine is also faster (Nair et al. 2008; Accorinte Mde et al. 2008; Asgary et al. 2008). Histologic studies and in vitro MTA research also report favourable results in relation to its biocompatibility, chemical and physical properties, sealing properties and antibacterial activity (Torabinejad and Parirokh 2010) with associated high clinical success rates (Li et al. 2015).

1.4 Caries Progression and Lesion Depth

Dental caries as a disease, results from an ecologic shift within the dental biofilm, from a balanced population of microorganisms to an acidogenic, acidoduric and cariogenic population. The shift in biofilm activity is developed and maintained by frequent consumption of fermentable dietary carbohydrates, which cause an imbalance between the de- and remineralization process. The resulting net loss of minerals within dental hard tissues leads to the formation of a carious lesion (Innes et al. 2016; Fejerskov et al. 2015). The carious process demineralizes and softens dentine, causing an inflammatory response in the pulp. When a lesion approaches the pulp, this response becomes heightened and increases in magnitude. It usually does not become severe until the carious lesion is very close to the pulp tissue (Bjørndal 2008; Siqueira Jr 2011). Classic research suggests that bacteria within 1.1 mm of the pulp have little impact on pulpal tissue and that the pulp only becomes inflamed when the carious lesion is within 0.5 mm of the pulp (Reeves and Stanley 1966). Predicting healing outcomes for pulps associated with deep carious lesions is notoriously difficult, but it is now understood that even cariously exposed pulps are not automatically associated with irreversible pulpitis. Indeed within one lesion the caries process can be active or arrested, with both processes having a different effect on the pulp (Bjørndal 2008). This outcome is related to the fact that the caries process can stop when the bacterial biofilm that sustains it is excluded from the oral environment promoting a biological shift, as a result of a reduction in nutrition. This then results in the softened dentine hardening. It is now accepted that the caries process stops when infected dentine is sealed off from the oral environment by a well-placed dental restoration, which deprives the remaining bacteria of nutrition and that complete removal of microorganisms/infected dentine is therefore not necessary even if it were possible to do so (Innes et al. 2016).

In the past caries progression and consequently lesion depth have been used as a measure for assessing pulpal health. The caries progression and extent were evaluated on bitewings radiographs, following a specific classification, with the depth of the lesion being used in several clinical studies to determine the subsequent treatment protocol regarding deep carious lesions (Bjørndal et al. 2010). However, this method has some limitations:

1. Caries progression towards the pulp is a three-dimensional process. The radiograph is only a two-dimensional representation and therefore unreliable to accurately assess the progression of caries.
2. The choice of treatment should be based on the pulpal diagnosis, as the reaction of the pulp to the carious lesion is an important factor predicting the potential for pulpal healing.
3. The caries progression itself or the depth of the lesion is secondary as pulpal healing does not depend on caries progression alone but also on the biofilm activity of the caries process and its effect on the pulp and if the pulp tissue is infected or not.

1.5   Pulpal Healing

An inflammatory reaction does not mean that the pulp is necessarily irreversibly damaged; inflammation is a normal healing response of the pulp (and other tissues) to a stimulus (Simon et al. 2011). Healing is a longitudinal process and whether healing occurs depends on the virulence of the microorganisms present and the healing capacity of the pulp. New observations regarding the pulp's healing processes in response to infected carious dentine have provided new insights into vital pulp therapy (Simon et al. 2011). Dentine can be considered a cellular tissue, in which the dentinal tubules contain cellular extensions of the odontoblasts that reside at the periphery of the pulp. Dentine and pulp, therefore, must be examined together as a pulp-dentinal complex (Pashley 1996). When the pulp is under microbial attack (caries), diffusion of microbes and microbial products towards the pulp is reduced by sclerosis of dentinal tubules and the development of tertiary dentine (Bjørndal 2008). These innate defensive mechanisms enable a resistance by the pulp to microbial attacks (Farges et al. 2013; Bjørndal et al. 2014). During the process of demineralization and formation of a carious lesion growth factors are released from the pulp-dentinal complex (Finkelman et al. 1990; Cassidy et al. 1997; Cooper et al.

2010, 2011) that where 'fossilized' in the dentine matrix during its initial formation. The release of these factors and their diffusion towards the pulp promote pulp repair and regeneration (Smith et al. 2012, 2016). Ongoing research continues to uncover new factors and their associated positive effects on the pulp (Tomson et al. 2017).

1.6   Conclusion

As the pulp is more resilient to microbial attacks than previously thought, it logically follows that caries progression and lesion depth should not dictate treatment modalities. Instead, observed clinical symptoms are more important in predicting pulpal healing potential and therefore are better suited to direct the treatment of choice.

1.7   Inflammation of the Pulp

There are different degrees of pulpitis, and in the classic concept, the process is classified as either reversible pulpitis (when there is no prolonged reaction to a cold stimulus) or irreversible pulpitis (when the patient experiences mild to strong pain that lasts for more than a few seconds, after a cold stimulus). Usually the treatment of choice following irreversible pulpitis is pulpectomy, which involves removal of all tissue from the pulp chamber and the root canal system. However, it is questionable if this is the best course of action in cases of so-called irreversible pulpitis. Indeed a lingering pain after a stimulus, usually associated with irreversible pulpitis, may not necessarily reflect an irreversible state of inflammation of the entire pulp.

Often, if symptoms of lingering pain after a cold/hot stimulus are present, only pulp tissue occupying the pulp chamber is irreversibly inflamed, while the pulp tissue in the root remains relatively uninflamed (Ricucci et al. 2014). Pulps demonstrating symptoms of irreversible pulpitis have a limited chance to revert to normal if only the irritant stimulus is removed. In these cases the intervention should include removal of the inflamed coronal pulp tissue so that the remaining uninflamed tissue can recover and heal (Ricucci et al. 2014). With the appropriate minimally invasive intervention, presumably, many pulps diagnosed with irreversible pulpitis have the potential to heal, and research has shown that this strategy is successful as teeth diagnosed with irreversible pulpitis have been successfully treated with a pulpotomy (Taha et al. 2017; Qudeimat et al. 2017; Asgary et al. 2014).

Careful clinical pulpal diagnosis, including a detailed report of the patient's complaints (Bender 2000), could be a better alternative to indicate the status of the pulp. In order to determine the best treatment approach of each case, the extent of pulpal inflammation has to be determined and reflected in the diagnosis. All clinical relevant information including a through patient pain history is of paramount importance. By careful examination and a thorough anamnesis, cases with extensive irreversible pulpitis (treated with extraction or pulpectomy) could potentially be separated from cases which are not extensively inflamed but which have traditionally been diagnosed as being irreversible as well. In these cases the inflammation is most probably confined to the pulp chamber and the remaining pulp can therefore be considered to be reversibly inflamed, because part of the pulp remains vital (Ricucci et al. 2014). If this residual pulp vitality is preserved, then the prognosis for survival of the tooth is improved (Aguilar and Linsuwanont 2011). The role of percussion as a diagnostic tool may also be critical. A positive outcome when using percussion indicates inflammation at the periapex (apical periodontitis). This does not mean, however, that microbes are necessarily present in the periapex. The infection could be limited to the coronal pulp whereby diffusing microbial metabolites cause an inflammatory process in the region of the periapex. The inflammation can also be sterile as a result of cellular damage caused by mechanical trauma/force/overburdening. When the trauma subsides, the cellular damage is resolved, and the pulp and periapical tissues heal, and there is no more pain. This means that acute apical periodontitis can also be considered reversible or irreversible.

The patient's account of symptoms can give an accurate impression of the pulpal condition of the tooth in question. A properly conducted clinical pulpal examination can now accurately reflect the histological condition of the pulp, contradicting older research (Ricucci et al. 2014). Research shows that clinical symptoms with regard to the inflammatory condition of the pulp correspond well with histological changes with a clinical diagnosis of normal/reversible and irreversible pulpitis corresponding to 96.6% and 84.4% of cases with the actual histological state of the pulp (Ricucci et al. 2014). Upon examination it has become apparent that in both diagnostic situations the pulpal inflammation was confined to the pulp chamber only. Pulpal tissue in the root canals however was not inflamed (Aguilar and Linsuwanont 2011).

1.8   Conclusion

The development of a new more detailed system for diagnosing different stages of pulpits for the correct assessment of pulpal condition would be helpful, and it has been shown that this is important in the prediction of treatment outcomes (Bjørndal et al. 2010). The fact that the regenerative potential of the pulp-dentinal complex is evident in teeth with symptoms indicative of irreversible pulpitis indicates that the current classification of pulpitis may need to be revised (Ricucci et al. 2014). Probably cases traditionally deemed irreversible may in fact still be salvageable, thereby shifting the balance of what was irreversible towards reversible, when the appropriate treatment is applied (Taha et al. 2017).

1.9   Minimal Intervention Treatment of Deep Carious Lesions

1.9.1   Treatment Options for Deep Carious Lesions

1.9.1.1 Partial Caries Removal
Root canal treatment should be avoided when treating deep carious lesions, and instead partial (or selective) caries removal (PCR) strategies should be used to

prevent unnecessary pulpal exposures (Leksell et al. 1996). The PCR procedure is performed on teeth with deep carious lesions approximating the pulp, but without signs or symptoms of pulp degeneration. During PCR the periphery of the cavity is cleaned and should consist of 'sound' enamel, and the adjacent peripheral dentine should be hard to allow for the best adhesive seal during the restoration procedure (Innes et al. 2016). The caries surrounding the pulp is left in situ to avoid pulp exposure before being 'sealed' by the restoration. This means that within the PCR procedure only the biofilm covering the dentine surface in the cavity is removed rather than all 'infected dentine' (Gruythuysen et al. 2010). The residual bacterial population in proximity to the pulp do not appear to multiply in sealed lesions, and several studies involving microbiological monitoring indicate a substantial reduction in cultivable flora (Bjørndal and Larsen 2000; Paddick et al. 2005), and it has been shown that sealing in bacteria has no detrimental effects on the pulp (Ricketts et al. 2013). It appears that the microbial flora ecologically changes to a less cariogenic composition due to being isolated from the oral environment by the restoration and tubular sclerosis, as nutrients become limited (Bjørndal and Larsen 2000; Paddick et al. 2005).

1.9.1.2 Stepwise Excavation

Stepwise excavation (SW) procedures entail the removal of caries in two steps in order to reduce the risk of pulp exposure. During the first step carious dentine is removed peripherally, followed by provisionally sealing of the cavity, leaving infected soft dentine in place until the second intervention, weeks or months later. This allows time for the lesion to remineralise and sclerose as well as for the formation of tertiary dentine. This is critical as it reduces (but does not eliminate) the risk of pulp exposure and postoperative complications after the second excavation procedure. This approach is performed after some time to completely excavate the caries, followed by definitive cavity restoration (Bjørndal 2011).

A recent review concluded that partial caries removal has a better prognosis when treating deep carious lesions, as pulpal exposure does occur more often when the two-step SW procedure is performed (Maltz et al. 2018). Adjusted survival rates in a study comparing both techniques were 91% for PCR and 69% for SW. These results indicate that it is potentially better to avoid reopening a cavity and performing a second excavation for pulp vitality to be preserved (Maltz et al. 2012a, b, 2013; Hoefler et al. 2016). It is difficult to evaluate the restoration failure after the different approaches; however, it appears that the risk of failure was similar for complete and incompletely excavated teeth (Schwendicke et al. 2013). Evidently, the burden on patients is however less with a one-visit treatment.

1.10 Conclusion

The carious dentine that has been sealed in a one-step procedure does not affect pulp vitality, and research now suggests that the procedure of reopening the cavity in a second step for more carious dentine removal is not necessary.

1.11 When Do We Need to Treat the Pulp Directly?

In a recently published study on IPT (Hashem et al. 2015), a new classification based on clinical symptoms was introduced:

- *Mild reversible pulpitis*: sensitivity to hot, cold and sweet lasting up to 15–20 s and settling spontaneously
- *Severe reversible pulpitis*: increased pain for more than several minutes and needing oral analgesics

Both classifications are normally related to the clinical diagnosis of irreversible pulpitis, but when cases exhibiting irreversible symptoms were treated with PCR, the first group had a success rate of around 90.25% and the second group 68%, after 1 year (Hashem et al. 2015). This indicates that in pulps with severe reversible pulpitis, healing was less predictable. These pulps could perhaps benefit from direct intervention with a partial or total pulpotomy procedure to remove inflamed tissue and preserve partial vitality.

Often a pulpotomy is performed as an emergency measure to relieve pain when a tooth is diagnosed clinically with irreversible pulpitis (Eren et al. 2018). However, if pulp tissue in root canals is not inflamed/infected, removal of the infected pulp tissue from the pulp chamber should enable the remaining tissue in the root to remain healthy and viable when it is covered with a biocompatible material. It has been shown that after pulpotomies using MTA, root canals do not show signs of calcific obliteration, and there were no signs of apical pathology evident radiographically after a 2-year period (Simon et al. 2013). It seems that pulpotomies of teeth with the clinical pulpal diagnosis of irreversible pulpitis have comparable outcomes to 'complete' root canal treatments (pulpectomy) (Simon et al. 2013; Asgary et al. 2013; Alqaderi et al. 2016).

If the treatment of choice is pulpectomy and not pulpotomy, it is not yet completely clear how far instrumentation and removal of pulpal tissue should extend. Should instrumentation be extended to the apical foramen or to 'stay short' and intentionally leave a vital apical pulp stump (Wu et al. 2000). The literature indicates that leaving an apical pulp stump has advantages. The remaining viable tissue in the canal above the apical constriction can withstand the trauma of instrumentation and irrigation better than the periapical tissue near the constriction. Furthermore, less deep instrumentation reduces the technical risk of ledging in the often tortuous apical portion of the root and prevents overfilling and extrusion of root canal fill material in the apical portion, which is associated with lower clinical success rates.

1.12 Conclusion

Pulpotomies have a high success rate. How much tissue to remove and when to implement the appropriate measure depends on the extent of pulpal inflammation. This can be ascertained by the clinical symptoms observed, and therefore a new pulpal diagnosis system is needed to differentiate between the different stages of pulpitis.

1.13 Pulpal Diagnosis

1.13.1 Pulpitis: Symptom Assessment and Pulpal Diagnosis: A New Philosophy

It has become clear that it is time to re-evaluate pulpitis and conventional root canal treatment procedures. Caries progression should not dictate treatment modalities, but observed clinical symptoms reflect the state of the pulp and therefore need to indicate the choice of treatment. Many pulps diagnosed with irreversible pulpitis have the potential to heal if the appropriate minimally invasive treatments are implemented. This means that lingering pain after a stimulus, normally recognized as indicative of irreversible pulpitis, does not necessarily reflect an irreversible state of inflammation of the entire pulp, and often only pulp tissue located in the pulp chamber is irreversibly inflamed when these symptoms are present. PCR or coronal pulpotomy can provide an excellent less invasive alternative treatment which allows the remaining uninflamed/reversibly inflamed pulp tissue to regenerate and heal (Taha et al. 2017).

1.13.2 A New Proposal for Clinical Pulp Diagnosis Terminology and Associated Treatment Modalities (Wolters et al. 2017)

1.13.2.1 Initial Pulpitis

Heightened but not lengthened response to a cold stimulus, not sensitive to percussion and no spontaneous pain.

Therapy: Indirect pulp therapy (van der Sluis et al. 2013).

1.13.2.2 Mild Pulpitis

Heightened and lengthened reaction to cold, warmth and sweet stimuli that can last up to 20 s but then subsides. The tooth is possibly percussion sensitive, but there is no spontaneous pain. Symptoms in agreement with histological findings imply that there is limited local pulpal inflammation confined to the crown pulp.

Therapy: Indirect pulp therapy (van der Sluis et al. 2013; Asgary et al. 2015).

1.13.2.3 Moderate Pulpitis

Clear symptoms, strong, heightened and prolonged reaction to a cold stimulus, which can last for minutes. Possibly percussion sensitive and dull spontaneous pain that can be more or less suppressed with pain medication. Symptoms in agreement with histological findings imply that there is extensive local pulpal inflammation confined to the crown.

Therapy: Coronal pulpotomy—partial/complete (Fig. 1.1)

1.13.2.4 Severe Pulpitis

Severe sharp to dull pain symptoms. Pain medication does not give much relief, and the patient has difficulty sleeping because of the pain (gets worse when lying down). Strongly painful reaction to cold and warm stimuli is present. The tooth is very sensitive to touch and percussion. Symptoms are in agreement with histological

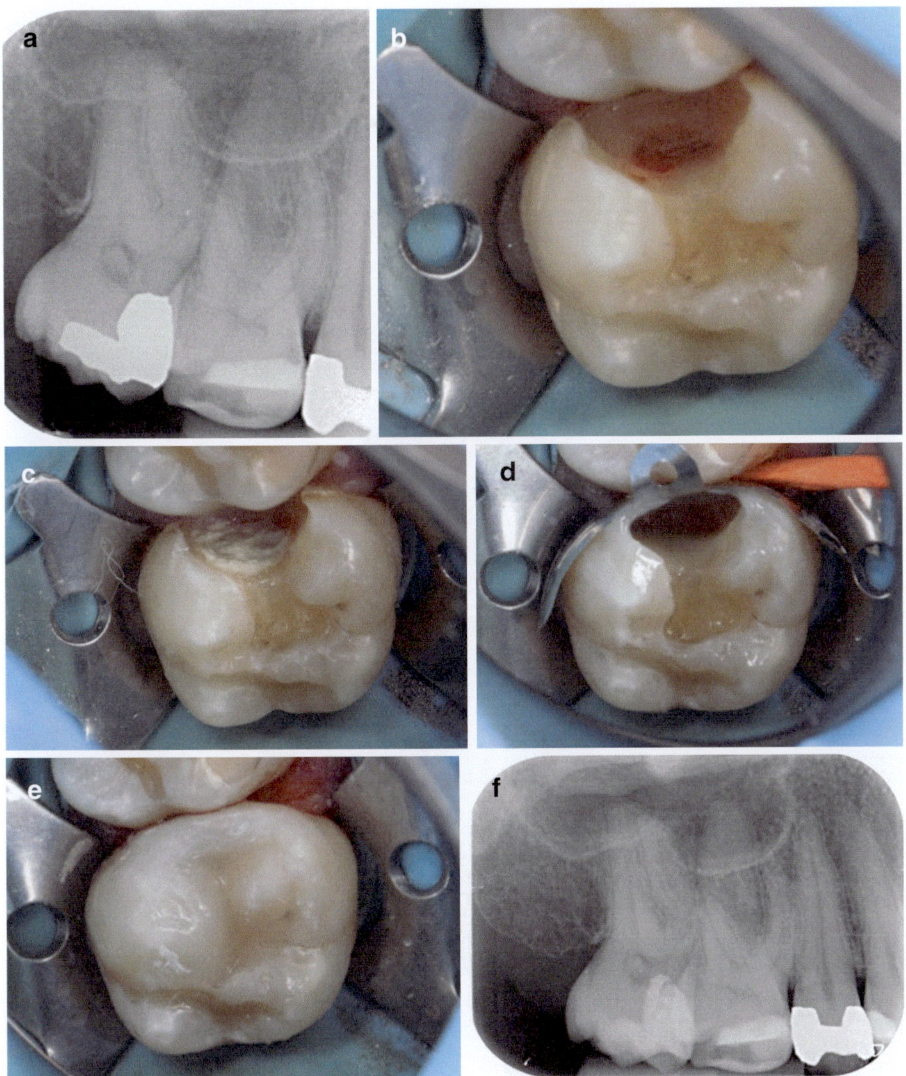

Fig. 1.1 (**a–f**) Partial pulpotomy treatment of a molar (Ng et al. 2008) exhibiting symptoms of moderate pulpitis. After partial removal of inflamed/infected tissue, the remaining tissue is covered with MTA and restored with resin-based composite. After 1 year the tooth responds normally to a cold stimulus (Figures courtesy of M. Marques, private practice, Netherlands)

findings which imply that there is extensive local pulpal inflammation in the crown pulp that possibly extends into the root canals.

Therapy: Coronal pulpotomy—if the haemorrhage is controlled and there is no prolonged bleeding of pulp stumps in the orifices of the canals, these are covered with MTA, followed by restoration (Alqaderi et al. 2016). If one or more of the pulp stumps continues bleeding after rinsing with 2 mL 2% NaOCl, a partial pulpectomy can be carried out. This means removing more of the inflamed tissue until approximately 3–4 mm from the radiographic apex remains. When bleeding ceases the vital short pulp stump is left in situ, and the rest of the root canal is filled with gutta-percha and cement at this working length. If bleeding does not stop, then a full pulpectomy should be performed in order to remove all inflamed tissue from the canal (Matsuo et al. 1996) (Fig. 1.2).

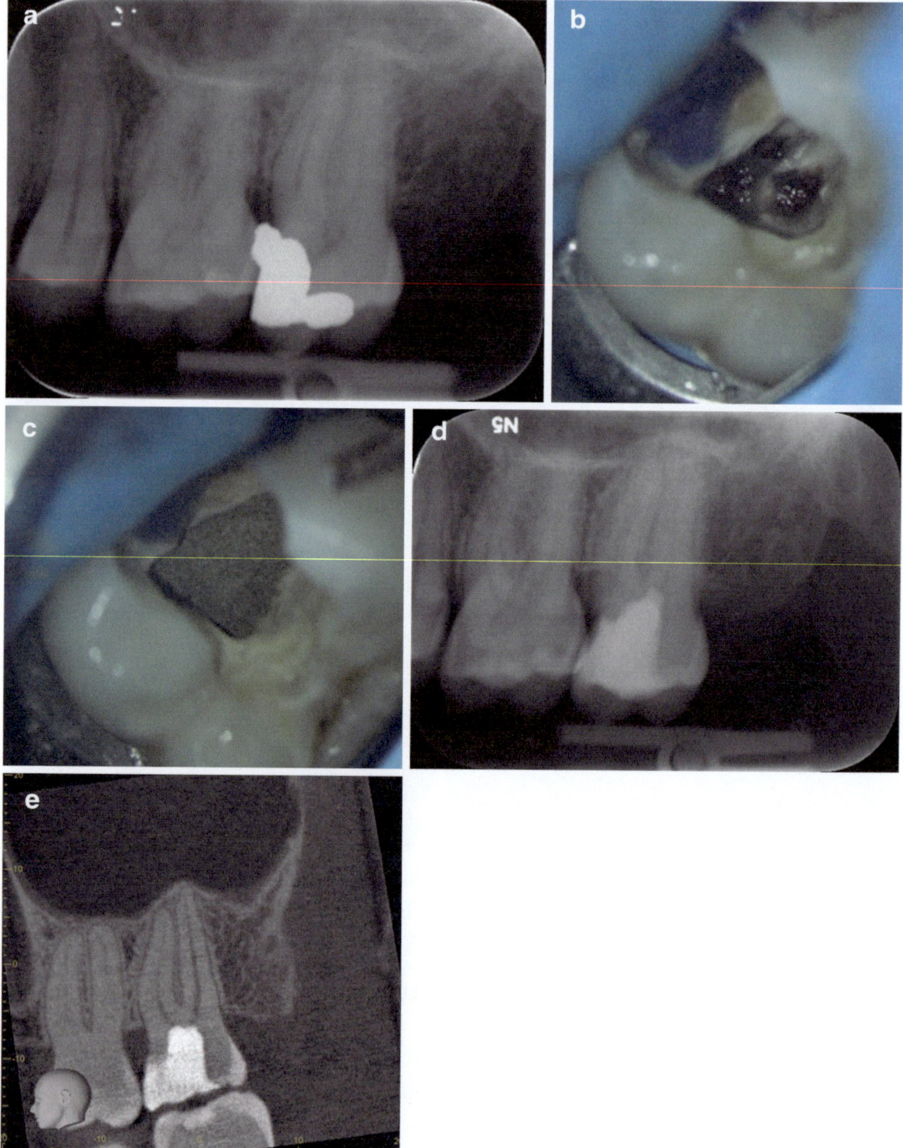

Fig. 1.2 (**a–e**) Coronal pulpotomy treatment of a molar (Wang et al. 2010) exhibiting symptoms of severe pulpitis. After removal of the crown pulp, the canal orifices are covered with MTA, and the tooth is restored with composite. After 15 months recall the tooth shows no signs of periapical pathosis (Figures courtesy of M. Marques, private practice, Netherlands)

1.14 Conclusion

The minimally invasive endodontic approach has several benefits:

- Maintaining the viability of the pulp as long as possible to induce a biological response to prevent apical periodontitis and improving the success rate of vital pulp treatment
- Saving tooth structure and consequently increasing tooth survival
- Saving time and cost for both the patient and/or society
- Reducing pain and discomfort for the patient with these less invasive treatments and keeping teeth functional for longer

References

Abella F, Patel S, Duran-Sindreu F, Mercadé M, Bueno R, Roig M (2012) Evaluating the periapical status of teeth with irreversible pulpitis by using cone-beam computed tomography scanning and periapical radiographs. J Endod 38(12):1588–1591. https://doi.org/10.1016/j.joen.2012.09.003

Accorinte Mde L, Holland R, Reis A, Bortoluzzi MC, Murata SS, Dezan E Jr, Souza V, Alessandro LD (2008) Evaluation of mineral trioxide aggregate and calcium hydroxide cement as pulp-capping agents in human teeth. J Endod 34(1):1–6

Aguilar P, Linsuwanont P (2011) Vital pulp therapy in vital permanent teeth with cariously exposed pulp: a systematic review. J Endod 37(5):581–587. https://doi.org/10.1016/j.joen.2010.12.004

Al-Nuaimi N, Patel S, Davies A, Bakhsh A, Foschi F, Mannocci F (2018) Pooled analysis of 1-year recall data from three root canal treatment outcome studies undertaken using cone beam computed tomography. Int Endod J 51:e216. https://doi.org/10.1111/iej.12844

Alqaderi H, Lee CT, Borzangy S, Pagonis TC (2016) Coronal pulpotomy for cariously exposed permanent posterior teeth with closed apices: a systematic review and meta-analysis. J Dent 44:1–7. https://doi.org/10.1016/j.jdent.2015.12.005

Asgary S, Eghbal MJ, Parirokh M, Ghanavati F, Rahimi H (2008) A comparative study of histologic response to different pulp capping materials and a novel endodontic cement. Oral Surg Oral Med Oral Pathol Oral Radiol Endod 106(4):609–614. https://doi.org/10.1016/j.tripleo.2008.06.006

Asgary S, Eghbal MJ, Ghoddusi J, Yazdani S (2013) One-year results of vital pulp therapy in permanent molars with irreversible pulpitis: an ongoing multicenter, randomized, non-inferiority clinical trial. Clin Oral Investig 17(2):431–439. https://doi.org/10.1007/s00784-012-0712-6

Asgary S, Fazlyab M, Sabbagh S, Eghbal MJ (2014) Outcomes of different vital pulp therapy techniques on symptomatic permanent teeth: a case series. Iran Endod J 9(4):295–300

Asgary S, Eghbal MJ, Fazlyab M, Baghban AA, Ghoddusi J (2015) Five-year results of vital pulp therapy in permanent molars with irreversible pulpitis: a non-inferiority multicenter randomized clinical trial. Clin Oral Investig 19(2):335–341. https://doi.org/10.1007/s00784-014-1244-z

Baume LJ, Holz J (1981) Long term clinical assessment of direct pulp capping. Int Dent J 31(4):251–260

Bender IB (2000) Reversible and irreversible painful pulpitides: diagnosis and treatment. Aust Endod J 26(1):10–14

Bjørndal L (2008) The caries process and its effect on the pulp: the science is changing and so is our understanding. Pediatr Dent 30(3):192–196

Bjørndal L (2011) In deep cavities stepwise excavation of caries can preserve the pulp. Evid Based Dent 12(3):68. https://doi.org/10.1038/sj.ebd.6400803

Bjørndal L, Larsen T (2000) Changes in the cultivable flora in deep carious lesions following a stepwise excavation procedure. Caries Res 34(6):502–508

Bjørndal L, Reit C, Bruun G, Markvart M, Kjaeldgaard M, Näsman P, Thordrup M, Dige I, Nyvad B, Fransson H, Lager A, Ericson D, Petersson K, Olsson J, Santimano EM, Wennström A, Winkel P, Gluud C (2010) Treatment of deep caries lesions in adults: randomized clinical trials comparing stepwise vs. direct complete excavation, and direct pulp capping vs. partial pulpotomy. Eur J Oral Sci 118(3):290–297. https://doi.org/10.1111/j.1600-0722.2010.00731.x

Bjørndal L, Demant S, Dabelsteen S (2014) Depth and activity of carious lesions as indicators for the regenerative potential of dental pulp after intervention. J Endod 40(4 Suppl):S76–S81. https://doi.org/10.1016/j.joen.2014.01.016

Bogen G, Kuttler S (2009) Mineral trioxide aggregate obturation: a review and case series. J Endod 35(6):777–790. https://doi.org/10.1016/j.joen.2009.03.006

Brynolf I (1967) Histological and roentgenological study of periapical region of human upper incisors. Odontol Revy 18(Suppl 11)

Cao Y, Song M, Kim E, Shon W, Chugal N, Bogen G, Lin L, Kim RH, Park NH, Kang MK (2015) Pulp-dentine regeneration: current state and future prospects. J Dent Res 94(11):1544–1551. https://doi.org/10.1177/0022034515601658

Cassidy N, Fahey M, Prime SS, Smith AJ (1997) Comparative analysis of transforming growth factor-beta isoforms 1-3 in human and rabbit dentine matrices. Arch Oral Biol 42(3):219–223

Chavez de Paz LE (2007) Redefining the persistent infection in root canals: possible role of biofilm communities. J Endod 33(6):652–662

Cooper PR, Takahashi Y, Graham LW, Simon S, Imazato S, Smith AJ (2010) Inflammation-regeneration interplay in the dentine-pulp complex. J Dent 38(9):687–697. https://doi.org/10.1016/j.jdent.2010.05.016

Cooper PR, McLachlan JL, Simon S, Graham LW, Smith AJ (2011) Mediators of inflammation and regeneration. Adv Dent Res 23(3):290–295. https://doi.org/10.1177/0022034511405389

van der Sluis L, Kidd E, Gruythuysen R, Peters L (2013) Preventive endodontics - an argument for avoiding root canal treatment. ENDO 4:259–274

Dominguez MS, Witherspoon DE, Gutmann JL, Opperman LA (2003) Histological and scanning electron microscopy assessment of various vital pulp-therapy materials. J Endod 29(5):324–333

Drake DR, Wiemann AH, Rivera EM, Walton RE (1994) Bacterial retention in canal walls in vitro: effect of smear layer. J Endod 20(2):78–82

Eren B, Onay EO, Ungor M (2018) Assessment of alternative emergency treatments for symptomatic irreversible pulpitis: a randomized clinical trial. Int Endod J 51:e227. https://doi.org/10.1111/iej.12851

European Society of Endodontology (2006) Quality guidelines for endodontic treatment: consensus report of the European Society of Endodontology. Int Endod J 39(12):921–930

Farges JC, Alliot-Licht B, Baudouin C, Msika P, Bleicher F, Carrouel F (2013) Odontoblast control of dental pulp inflammation triggered by cariogenic bacteria. Front Physiol 4:326. https://doi.org/10.3389/fphys.2013.00326

Fejerskov O, Nyvad B, Kidd EA (2015) Pathology of dental caries. In: Fejerskov O, Nyvad B, Kidd EAM (eds) Dental caries: the disease and its clinical management, 3rd edn. Wiley Blackwell, Oxford, pp 7–9

Finkelman RD, Mohan S, Jennings JC, Taylor AK, Jepsen S, Baylink DJ (1990) Quantitation of growth factors IGF-I, SGF/IGF-II, and TGF-beta in human dentine. J Bone Miner Res 5(7):717–723

Flemming HC, Wingender J (2010) The biofilm matrix. Nat Rev Microbiol 8(9):623–633. https://doi.org/10.1038/nrmicro2415

Gruythuysen RJ, van Strijp AJ, Wu MK (2010) Long-term survival of indirect pulp treatment performed in primary and permanent teeth with clinically diagnosed deep carious lesions. J Endod 36(9):1490–1493. https://doi.org/10.1016/j.joen.2010.06.006

Haapasalo M, Shen Y, Ricucci D (2011) Reasons for persistent and emerging post-treatment endodontic disease. Endod Topics 18:31–50. https://doi.org/10.1111/j.1601-1546.2011.00256.x

Hashem D, Mannocci F, Patel S, Manoharan A, Brown JE, Watson TF, Banerjee A (2015) Clinical and radiographic assessment of the efficacy of calcium silicate indirect pulp capping: a randomized controlled clinical trial. J Dent Res 94(4):562–568. https://doi.org/10.1177/0022034515571415

Hoefler V, Nagaoka H, Miller CS (2016) Long-term survival and vitality outcomes of permanent teeth following deep caries treatment with step-wise and partial-caries-removal: a systematic review. J Dent 54:25–32. https://doi.org/10.1016/j.jdent.2016.09.009

Innes NPT, Frencken JE, Bjørndal L, Maltz M, Manton DJ, Ricketts D, Van Landuyt K, Banerjee A, Campus G, Doméjean S et al (2016) Managing carious lesions: consensus recommendations on terminology. Adv Dent Res 28(2):49–57. https://doi.org/10.1177/0022034516639276

Kundzina R, Stangvaltaite L, Eriksen HM, Kerosuo E (2017) Capping carious exposures in adults: a randomized controlled trial investigating mineral trioxide aggregate versus calcium hydroxide. Int Endod J 50(10):924–932. https://doi.org/10.1111/iej.12719

Leksell E, Ridell K, Cvek M, Mejàre I (1996) Pulp exposure after stepwise versus direct complete excavation of deep carious lesions in young posterior permanent teeth. Endod Dent Traumatol 12(4):192–196

Li Z, Cao L, Fan M, Xu Q (2015) Direct pulp capping with calcium hydroxide or mineral trioxide aggregate: a meta-analysis. J Endod 41(9):1412–1417. https://doi.org/10.1016/j.joen.2015.04.012

Liu R, Kaiwar A, Shemesh H, Wesselink PR, Hou B, Wu MK (2013) Incidence of apical root cracks and apical dentineal detachments after canal preparation with hand and rotary files at different instrumentation lengths. J Endod 39(1):129–132. https://doi.org/10.1016/j.joen.2012.09.019

Maltz M, Garcia R, Jardim JJ, de Paula LM, Yamaguti PM, Moura MS, Garcia F, Nascimento C, Oliveira A, Mestrinho HD (2012a) Randomized trial of partial vs. stepwise caries removal: 3-year follow-up. J Dent Res 91(11):1026–1031. https://doi.org/10.1177/0022034512460403

Maltz M, Henz SL, de Oliveira EF, Jardim JJ (2012b) Conventional caries removal and sealed caries in permanent teeth: a microbiological evaluation. J Dent 40(9):776–782. https://doi.org/10.1016/j.jdent.2012.05.011

Maltz M, Jardim JJ, Mestrinho HD, Yamaguti PM, Podestá K, Moura MS, de Paula LM (2013) Partial removal of carious dentine: a multicenter randomized controlled trial and 18-month follow-up results. Caries Res 47(2):103–109. https://doi.org/10.1159/000344013

Maltz M, Koppe B, Jardim JJ, Alves LS, de Paula LM, Yamaguti PM, Almeida JCF, Moura MS, Mestrinho HD (2018) Partial caries removal in deep caries lesions: a 5-year multicenter randomized controlled trial. Clin Oral Investig 22:1337. https://doi.org/10.1007/s00784-017-2221-0

Marquis VL, Dao T, Farzaneh M, Abitbol S, Friedman S (2006) Treatment outcome in endodontics: the Toronto Study. Phase III: initial treatment. J Endod 32(4):299–306

Matsuo T, Nakanishi T, Shimizu H, Ebisu S (1996) A clinical study of direct pulp capping applied to carious-exposed pulps. J Endod 22(10):551–556

Molander A, Reit C, Dahlén G, Kvist T (1998) Microbiological status of root-filled teeth with apical periodontitis. Int Endod J 31(1):1–7

Murray PE, Garcia-Godoy F, Hargreaves KM (2007) Regenerative endodontics: a review of current status and a call for action. J Endod 33(4):377–390

Nair PN, Duncan HF, Pitt Ford TR, Luder HU (2008) Histological, ultrastructural and quantitative investigations on the response of healthy human pulps to experimental capping with mineral trioxide aggregate: a randomized controlled trial. Int Endod J 41(2):128–150

Ng YL, Mann V, Rahbaran S, Lewsey J, Gulabivala K (2008) Outcome of primary root canal treatment: systematic review of the literature -- Part 2. Influence of clinical factors. Int Endod J 41(1):6–31

Ørstavik D, Qvist V, Stoltze K (2004) A multivariate analysis of the outcome of endodontic treatment. Eur J Oral Sci 112(3):224–230

Paddick JS, Brailsford SR, Kidd EA, Beighton D (2005) Phenotypic and genotypic selection of microbiota surviving under dental restorations. Appl Environ Microbiol 71(5):2467–2472

Pashley DH (1996) Dynamics of the pulpo-dentine complex. Crit Rev Oral Biol Med 7(2):104–133

Pashley DH, Tao L, Boyd L, King GE, Horner JA (1988) Scanning electron microscopy of the substructure of smear layers in human dentine. Arch Oral Biol 33(4):265–270

Peterson BW, He Y, Ren Y, Zerdoum A, Libera MR, Sharma PK, van Winkelhoff A-J, Neut D, Stoodley P, van der Mei HC, Busscher HJ (2015) Viscoelasticity of biofilms and their recalcitrance to mechanical and chemical challenges. FEMS Microbiol Rev 39(2):234–245. https://doi.org/10.1093/femsre/fuu008

Qudeimat MA, Alyahya A, Hasan AA (2017) Mineral trioxide aggregate pulpotomy for permanent molars with clinical signs indicative of irreversible pulpitis: a preliminary study. Int Endod J 50(2):126–134. https://doi.org/10.1111/iej.12614

Reeves R, Stanley HR (1966) The relationship of bacterial penetration and pulpal pathosis in carious teeth. Oral Surg Oral Med Oral Pathol 22(1):59–65

Ricketts D, Lamont T, Innes NP, Kidd E, Clarkson JE (2013) Operative caries management in adults and children. Cochrane Database Syst Rev 3:CD003808. https://doi.org/10.1002/14651858.CD003808.pub3

Ricucci D, Loghin S, Siqueira JF Jr (2014) Correlation between clinical and histologic pulp diagnoses. J Endod 40(12):1932–1939. https://doi.org/10.1016/j.joen.2014.08.010

Saoud TM, Martin G, Chen YH, Chen KL, Chen CA, Songtrakul K, Malek M, Sigurdsson A, Lin LM (2016) Treatment of mature permanent teeth with necrotic pulps and apical periodontitis using regenerative endodontic procedures: a case series. J Endod 42(1):57–65. https://doi.org/10.1016/j.joen.2015.09.015

Schwendicke F, Dörfer CE, Paris S (2013) Incomplete caries removal: a systematic review and meta-analysis. J Dent Res 92(4):306–314. https://doi.org/10.1177/0022034513477425

Shemesh H, Wesselink PR, Wu MK (2010) Incidence of dentineal defects after root canal filling procedures. Int Endod J 43(11):995–1000. https://doi.org/10.1111/j.1365-2591.2010.01740.x

Simon SR, Berdal A, Cooper PR, Lumley PJ, Tomson PL, Smith AJ (2011) Dentine-pulp complex regeneration: from lab to clinic. Adv Dent Res 23(3):340–345. https://doi.org/10.1177/0022034511405327

Simon S, Perard M, Zanini M, Smith AJ, Charpentier E, Djole SX, Lumley PJ (2013) Should pulp chamber pulpotomy be seen as a permanent treatment? Some preliminary thoughts. Int Endod J 46(1):79–87. https://doi.org/10.1111/j.1365-2591.2012.02113.x

Siqueira JF Jr (2011) Treatment of endodontic infections. Quintessence Publishing, London

Sjogren U, Hagglund B, Sundqvist G, Wing K (1990) Factors affecting the long-term results of endodontic treatment. J Endod 16(10):498–504

Smith AJ, Scheven BA, Takahashi Y, Ferracane JL, Shelton RM, Cooper PR (2012) Dentine as a bioactive extracellular matrix. Arch Oral Biol 57(2):109–121. https://doi.org/10.1016/j.archoralbio.2011.07.008

Smith AJ, Duncan HF, Diogenes A, Simon S, Cooper PR (2016) Exploiting the bioactive properties of the dentine-pulp complex in regenerative endodontics. J Endod 42(1):47–56. https://doi.org/10.1016/j.joen.2015.10.019

Stewart PS, Franklin MJ (2008) Physiological heterogeneity in biofilms. Nat Rev Microbiol 6(3):199–210. https://doi.org/10.1038/nrmicro1838

Taha NA, Ahmad MB, Ghanim A (2017) Assessment of mineral trioxide aggregate pulpotomy in mature permanent teeth with carious exposures. Int Endod J 50(2):117–125. https://doi.org/10.1111/iej.12605

Tomson PL, Lumley PJ, Smith AJ, Cooper PR (2017) Growth factor release from dentine matrix by pulp-capping agents promotes pulp tissue repair-associated events. Int Endod J 50(3):281–292. https://doi.org/10.1111/iej.12624

Torabinejad M, Parirokh M (2010) Mineral trioxide aggregate: a comprehensive literature review-part II: leakage and biocompatibility investigations. J Endod 36(2):190–202. https://doi.org/10.1016/j.joen.2009.09.010

Violich DR, Chandler NP (2010) The smear layer in endodontics - a review. Int Endod J 43(1):2–15. https://doi.org/10.1111/j.1365-2591.2009.01627.x

Wang Z, Pan J, Wright JT, Bencharit S, Zhang S, Everett ET, Teixeira FB, Preisser JS (2010) Putative stem cells in human dental pulp with irreversible pulpitis: an exploratory study. J Endod 36(5):820–825. https://doi.org/10.1016/j.joen.2010.02.003

Wang Z, Shen Y, Ma J, Haapasalo M (2012) The effect of detergents on the antibacterial activity of disinfecting solutions in dentine. J Endod 38(7):948–953. https://doi.org/10.1016/j.joen.2012.03.007

Wang J, Chen W, Jiang Y, Liang J (2013) Imaging of extraradicular biofilm using combined scanning electron microscopy and stereomicroscopy. Microsc Res Tech 76(9):979–983. https://doi.org/10.1002/jemt.22257

Wolters WJ, Duncan HF, Tomson PL, Karim IE, McKenna G, Dorri M, Stangvaltaite L, van der Sluis LWM (2017) Minimally invasive endodontics: a new diagnostic system for assessing pulpitis and subsequent treatment needs. Int Endod J 50(9):825–829. https://doi.org/10.1111/iej.12793

Wu MK, Wesselink PR, Walton RE (2000) Apical terminus location of root canal treatment procedures. Oral Surg Oral Med Oral Pathol Oral Radiol Endod 89(1):99–103

Wu MK, Dummer PM, Wesselink PR (2006) Consequences of and strategies to deal with residual post-treatment root canal infection. Int Endod J 39(5):343–356

Wu MK, Shemesh H, Wesselink PR (2009) Limitations of previously published systematic reviews evaluating the outcome of endodontic treatment. Int Endod J 42(8):656–666. https://doi.org/10.1111/j.1365-2591.2009.01600.x

Current and Future Views on Pulpal Pain and Neurogenesis

2

Fionnuala T. Lundy, Ikhlas El karim, and Ben A. Scheven

2.1 Introduction

2.1.1 A Brief Overview of Neurogenesis

Neurogenesis refers to the formation (or birth) of new neurons and involves a multistep process of proliferation, migration and differentiation of neural precursors followed by integration of new neurons/neural tissues (for review see (Braun and Jessberger 2014)). A fundamental principle of neurogenesis is the presence of neural stem cells (NSC) residing in a regulatory neurogenic microenvironment, also referred to as the neural stem cell niche. During embryonic development, neuroepithelial stem cells are typically located in the neuroectodermally derived neural tube, which give rise to radial glial cells. Radial glial cells are capable of differentiating to neural and glial precursors as well as playing a role in guiding migration of newly formed neural cells. Thus radial glial cells resemble NSC (Xu et al. 2017), and although multiple types of NSC may exist and differences and similarities have been described for embryonic and adult NSC, it is generally accepted that glial-like NSCs contribute to both embryonic and adult neurogenesis (Kriegstein and Alvarez-Buylla 2009).

The presence of NSC and the process of neurogenesis have been confirmed in adult brain tissue across the animal kingdom including vertebrae and mammals through various labelling and tracing studies (Jessberger and Gage 2014). NSC have

F. T. Lundy (✉) · I. El karim
Wellcome-Wolfson Institute of Experimental Medicine, School of Medicine, Dentistry and Biomedical Sciences, Queen's University Belfast, Belfast, Northern Ireland
e-mail: f.lundy@qub.ac.uk; i.elkarim@qub.ac.uk

B. A. Scheven
School of Dentistry, Institute of Clinical Sciences, College of Medical and Dental Sciences, University of Birmingham, Birmingham, UK
e-mail: b.a.scheven@bham.ac.uk

© Springer Nature Switzerland AG 2019
H. F. Duncan, P. R. Cooper (eds.), *Clinical Approaches in Endodontic Regeneration*,
https://doi.org/10.1007/978-3-319-96848-3_2

been isolated from adult brain tissues and can be cultured as typical neurospheres and differentiated under neurogenic conditions towards both neuronal and glial cell (astrocyte and oligodendrocyte) phenotypes. As neurogenesis is not restricted to embryonic and perinatal developmental stages, adult brain has a greater plasticity than originally thought with roles in the maintenance and function of the nervous system. Adult neurogenesis is traditionally considered in the context of the brain where they reside in discrete canonical neurogenic regions of the brain, namely, the subgranular zone (SGZ) of the dentate gyrus (DG) in the hippocampus and the subventricular zone (SVZ) of the lateral ventricle (LV). Neurogenesis has been implicated in learning and memory retention and responds to various environmental stimuli, assaults or disease (e.g. physical activity, brain trauma, stroke). However, the contribution of endogenous NSC in the repair of the CNS appears limited due to intrinsic inhibitory factors and hurdles preventing efficient migration of neural precursors, maturation and functional integration at sites of injury. It is not clear to what extent NSC are present in human brains and their precise physiological role and potential in humans.

Neurogenesis in the peripheral nervous system (PNS) has attracted less attention, but evidence of glial-like neural precursors in sensory ganglia such as the dorsal root ganglion (DRG) suggests that neurogenesis may contribute to PNS regeneration following injury (see also below). An emerging paradigm is that besides the canonical adult brain NSC, neural tissues may contain endogenous (parenchymal) cells with NSC-like properties which may potentially be activated following tissue damage. Candidates for such local NSC include ventricular ependymal cells, olfactory bulb neuroepithelium and neural crest-derived multipotent cells which may persist in specific adult organs.

It is noteworthy that dental mesenchymal stem cells have been ascribed a glial cell origin (Kaukua et al. 2014), which together with their known neural crest origin would underscore the NSC-like nature of these cells. In fact, dental pulp stem cells (DPSC) share a variety of neuronal lineage markers including nestin and glial fibrillary acidic protein (GFAP) and the neurotrophin receptor p75NTR (CD271).

2.2 Dental Neurogenesis and Tooth Innervation

Nervous innervation of the dental pulp plays a pivotal role in the regulation of tooth function including dentinogenesis, pulpal vasculogenesis, blood flow and inflammation (Holland 1996; Olgart et al. 1991). However, the developmental and functional relationship of pulpal nerve fibres with dentinogenesis is complex and not well understood (Holland 1996). Neurotrophic factors (NTFs), which play an essential role in the neuroprotection, survival and activity of neurons, such as nerve growth factor (NGF) and glial cell-derived neurotrophic factor (GDNF), have also been directly implicated in dentinogenesis and dental repair responses (see also (Mitsiadis and Luukko 1995; Gale et al. 2011)). It is also well established that various NTFs can be produced by nonneuronal mesenchymal cells of the dental pulp thereby underlining the potential role of dental pulp stromal/stem cells in various aspects of pulpal homeostasis including regulation of pulpal nerves and possibly sensory function such as pain detection and dentine formation.

Tooth development is a complex and finely tuned process involving an intricate reciprocal interplay between the embryonic oral epithelium and ectomesenchyme (Nanci 2012). It is accepted that the oral epithelium is critical for tooth initiation and instructing the underlying ectomesenchyme to become committed to tooth formation. Developing nerves are closely associated with the consecutive stages of tooth formation according to tightly interlinked spatio-temporally dependent processes. In general, developing nerves are guided to specific targets by environmental local factors. At an early stage in embryonic development, nerve fibres outgrowing from the trigeminal ganglion invade the mandibular process and become located close to the odontogenic regions near the oral epithelium suggesting an association and possible role of neurons in tooth induction (Kollar and Lumsden 1979). However, in vitro "recombination" tissue culture experiments suggested that trigeminal ganglion nerves were not necessary for tooth initiation (Lumsden and Buchanan 1986). There remains much to learn about the molecular and cellular processes underlying tooth induction and development, and it cannot be excluded that the invading and condensing ectomesenchyme exerts an early influence over the oral epithelium, prior to acquiring its odontogenic capability inducing, controlling and directing the ingrowing pioneer axons.

Trigeminal nerve fibres first form a plexus near the condensed mesenchyme underlying the primary epithelial band; these remain outside the tooth germ and developing dental papilla but move into the dental follicle during the late cap/early bell phase. Axons enter the dental papilla during the late bell stage, which coincides with the start of hard dental tissue differentiation and mineralisation. Thus dental innervation is closely correlated with the onset and progression of amelogenesis and dentinogenesis. Local regulatory signalling factors affecting axon guidance and innervation are produced during the reciprocal epithelial-mesenchymal interactions that characterise tooth development (Hildebrand et al. 1995; Fried et al. 2000; Luukko and Kettunen 2014). Thus it is regarded that the developing tooth regulates its own innervation. Candidates for dental axon directing factors include NTFs such as NGF and brain-derived neurotrophic factor (BDNF) as well as members of the semaphorin family (Luukko and Kettunen 2014; Løes et al. 2001), specifically, Sema3A, whose expression is induced in the dental mesenchyme at an early stage in tooth development and is considered to play a crucial role in dental axon navigation and patterning. Interestingly, Sema3A has recently been identified as an osteoblast-inducing factor with potential role in reparative dentine formation in response to tooth injury in a rat dental exposure model (Yoshida et al. 2016).

2.3   The Innervation of the Dental Pulp

The dental pulp is a small but complex sensory organ capable of neurogenic changes that are intimately involved in the aetiology of endodontic disease. The mature dental pulp is innervated by both sensory and autonomic nerve fibres of the PNS. The extent of sensory innervation of the dental pulp is readily apparent to patients who have experienced dentine sensitivity or toothache (Chung et al. 2013), and there has been extensive research interest in pulpal sensory nerves as targets for dental pain relief. The autonomic innervation of the dental pulp has been less well studied, but there is mounting evidence for an important role for the autonomic nerves in the regulation of pulpal blood flow and in the recruitment of inflammatory cells during chronic inflammation (Haug and Heyeraas 2006).

The sensory innervation of the dental pulp consists of both A-fibres and C-fibres, whilst the autonomic innervation consists of sympathetic and parasympathetic fibres. In terms of nerve fibre abundance within the dental pulp, the sensory nerves are much more abundant than sympathetic nerves, and it is thought that parasympathetic nerves are the least abundant of all. A brief description of the various nerve fibre types and their distribution in the dental pulp is provided in Table 2.1. It is important to note, however, that it is impossible to present a complete anatomical or biochemical description of pulpal nerves, because neuronal phenotype can alter, especially

Table 2.1 Innervation of the dental pulp

Nerve fibre type	Subclassification	Myelinated	Distribution
Sensory			
A-fibre	A-beta (Aβ)	Yes	Pulp proper, sub-odontoblast layer, odontoblast layer, predentine and dentinal tubules
	A-delta fast (Aδ-f)	Yes	Pulp proper, sub-odontoblast layer, odontoblast layer, predentine and dentinal tubules
	A-delta slow (Aδ-s)	No/lightly/thinly	Pulp proper (including blood vessels), sub-odontoblast layer
C-fibre	Nociceptive C-fibres	No	Pulp proper, sub-odontoblast layer
	Glial-derived neurotrophic factor-regulated C-fibres	No	Pulp proper (including blood vessels)
	Polymodal C-fibres	No	Pulp proper (including blood vessels) and immunocompetent cells
Autonomic			
Sympathetic	Sympathetic	No	Pulp proper (including blood vessels) and immunocompetent cells
Parasympathetic[a]	Parasympathetic	Unknown	Pulp proper (including blood vessels) and immunocompetent cells but unknown

Myelinated and unmyelinated sensory nerves, as well as unmyelinated autonomic nerves, are distributed throughout the dental pulp. Axon diameter tends to determine whether nerves are myelinated or unmyelinated. Larger-diameter axons tend to be myelinated, whereas smaller-diameter axons tend to be unmyelinated. Myelinated axons have faster conduction velocities compared with unmyelinated axons. Fast-conducting A-delta fibres evoke a rapid, sharp pain sensation, whereas slow-conducting C-fibres evoke slow, dull, throbbing pain

[a]To date there is limited evidence for parasympathetic innervation of the dental pulp, apart from the presence of certain neuropeptides, such as vasoactive intestinal polypeptide, that tend to be associated with parasympathetic innervation ((Rodd and Boissonade 2002), (El Karim et al. 2006a) (Figure 1A), (Caviedes-Bucheli et al. 2008))

during pulpal injury or infection. Indeed during tissue injury/inflammation, sprouting of nerve fibres has been reported in the dental pulp along with biochemical changes in neurotransmitter levels, many of which return to homeostatic conditions following the resolution phase, which is discussed in detail later in this chapter.

There are over 900 axons entering the average human premolar tooth (Reader and Foreman 1981), from the trigeminal ganglion, the majority of which enter the root through the main apical foramen. Axons course through the radicular pulp and then branch extensively in the coronal region. A general assumption can be made for DRG nerves are that the size of their cell body or soma is positively correlated with the size of the axons (Lawson and Waddell 1991). However the majority of the nerves innervating the dental pulp have medium or large somata (Fried et al. 1989), but it is known that their axons are shorter than those from the DRG. When the degree of branching of the trigeminal nerves within the teeth is taken into consideration, it is apparent that the extensive peripheral branching of trigeminal nerves within the tooth could explain this apparent anomaly. Indeed it is understood that a single pulpal axon can innervate up to 100 dentinal tubules (Gunji 1982). Therefore the total amount of axoplasm, which is determined by both the length of the axon and its degree of terminal branching of trigeminal nerves, is likely to fit with the correlation previously proposed for DRG nerves.

In morphological terms the vast majority (approximately 70–90%) of sensory dental pulp axons are unmyelinated or C-fibre type, with most of the remainder belonging to the Aδ range and only very few Aβ fibres (Cadden et al. 1983). Despite the fact that the majority of pulpal nerves are unmyelinated, their parent axons entering the apical foramen tend to be myelinated. Thus it would appear that many pulpal axons lose their myelin sheath as they travel from the radicular to the coronal pulp, branching and tapering. Evidence supporting this phenomenon has come from immunohistochemical studies showing that unmyelinated dental pulp axons are immunoreactive for markers of myelination such as neurofilament (Henry et al. 2012); however, the existence of "conventional" unmyelinated C-fibres and "conventional" myelinated Aδ fibres within the dental pulp cannot be discounted. It is recognised that axons may also branch to the dental pulp of a neighbouring tooth (Atkinson and Kenyon 1990), which offers clinicians an anatomical explanation for the difficultly some patients may have in localising pain to the correct tooth.

2.4 Insights into the Cellular and Molecular Mechanisms of Dental Nociception

According to the International Association for the Study of Pain, pain constitutes an "unpleasant sensory and emotional experience associated with actual or potential tissue damage" (Loeser and Treede 2008). Pain generally serves as a protective mechanism and as an alarm system for a variety of pathological conditions. The terminology that has been widely used to define the process of peripheral detection, transduction and processing of noxious stimuli is "nociception", which describes the neural mechanisms and pathways in both the peripheral and central nervous systems.

The perception of pain in the dental pulp depends of course on the nature of the stimulus but also to a large extent on the type (morphology) of the nerve fibres present and the pro-inflammatory/antinociceptive balance of the neurotransmitters within them. Although primary sensory neurons have conventionally been classified primarily on their morphology (as outlined in Table 2.1), they can also be classified based on their neurochemistry (expression of receptors/channels and neurotransmitters). These receptors or channels play a vital role in the detection of various noxious stimuli which the nociceptive neuron then converts into electrical signals for transmission to the central nervous system (CNS). Membrane proteins belonging to the transient receptor potential (TRP) family constitute a major group of ion channels present on nociceptive sensory neurons, along with other channels such as acid sensing ion channels (ASIC), potassium, sodium and ligand-gated ion channels.

Many of these sensory receptors and channels are also present on odontoblasts, the specialised cells of the dental pulp that are localised between the dentine and pulp and play a primary role in dentine synthesis. The anatomical location of odontoblasts places them in the unique position as the target cells for a range of external stimuli that may reach the dental pulp tissue if the enamel and dentine have been damaged by caries or by trauma (Ruch 1998). Recent work has elucidated a role for odontoblasts as sensory cells, with the ability to detect a wide range of stimuli as a result of expressing several classes of ion channels including K+ channels (Magloire et al. 2003), voltage-gated sodium channels (Allard et al. 2006) and TRP channels (El Karim et al. 2011). Indeed it has been shown that odontoblasts form a syncytium that is directionally independent via symmetric gap junction channels in the odontoblast layer (Ikeda and Suda 2013). $P2X_3$-positive nerve fibres have been detected in the sub-odontoblast layer of the human dental pulp, in close proximity to odontoblasts (Alavi et al. 2001), and thus ATP has been proposed as a means by which odontoblasts could directly transmit to the nervous system (Liu et al. 2015; Solé-Magdalena et al. 2018). The TRP family of ion channels are an example of non-selective cation channels, and in addition to their expression on nociceptive sensory neurons, they are found on a wide range of cell types, including odontoblasts. They are activated by a diverse range of stimuli including those of thermal, chemical and mechanical origin (Ramsey et al. 2006). TRP channels are grouped into six mammalian subfamilies based on their sequence homology: the vanilloid (TRPV), ankyrin (TRPA), melastatin (TRPM), canonical or classical (TRPC), polycystin (TRPP) and mucolipin (TRPML) subfamilies. To date the TRPV and TRPA families have been most intensely studied in humans and are described briefly below.

The TRPV1 channel was the first mammalian TRP to be cloned in 1997 (Caterina et al. 1997) and is sensitive to the vanilloid compound capsaicin (8-Methyl-N-vanillyl-trans-6-nonenamide), the active ingredient of hot chilli peppers. TRPV1 is also responsive to heat (with an activation threshold >43 °C) and acidic pH (with an activation threshold < pH 5.5). Other members of the TRPV family, such as TRPV2, TRPV3 and TRPV4, respond to increases in temperature with varying activation thresholds (Caterina et al. 1999; Smith et al. 2002; Güler et al. 2002). Mice lacking the functional TRPV1 gene ($Trpv1^{-/-}$) exhibit a dramatic attenuation of acute noxious heat sensitivity (Caterina et al. 2000), supporting a role for TRPV1 in thermosensation. Furthermore, the sensitivity of TRPV1 to noxious heat can be greatly enhanced by inflammatory agents, providing a mechanism through which tissue injury can produce thermal hypersensitivity (Julius and Basbaum 2001).

At the other end of the temperature spectrum is the TRPA1 channel (the only member of the TRPA family), which is activated by temperatures lower that 17 °C, considered to be painfully cold (Story et al. 2003). TRPA1 channels are expressed on distinct subpopulation of small-diameter sensory neurons that also express TRPV1. In addition to their activation by cold temperatures, TRPA1 is also activated by natural isothiocyanate-containing compounds such as horseradish, mustard oil and wasabi (Jordt et al. 2004). A thermosensitive channel from the TRPM family, namely, TRPM8, responds to cool (<27 °C) temperatures and can be activated by cooling-mimetic compounds such as menthol (McKemy et al. 2002; Peier et al. 2002).

In the quest to discover endogenous chemical activators of TRP channels, arachidonic acid and its metabolites have been shown to be agonists for TRPV4, TRPA1 and TRPV1 (Watanabe et al. 2003; Redmond et al. 2014; Hargreaves and Ruparel 2016; Sisignano et al. 2014); however, additional endogenous activators undoubtedly remain to be discovered. In addition to their thermo-responsive properties, TRPV2 and TRPV4 have also been reported to respond to mechanical or osmotic stimuli (Liedtke et al. 2000; Muraki et al. 2007).

2.5 Pain-Signalling Mechanisms in Health and Disease

The detection of noxious stimuli by membrane channels such as TRPs represents only the first stage in transmission of a pain signal to the CNS. Noxious stimuli detected by TRPs are converted into electrical activity, which, if sufficiently large, begins to drive action potentials along the axon to the CNS. Synaptic communication plays an important role in pain perception, as nerves innervating the teeth and orofacial tissues have cell bodies located in the trigeminal ganglion, peripheral axons that innervate the orofacial tissues and central axons that enter the CNS to synapse with nociceptive second-order neurons. The detection of dental pain by the CNS is a protective response aimed at reducing the likelihood of exacerbating the damaged tissue. Very often, however, the inflammatory milieu in the local dental pulp tissue alters the expression of channels and receptors on the sensory nerve terminals, by a process known as neuronal plasticity. Nociceptive nerves within the dental pulp are therefore not static detectors but are highly plastic and have the ability to change depending on micro-environmental conditions such as those occurring during injury or inflammation.

2.6 Inflammatory Pain in the Dental Pulp

Inflammation in the dental pulp, like other soft tissues, has both cellular and vascular components. Activation of these components results in vasodilation and in inflammatory cell infiltration to the site of injury/infection. The fact that the dental

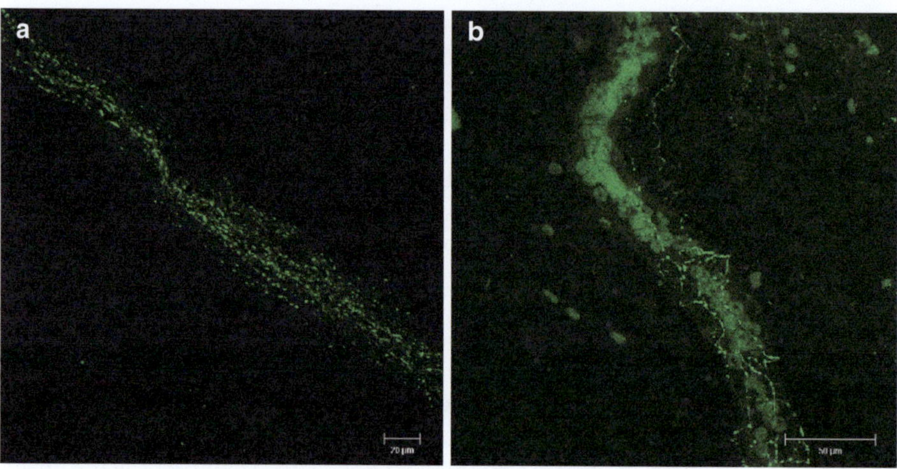

Fig. 2.1 Vasoactive intestinal polypeptide (VIP) and neuropeptide Y (NPY) expression in the dental pulp. (**a**) Free-running nerve fibres immunoreactive for VIP in the central pulp region of a moderately carious tooth (Reprinted from El Karim et al. (El Karim et al. 2006a)). (**b**) Nerve fibre immunoreactive for NPY, characteristically encircling a blood vessel in the pulp of a noncarious tooth (Reprinted from El Karim et al. (El Karim et al. 2006b))

pulp is a highly innervated tissue places pulpal nerves in the ideal position to respond to injury by mounting a so-called neurogenic inflammatory response, which is characterised by the release of neuropeptides such as substance P, calcitonin gene-related peptides (CGRP) and neuropeptide Y (Awawdeh et al. 2002; Lundy and Linden 2004; El Karim et al. 2006b) (Fig. 2.1b). Neuropeptides are released by an axonal reflex following activation of sensory neurons by both external and internal stimuli. They orchestrate inflammation in many aspects including increased vascular permeability, plasma extravasation and oedema formation (Lundy and Linden 2004). The cellular infiltrates accompanying these vascular changes result in recruitment and infiltration of immune cells and subsequent production of master inflammatory cytokines such as tumour necrosis factor-alpha (TNF-α), interleukin-1 beta (IL-1β), interleukin-8 (IL-8) and neurotrophic factors such as NGF (Julius and Basbaum 2001). These Inflammatory mediators are capable of modulating nociceptive TRP channels, thereby enabling diverse mechanisms to allow robust and sustained activation of these channels during injury, inflammation and various disease processes. A simplified scheme for TRP involvement in pathological conditions has previously been proposed (Mickle et al. 2016). Pathological conditions can lead to (1) local thermoactivation of TRPV1 and TRPA1, or activation via mild-to-moderate acidic or oxidative stress conditions; (2) prolonged channel activation, due to reduced desensitisation; (3) enhanced channel activation, due to increases in the expression and surface trafficking of TRPV1 and TRPA1 proteins; (4) cross-sensitisation of channel activation (by Ca^{2+} and other intracellular signal transduction molecules); and (5) increased gene

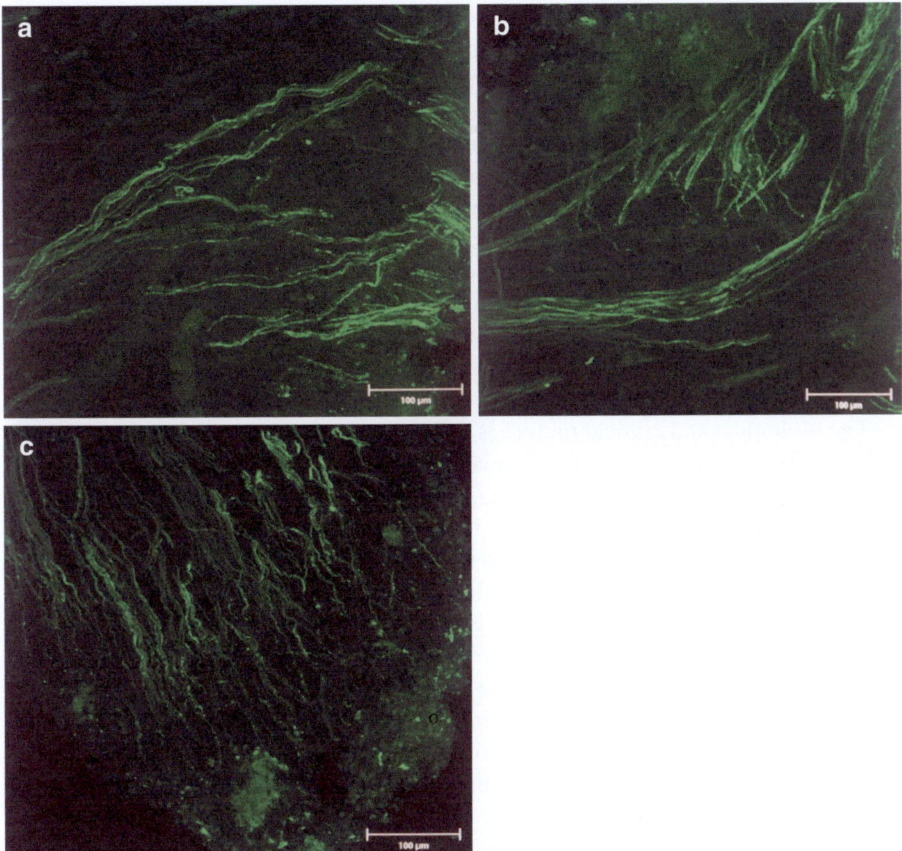

Fig. 2.2 Protein gene product 9.5 (PGP 9.5) staining in the dental pulp of a carious tooth. (**a**) Coronal region of the dental pulp showing intense staining of nerve bundles in the sub-odontoblastic and pulp proper regions. (**b**) Long nerve bundles in the pulp proper region. (**c**) Long nerves and nerve bundles in the radicular pulp

expression and mRNA translation for these channels. Together, these processes result in increased nociceptive excitation and prolonged nociceptor firing, providing complexity that offers both opportunities and challenges for targeting pain (Mickle et al. 2016).

Within the dental pulp neuronal sprouting (Fig. 2.2) has been shown to be associated with caries-induced pulpal inflammation (Rodd and Boissonade 2000). Expression of nociceptive ion channels including TRPV1, TRPA1 and NaV1 was shown to be upregulated in caries-induced pulp inflammation (Luo et al. 2008). The role of neurotrophic factors such as NGF and other cytokines in increasing trigeminal neuronal sensitisation has been demonstrated (Diogenes et al. 2007), and this combined with the high expression levels of these cytokines in teeth with painful pulpitis; these data further support their role in tooth pain signalling.

The neuronal inflammatory features described above occur to varying degrees during pulpal inflammation. In the situation where inflammation is limited and confined to a small space as in reversible pulpitis, there is generally increased pulpal innervation and neuronal sprouting leading to increased pain sensitivity to stimuli such as cold (thermosensitive ion channels) or an air blast (mechanosensitive ion channels). The pain in this clinical situation is usually sharp, localised and only develops in response to the stimulus but disappears immediately after removal of such stimulus. The nerve fibres responsible for this type of pain are usually the A-delta fibres. There is no clear evidence however to suggest that the mild to moderate inflammation associated with reversible pulpitis affect A-delta fibres exclusively, but as these fibres are mostly located in the peripheral zone of the dental pulp and extend to the inner dentine, then they are considered more likely to be affected by early inflammatory changes in the dental pulp.

The biological and clinical picture is however more complex in relation to severe pulpal inflammation or so-called irreversible pulpitis. In this scenario the dental pulp is generally invaded by bacteria, and a severe inflammatory response has extended deep into the pulpal tissues, involving the deeply seated C-fibres (Närhi et al. 1992). Here the nerve fibres (as in the case of reversible pulpitis) are sensitised by inflammatory mediators, and together with increased neuronal sprouting, this results in both hyperalgesia and allodynia in response to external stimuli. In this scenario, however, the nature of pain developed varies from sharp to a dull ache and is usually severe. Characteristically, the pain will usually linger after removal of the stimulus. Pain has also been shown to develop spontaneously when the pulp is severely inflamed, and this is likely to be due to continuous activation of pulpal nociceptors by the components of the inflammatory milieu and the increase intrapulpal pressure created by the severe inflammatory response (Heyeraas and Berggreen 1999). In painful, inflammatory conditions such as pulpitis (Fig. 2.3), ion channels such as TRPA1 (cold receptor) and TRPV1 (heat receptor) were found to be directly activated by tissue injury products and the acidic pH of the inflammatory environment (Bautista et al. 2013; Taylor-Clark et al. 2009; Morales-Lázaro et al. 2013). It also likely that bacteria and bacterial products found in irreversible pulpitis may directly activate these channels to produce spontaneous pain (Meseguer et al. 2014).

Although it is reasonable to suggest that pain severity correlates with the level of inflammation and degree of neuronal sensitisation, traditionally, it was thought that there was a poor relationship between clinical signs and symptoms and the histological state of the pulp in mature teeth (Seltzer et al. 1963; Dummer et al. 1980). However, this convention has recently been questioned, as a more recent histological study of the dental pulp in health and disease has shown that there is a good correlation between clinical symptoms of pulpitis and the corresponding histological state of a diseased pulp (Ricucci et al. 2014). This has led to the rethinking of the current diagnostic system for pulpitis and in turn has challenged the concept of irreversible pulpitis (Wolters et al. 2017). Subsequently it has been proposed that pulpitis should be classified according to the degree of inflammation as initial, mild, moderate and severe rather than simply reversible or irreversible.

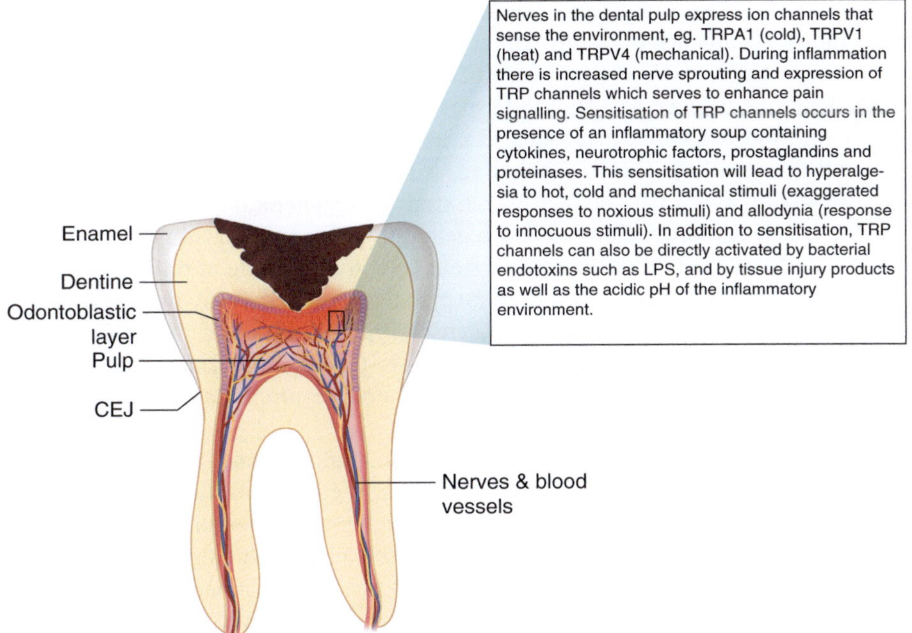

Fig. 2.3 Inflammation within the dental pulp leads to increased nerve sprouting and activation or modulation of ion channel function

Pain is subjective however, and there are other factors which need to be considered in the pain signalling pathway including, but not limited to, psychological factors and previous pain experience. Therefore, diagnosis of pulpal pain is always considered by a combined approach involving pain history, clinical investigations (sensibility thermal tests and electric pulp testing) and radiographic examination. Even with a combined approach, the validity of the currently employed clinical tests to determine the actual status of the dental pulp has been questioned. A recent systematic review of the literature on the diagnostic accuracy of signs/symptoms and current tests used to determine the condition of the pulp, concluded that the overall evidence was insufficient to support the accuracy of such tests (Mejre et al. 2012). Therefore, the current diagnostic procedures do not reliably identify the inflammatory status of the pulp, and further research is required to improve pulpal diagnosis and guide novel and targeted therapeutic strategies for repair.

2.7 Tooth Innervation and Repair

The current understanding that the dental mesenchyme controls pulpal innervation during tooth development strongly suggests that mesenchymal factors are central to regulating axonal repair and regeneration in the dental pulp. Unlike the CNS, the PNS has a substantial capacity for repair and regeneration, in particular when the nerve axon is severed whilst still attached to an intact neuronal cell body. Following PNS injury, a sequence of events will occur that allow (de)myelination of the damaged axons and growth and guidance of new axon endings, a process also called sprouting or neuritogenesis, involving specific inputs by supporting glial (Schwann cells) and immune cells (macrophages), as well as neuroprotective and neuroregenerative signalling factors including NTFs (e.g. NGF, GDNF) and IGF-I (Frostick et al. 1998; Ishii et al. 1994). Extensive regeneration has been described for the DRG, and apart from axonal regeneration from pre-existing neurons, the presence of local neural progenitor or stem cells that are able to differentiate into neurons and glia has been recognised (see also above). This may present a model for a neural stem cell niche within the sensory ganglia with intrinsic self-regenerating capability (Czaja et al. 2012). Likewise, the trigeminal ganglion with its dental sensory nerves contains similar regenerative properties (Holland 1996; Arthur et al. 2009).

Accumulating evidence indicates that postnatal pulp mesenchyme is also able to secrete a range of NTFs and other neurovascular regulatory factors such as PDGF and VEGF that may be involved in dental pulp homeostasis, neuronal function, reinnervation and repair. In fact, expression of growth factors including NGF and VEGF is significantly increased after tooth injury or orthodontic treatment (Mitsiadis et al. 2017). Notably numerous signalling molecules are sequestered within the dentine matrix during dentinogenesis which could be released during tooth caries and contribute to pulpal repair, neural repair and reinnervation and reparative dentinogenesis (Smith et al. 2012).

2.8 Neurogenic and Neurotrophic Properties of DPSC: Exploitation for Nerve Repair

The neural crest origin of DPSC has led to a considerable interest in using these cells for various cell therapeutic applications in dental and non-dental neuronal repair. In fact, a significant number of studies have now provided evidence for the potential and advantageous beneficial effects of DPSC for repairing nerve injuries and various neurodegenerative conditions relating to, for example, ischemic stroke or Parkinson's disease (see recent review (Mead et al. 2016)). The mechanisms underlying the therapeutic effects of DPSC are not yet fully understood but appear multifaceted encompassing both cell differentiation or replacement as well stimulating endogenous repair through secretion of growth-promoting and anti-inflammatory signalling molecules and NTFs (Sakai et al. 2012; Mead et al. 2017).

The multipotentiality of neural crest-derived DPSC was proposed to go beyond the classical trio of mesenchymal (osteogenic, chondrogenic and adipogenic) cell lineages and extend to neurogenic differentiation (Huang et al. 2009). This notion was originally highlighted in the seminal Gronthos' study (Gronthos et al. 2000) whereby DPSC were isolated from adult human molars and shown to be able to acquire neuronal characteristics after culture in neurogenic medium. Neuronal phenotypic differentiation from heterogeneous DPSC as well as selected and more defined subpopulations have been reported in several studies including the use of promising neurosphere assays (Huang et al. 2009; Arthur et al. 2008; Gervois et al. 2015). Whether all neural-like cells detected in culture were in fact bona fide, functional neurons remain a matter of debate (Mead et al. 2016, 2017).

Evidence has also been presented as to the glial differentiation ability of DPSC as they have been differentiated in Schwann-like cells in media containing a combination of various differentiation-inducing factors such as retinoic acid, forskolin and PDGF (Martens et al. 2014). Interestingly, these differentiated pulpal cells not only displayed Schwann-like markers such as GFAP, they also secreted significantly higher quantities of NTFs compared with "native" undifferentiated DPSC. The DPSC-derived Schwann cells also were able to promote DRG neurite outgrowth in an indirect, paracrine manner (Martens et al. 2014). Thus differentiation into glial cells could be one of the core mechanisms by which DPSC exert their therapeutic effects.

Notwithstanding cell differentiation, the paracrine action of MSC/DPSC has gained substantial support as a crucial mode of action in neural repair (Mead et al. 2017). DPSC produce relatively high levels of NTFs including NGF, BDNF and GDNF which may exceed the levels secreted by other MSC such as BMMSC and adipose-derived stem cells suggesting that DPSC may provide an advantageous cell therapy for nerve repair compared with other MSCs (Mead et al. 2014a, b). In the optic nerve crush injury model, where due to disruption of retrograde neurotrophic support the retinal ganglion cells (RGC) degenerate, intravitreally injected DPSC were able to provide significant RGC neuroprotection and promote optic nerve regeneration (Mead et al. 2014b, 2013). DPSC proved to be more efficacious than BMSC, a remarkable therapeutic effect that was similarly observed in an experimental glaucomatous eye model featuring cytokine-induced elevated eye pressure and associated RGC neurodegeneration (Mead et al. 2016). One of the future challenges is to explore whether the secretomes and extracellular vesicles including exosomes from DPSC/MSC are just as effective as whole cell therapy in promoting neuronal repair and neurogenesis. Such research will undoubtedly lead to more controlled and potentially "off-the-shelf" cell-free, therapeutic approaches.

Indeed, emerging evidence indicates that DPSC display an effective and promising therapeutic neurotropic and neurogenic capacity which is in line with the putative role of the dental ectomesenchyme in dental innervation during tooth development. On the other hand, dental neurons and pulpal-derived NTFs may be involved in the regulation of dentinogenesis and tooth repair. Future research is warranted to develop and harness DPSC for a wide range of nerve repair applications, including dental clinical applications to promote pulpal health and vitality. It is also tempting to speculate that DPSC-based therapies may possibly offer a strategy to relieve dental pain or hypersensitivity through the analgesic action of NTFs, such as GDNF, or stimulation of reparative dentine formation thereby sealing off of dentinal tubules (Mitsiadis and Luukko 1995; Boucher and McMahon 2001; Scheven et al. 2009).

Conclusion

Scientific discoveries over the last few decades have greatly improved our understanding of aspects of dental pain and neurogenesis. The discovery of TRP channels and their modulation during inflammation was a major step in our understanding of the molecular mechanisms of pulpal pain, paving the way for novel therapeutic targets for pain relief. Emerging evidence regarding the neurogenic potential of DPSCs and their neural crest origin makes these cells ideal for neuronal regeneration, not only for regenerative endodontics but also for other PNS applications. Human neuronal models, based on cells differentiated from dental pulp stem cells (Clarke et al. 2017), are also proving useful for in vitro PNS research, with the potential for providing an alternative to animal models.

References

Alavi AM, Dubyak GR, Burnstock G (2001) Immunohistochemical evidence for ATP receptors in human dental pulp. J Dent Res 80(2):476–483

Allard B, Magloire H, Couble ML, Maurin JC, Bleicher F (2006) Voltage-gated sodium channels confer excitability to human odontoblasts: possible role in tooth pain transmission. J Biol Chem 281(39):29002–29010

Arthur A, Rychkov G, Shi S, Koblar SA, Gronthos S (2008) Adult human dental pulp stem cells differentiate toward functionally active neurons under appropriate environmental cues. Stem Cells 26(7):1787–1795

Arthur A, Shi S, Zannettino AC, Fujii N, Gronthos S, Koblar SA (2009) Implanted adult human dental pulp stem cells induce endogenous axon guidance. Stem Cells 27(9):2229–2237

Atkinson ME, Kenyon C (1990) Collateral branching innervation of rat molar teeth from trigeminal ganglion cells shown by double labeling with fluorescent retrograde tracers. Brain Res 508:289–292

Awawdeh L, Lundy FT, Shaw C, Lamey P-J, Linden GJ, Kennedy JG (2002) Quantitative analysis of substance P, neurokinin A and calcitonin gene-related peptide in pulp tissue from painful and healthy human teeth. Int Endod J 35:30–36

Bautista DM, Pellegrino M, Tsunozaki M (2013) TRPA1: a gatekeeper for inflammation. Annu Rev Physiol 75:181–200

Boucher TJ, McMahon SB (2001) Neurotrophic factors and neuropathic pain. Curr Opin Pharmacol 1(1):66–72

Braun SM, Jessberger S (2014) Adult neurogenesis: mechanisms and functional significance. Development 141(10):1983–1986

Cadden SW, Lisney SJ, Matthews B (1983) Thresholds to electrical stimulation of nerves in cat canine tooth-pulp with A beta-, A delta- and C-fibre conduction velocities. Brain Res 261(1):31–41

Caterina MJ, Schumacher MA, Tominaga M, Rosen TA, Levine JD, Julius D (1997) The capsaicin receptor: a heat-activated ion channel in the pain pathway. Nature 389:816–824

Caterina MJ, Rosen TA, Tominaga M, Brake AJ, Julius D (1999) A capsaicin-receptor homologue with a high threshold for noxious heat. Nature 398(6726):436–441

Caterina MJ, Leffler A, Malmberg AB, Martin WJ, Trafton J et al (2000) Impaired nociception and pain sensation in mice lacking the capsaicin receptor. Science 288:306–313

Caviedes-Bucheli J, Muñoz HR, Azuero-Holguín MM, Ulate E (2008) Neuropeptides in dental pulp: the silent protagonists. J Endod 34(7):773–788

Chung G, Jung SJ, Oh SB (2013) Cellular and molecular mechanisms of dental nociception. J Dent Res 92(11):948–955

Clarke R, Monaghan K, About I, Griffin CS, Sergeant GP, El Karim I, McGeown JG, Cosby SL, Curtis TM, McGarvey LP, Lundy FT (2017) TRPA1 activation in a human sensory neuronal model: relevance to cough hypersensitivity? Eur Respir J 50(3). [pii] 1700995

Czaja K, Fornaro M, Geuna S (2012) Neurogenesis in the adult peripheral nervous system. Neural Regen Res 7(14):1047–1054

Diogenes A, Akopian AN, Hargreaves KM (2007) NGF up-regulates TRPA1: implications for orofacial pain. J Dent Res 86(6):550–555

Dummer PM, Hicks R, Huws D (1980) Clinical signs and symptoms in pulp disease. Int Endod J 13(1):27–35

El Karim IA, Lamey PJ, Ardill J, Linden GJ, Lundy FT (2006a) Vasoactive intestinal polypeptide (VIP) and VPAC1 receptor in adult human dental pulp in relation to caries. Arch Oral Biol 51(10):849–855

El Karim IA, Lamey PJ, Linden GJ, Awawdeh LA, Lundy FT (2006b) Caries-induced changes in the expression of pulpal neuropeptide Y. Eur J Oral Sci 114(2):133–137

El Karim IA, Linden GJ, Curtis TM, About I, McGahon MK, Irwin CR, Lundy FT (2011) Human odontoblasts express functional thermo-sensitive TRP channels: implications for dentin sensitivity. Pain 152(10):2211–2223

Fried K, Arvidsson J, Robertson B, Brodin E, Theodorsson E (1989) Combined retrograde tracing and enzyme/immunohistochemistry of trigeminal ganglion cell bodies innervating tooth pulps in the rat. Neuroscience 33(1):101–109

Fried K, Nosrat C, Lillesaar C, Hildebrand C (2000) Molecular signaling and pulpal nerve development. Crit Rev Oral Biol Med 11(3):318–332

Frostick SP, Yin Q, Kemp GJ (1998) Schwann cells, neurotrophic factors, and peripheral nerve regeneration. Microsurgery 18(7):397–405

Gale Z, Cooper PR, Scheven BA (2011) Effects of glial cell line-derived neurotrophic factor on dental pulp cells. J Dent Res 90(10):1240–1245

Gervois P, Struys T, Hilkens P, Bronckaers A, Ratajczak J, Politis C, Brône B, Lambrichts I, Martens W (2015) Neurogenic maturation of human dental pulp stem cells following neurosphere generation induces morphological and electrophysiological characteristics of functional neurons. Stem Cells Dev 24(3):296–311

Gronthos S, Mankani M, Brahim J, Robey PG, Shi S (2000) Postnatal human dental pulp stem cells (DPSCs) in vitro and in vivo. Proc Natl Acad Sci U S A 97(25):13625–13630

Güler AD, Lee H, Iida T, Shimizu I, Tominaga M, Caterina M (2002) Heat-evoked activation of the ion channel, TRPV4. J Neurosci 22(15):6408–6414

Gunji T (1982) Morphological research on the sensitivity of dentin. Arch Histol Jap 45:45–67

Hargreaves KM, Ruparel S (2016) Role of oxidized lipids and TRP channels in orofacial pain and inflammation. J Dent Res 95(10):1117–1123

Haug SR, Heyeraas KJ (2006) Modulation of dental inflammation by the sympathetic nervous system. J Dent Res 85(6):488–495

Henry MA, Luo S, Levinson SR (2012) Unmyelinated nerve fibers in the human dental pulp express markers for myelinated fibers and show sodium channel accumulations. BMC Neurosci 13:29

Heyeraas KJ, Berggreen E (1999) Interstitial fluid pressure in normal and inflamed pulp. Crit Rev Oral Biol Med 10(3):328–336

Hildebrand C, Fried K, Tuisku F, Johansson CS (1995) Teeth and tooth nerves. Prog Neurobiol 45(3):165–222

Holland GR (1996) Experimental trigeminal nerve injury. Crit Rev Oral Biol Med 7(3):237–258

Huang GT, Gronthos S, Shi S (2009) Mesenchymal stem cells derived from dental tissues vs. those from other sources: their biology and role in regenerative medicine. J Dent Res 88(9):792–806

Ikeda H, Suda H (2013) Odontoblastic syncytium through electrical coupling in the human dental pulp. J Dent Res 92(4):371–375

Ishii DN, Glazner GW, Pu SF (1994) Role of insulin-like growth factors in peripheral nerve regeneration. Pharmacol Ther 62(1-2):125–144

Jessberger S, Gage FH (2014) Adult neurogenesis: bridging the gap between mice and humans. Trends Cell Biol 24(10):558–563

Jordt SE, Bautista DM, Chuang HH, McKemy DD, Zygmunt PM, Högestätt ED, Meng ID, Julius D (2004) Mustard oils and cannabinoids excite sensory nerve fibres through the TRP channel ANKTM1. Nature 427(6971):260–265

Julius D, Basbaum AI (2001) Molecular mechanisms of nociception. Nature 413:203–210

Kaukua N, Shahidi MK, Konstantinidou C, Dyachuk V, Kaucka M, Furlan A, An Z, Wang L, Hultman I, Ahrlund-Richter L, Blom H, Brismar H, Lopes NA, Pachnis V, Suter U, Clevers H, Thesleff I, Sharpe P, Ernfors P, Fried K, Adameyko I (2014) Glial origin of mesenchymal stem cells in a tooth model system. Nature 513(7519):551–554

Kollar EJ, Lumsden AG (1979) Tooth morphogenesis: the role of the innervation during induction and pattern formation. J Biol Buccale 7(1):49–60

Kriegstein A, Alvarez-Buylla A (2009) The glial nature of embryonic and adult neural stem cells. Annu Rev Neurosci 32:149–184

Lawson SN, Waddell PJ (1991) Soma neurofilament immunoreactivity is related to cell size and fibre conduction velocity in rat primary sensory neurons. J Physiol 435:41–63

Liedtke W, Choe Y, Martí-Renom MA, Bell AM, Denis CS, Sali A, Hudspeth AJ, Friedman JM, Heller S (2000) Vanilloid receptor-related osmotically activated channel (VR-OAC), a candidate vertebrate osmoreceptor. Cell 103(3):525–535

Liu X, Wang C, Fujita T, Malmstrom HS, Nedergaard M, Ren YF, Dirksen RT (2015) External dentin stimulation induces ATP release in human teeth. J Dent Res 94(9):1259–1266

Løes S, Kettunen P, Kvinnsland IH, Taniguchi M, Fujisawa H, Luukko K (2001) Expression of class 3 semaphorins and neuropilin receptors in the developing mouse tooth. Mech Dev 101(1-2):191–194

Loeser JD, Treede RD (2008) The Kyoto protocol of IASP basic pain terminology. Pain 137:473–477

Lumsden AG, Buchanan JA (1986) An experimental study of timing and topography of early tooth development in the mouse embryo with an analysis of the role of innervation. Arch Oral Biol 31:301–311

Lundy FT, Linden GJ (2004) Neuropeptides and neurogenic mechanisms in oral and periodontal inflammation. Crit Rev Oral Biol Med 15:82–98

Luo S, Perry GM, Levinson SR, Henry MA (2008) Nav1.7 expression is increased in painful human dental pulp. Mol Pain 4:16

Luukko K, Kettunen P (2014) Coordination of tooth morphogenesis and neuronal development through tissue interactions: lessons from mouse models. Exp Cell Res 325(2):72–77

Magloire H, Lesage F, Couble ML, Lazdunski M, Bleicher F (2003) Expression and localization of TREK-1 K+ channels in human odontoblasts. J Dent Res 82(7):542–545

Martens W, Sanen K, Georgiou M, Struys T, Bronckaers A, Ameloot M, Phillips J, Lambrichts I (2014) Human dental pulp stem cells can differentiate into Schwann cells and promote and guide neurite outgrowth in an aligned tissue-engineered collagen construct in vitro. FASEB J 28(4):1634–1643

McKemy DD, Neuhausser WM, Julius D (2002) Identification of a cold receptor reveals a general role for TRP channels in thermosensation. Nature 416(6876):52–58

Mead B, Logan A, Berry M, Leadbeater W, Scheven BA (2013) Intravitreally transplanted dental pulp stem cells promote neuroprotection and axon regeneration of retinal ganglion cells after optic nerve injury. Invest Ophthalmol Vis Sci 54(12):7544–7556

Mead B, Logan A, Berry M, Leadbeater W, Scheven BA (2014a) Paracrine-mediated neuroprotection and neuritogenesis of axotomised retinal ganglion cells by human dental pulp stem cells: comparison with human bone marrow and adipose-derived mesenchymal stem cells. PLoS One 9(10):e109305

Mead B, Logan A, Berry M, Leadbeater W, Scheven BA (2014b) Dental pulp stem cells, a paracrine-mediated therapy for the retina. Neural Regen Res 9(6):577–578

Mead B, Hill LJ, Blanch RJ, Ward K, Logan A, Berry M, Leadbeater W, Scheven BA (2016) Mesenchymal stromal cell-mediated neuroprotection and functional preservation of retinal ganglion cells in a rodent model of glaucoma. Cytotherapy 18(4):487–496

Mead B, Logan A, Berry M, Leadbeater W, Scheven BA (2017) Concise review: dental pulp stem cells: a novel cell therapy for retinal and central nervous system repair. Stem Cells 35(1):61–67

Mejre IA, Axelsson S, Davidson T et al (2012) Diagnosis of the condition of the dental pulp: a systematic review. Int Endod J 45:597–613

Meseguer V, Alpizar YA, Luis E, Tajada S, Denlinger B, Fajardo O, Manenschijn JA, Fernández-Peña C, Talavera A, Kichko T, Navia B, Sánchez A, Señarís R, Reeh P, Pérez-García MT, López-López JR, Voets T, Belmonte C, Talavera K, Viana F (2014) TRPA1 channels mediate acute neurogenic inflammation and pain produced by bacterial endotoxins. Nat Commun 5:3125

Mickle AD, Shepherd AJ, Mohapatra DP (2016) Nociceptive TRP channels: sensory detectors and transducers in multiple pain pathologies. Pharmaceuticals (Basel) 9(4). [pii] E72. Review

Mitsiadis TA, Luukko K (1995) Neurotrophins in odontogenesis. Int J Dev Biol 39(1):195–202

Mitsiadis TA, Magloire H, Pagella P (2017) Nerve growth factor signalling in pathology and regeneration of human teeth. Sci Rep 7(1):1327

Morales-Lázaro SL, Simon SA, Rosenbaum T (2013) The role of endogenous molecules in modulating pain through transient receptor potential vanilloid 1 (TRPV1). J Physiol 591(13):3109–3121. https://doi.org/10.1113/jphysiol.2013.251751

Muraki K, Shigekawa M, Imaizumi Y (2007) A new insight into the function of TRPV2 in circulatory organs. In: Liedtke WB, Heller S (eds) TRP Ion channel function in sensory transduction and cellular signaling cascades. CRC Press/Taylor & Francis, Boca Raton, FL

Nanci A (2012) Ten Cate Oral Histology. Mosby, St. Louis, MO

Närhi M, Jyväsjärvi E, Virtanen A, Huopaniemi T, Ngassapa D, Hirvonen T (1992) Role of intradental A- and C-type nerve fibres in dental pain mechanisms. Proc Finn Dent Soc 88(Suppl 1):507–516

Olgart L, Edwall L, Gazelius B (1991) Involvement of afferent nerves in pulpal blood-flow reactions in response to clinical and experimental procedures in the cat. Arch Oral Biol 36(8):575–581

Peier AM, Moqrich A, Hergarden AC, Reeve AJ, Andersson DA, Story GM, Earley TJ, Dragoni I, McIntyre P, Bevan S, Patapoutian A (2002) A TRP channel that senses cold stimuli and menthol. Cell 108(5):705–715

Ramsey IS, Delling M, Clapham DE (2006) An introduction to TRP channels. Annu Rev Physiol 68:619–647

Reader AI, Foreman DW (1981) An ultrastructural quantitative investigation of human intradental innervation. J Endod 7:493–499

Redmond WJ, Gu L, Camo M, McIntyre P, Connor M (2014) Ligand determinants of fatty acid activation of the pronociceptive ion channel TRPA1. PeerJ 2:e248

Ricucci D, Loghin S, Siqueira JF Jr (2014) Correlation between clinical and histologic pulp diagnoses. J Endod 40(12):1932–1939. https://doi.org/10.1016/j.joen.2014.08.010

Rodd HD, Boissonade FM (2000) Substance P expression in human tooth pulp in relation to caries and pain experience. Eur J Oral Sci 108(6):467–474

Rodd HD, Boissonade FM (2002) Comparative immunohistochemical analysis of the peptidergic innervation of human primary and permanent tooth pulp. Arch Oral Biol 47(5):375–385

Ruch JV (1998) Odontoblast commitment and differentiation. Biochem Cell Biol 76(6):923–938

Sakai K, Yamamoto A, Matsubara K, Nakamura S, Naruse M, Yamagata M, Sakamoto K, Tauchi R, Wakao N, Imagama S, Hibi H, Kadomatsu K, Ishiguro N, Ueda M (2012) Human dental pulp-derived stem cells promote locomotor recovery after complete transection of the rat spinal cord by multiple neuro-regenerative mechanisms. J Clin Invest 122(1):80–90

Scheven BA, Shelton RM, Cooper PR, Walmsley AD, Smith AJ (2009) Therapeutic ultrasound for dental tissue repair. Med Hypotheses 73(4):591–593

Seltzer S, Bender IB, Ziontz M (1963) The dynamics of pulp inflammation: correlations between diagnostic data and actual histologic findings in the pulp. Oral Surg Oral Med Oral Pathol 16:846–871

Sisignano M, Bennett DL, Geisslinger G, Scholich K (2014) TRP-channels as key integrators of lipid pathways in nociceptive neurons. Prog Lipid Res 53:93–107

Smith GD, Gunthorpe MJ, Kelsell RE, Hayes PD, Reilly P, Facer P, Wright JE, Jerman JC, Walhin JP, Ooi L, Egerton J, Charles KJ, Smart D, Randall AD, Anand P, Davis JB (2002) TRPV3 is a temperature-sensitive vanilloid receptor-like protein. Nature 418(6894):186–190

Smith AJ, Scheven BA, Takahashi Y, Ferracane JL, Shelton RM, Cooper PR (2012) Dentine as a bioactive extracellular matrix. Arch Oral Biol 57(2):109–121

Solé-Magdalena A, Martínez-Alonso M, Coronado CA, Junquera LM, Cobo J, Vega JA (2018) Molecular basis of dental sensitivity: the odontoblasts are multisensory cells and express multifunctional ion channels. Ann Anat 215:20–29

Story GM, Peier AM, Reeve AJ, Eid SR, Mosbacher J, Hricik TR, Earley TJ, Hergarden AC, Andersson DA, Hwang SW, McIntyre P, Jegla T, Bevan S, Patapoutian A (2003) ANKTM1, a TRP-like channel expressed in nociceptive neurons, is activated by cold temperatures. Cell 112(6):819–829

Taylor-Clark TE, Ghatta S, Bettner W, Undem BJ (2009) Nitrooleic acid, an endogenous product of nitrative stress, activates nociceptive sensory nerves via the direct activation of TRPA1. Mol Pharmacol 75:820–829

Watanabe H, Vriens J, Prenen J, Droogmans G, Voets T, Nilius B (2003) Anandamide and arachidonic acid use epoxyeicosatrienoic acids to activate TRPV4 channels. Nature 424(6947):434–438

Wolters WJ, Duncan HF, Tomson PL, El karim I, McKenna G, Dorri M, Stangvaltaite L, van der Sluis LWM (2017) Minimally invasive endodontics: a new diagnostic system for assessing pulpitis and subsequent treatment needs. Int Endod J 50(9):825–829

Xu W, Lakshman N, Morshead CM (2017) Building a central nervous system: the neural stem cell lineage revealed. Neurogenesis (Austin) 4(1):e1300037

Yoshida S, Wada N, Hasegawa D, Miyaji H, Mitarai H, Tomokiyo A, Hamano S, Maeda H (2016) Semaphorin 3A induces odontoblastic phenotype in dental pulp stem cells. J Dent Res 95(11):1282–1290

Current and Future Views on Pulpal Angiogenesis

3

Petra Hilkens, Ivo Lambrichts, and Annelies Bronckaers

3.1 Introduction

Dental pulp tissue has important functions in the maintenance of tooth vitality, providing nutrients and oxygen, innervation, pain sensation, an immune response and formation of reparative dentine after injury. It can be injured through trauma, excessive wear or invasion by cariogenic oral bacteria, which can ultimately lead to acute irreversible immune/inflammatory events and destruction of the pulp tissue. Preservation of pulp viability is a major challenge in endodontics, as devitalised teeth are more vulnerable and prone to tooth loss later. Treatment of immature teeth, in particular, remains to be a challenge as any factor that interferes with normal pulp physiology may conflict with the completion of root development. Adequate revascularisation is a determining factor in successful dental pulp tissue preservation. To understand the process of pulpal blood vessel formation, the general molecular mechanisms of neovascularisation during embryogenesis and adult life are first discussed.

3.2 The Principles of Blood Vessel Formation

Within the human body, an extensive network of arteries, veins and capillaries can be found which are responsible for the oxygen and nutrient supply, waste removal and transportation of a plethora of different cell types and molecules. Depending on its function and location, the vasculature also displays different tissue-specific and organ-specific features, which are already determined during embryonic development.

With regard to blood vessel growth and maturation, three different mechanisms can be distinguished, namely, vasculogenesis, angiogenesis and arteriogenesis.

P. Hilkens (✉) · I. Lambrichts · A. Bronckaers
Morphology Research Group, Biomedical Research Institute, Hasselt University,
Diepenbeek, Belgium
e-mail: petra.hilkens@uhasselt.be

© Springer Nature Switzerland AG 2019
H. F. Duncan, P. R. Cooper (eds.), *Clinical Approaches in Endodontic Regeneration*,
https://doi.org/10.1007/978-3-319-96848-3_3

3.2.1　Vasculogenesis

During embryonic development, the primitive vascular network is initially formed by vasculogenesis (Fig. 3.1a). This process comprises the recruitment of mesodermally

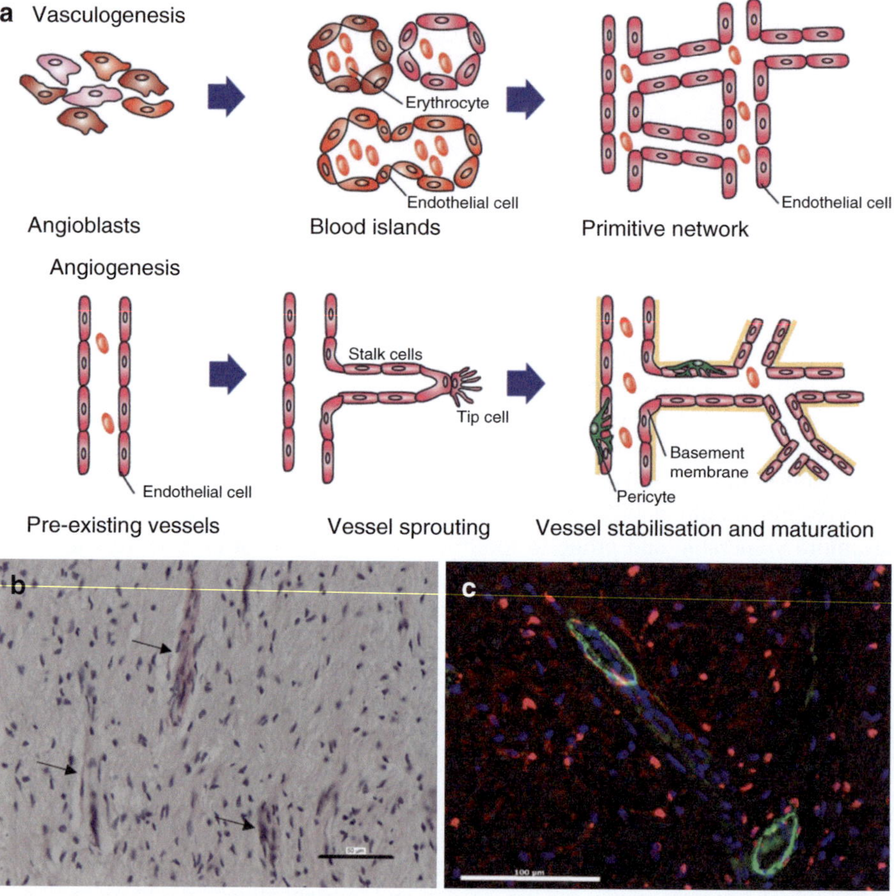

Fig. 3.1 (**a**) Schematic representation of vasculogenesis and angiogenesis. Vasculogenesis is defined as the formation of a primitive vascular network by mesodermally derived endothelial precursor cells, i.e. angioblasts. During embryonic development, angioblasts will first form primitive blood islands and differentiate into endothelial cells and erythrocytes. Subsequently, a primitive vascular plexus is formed which is further extended through angiogenesis. Angiogenesis comprises the formation of blood vessels out of pre-existing vessels during embryogenesis as well as in the adult human body. Specialised endothelial phenotypes will develop due to extensive growth factor signalling and give rise to immature blood vessels. Briefly, tip cells will migrate towards certain chemotactic stimuli, followed by the proliferation of stalk cells. The formation of intracellular vacuoles will eventually lead to the development of a vessel lumen. During the final phase of angiogenesis, i.e. blood vessel maturation, a stable vascular network emerges by anastomosis of adjacent sprouts, the formation of a basement membrane and the recruitment of pericytes. (**b**) Hematoxylin-eosin staining of human pulp tissue, indicating the presence of blood vessels (black arrows). Scale bar = 50 µm. (**c**) Immunofluorescent staining of human pulp tissue against VEGF (red) and CD146 (green). DAPI (blue) was used to stain the nuclei. This staining indicates a pronounced expression of CD146 in the pulp blood vessels, while the surrounding stromal cells express high amounts of VEGF. Scale bar = 100 µm

derived endothelial precursor cells or angioblasts that will coalesce. This begins in the yolk sack and will give rise to a primitive vascular plexus which provides the yolk sac circulation as well as the first primitive network inside the embryo, forming vessels such as the cardinal vein and the dorsal aorta. Subsequently, this network is enlarged by processes such as angiogenesis and arteriogenesis which are the key processes of blood vessel formation in adult life (Jain 2003; Swift and Weinstein 2009).

3.2.2 Angiogenesis

Generally speaking, angiogenesis can be defined as the formation of new capillaries from pre-existing blood vessels (Fig. 3.1a). Although the concept of angiogenesis entails both capillary sprouting and intussusception, i.e. the internal division of previously formed vessels, capillary sprouting is considered to be the most predominant form of vascular development within the adult human body (Swift and Weinstein 2009).

As any multistep biological process, the initiation and continuation of capillary sprouting are strongly coordinated by a myriad of growth factors, chemokines and other proteins. In general, these regulatory mechanisms are characterised by a distinct balance between activation and inhibition of blood vessel formation with the inhibiting factors being the most dominant, thus maintaining a quiescent state. In the presence of hypoxia or any other condition that requires oxygen and nutrients and thus new blood vessel formation, the excess production of stimulatory proteins causes a so-called 'angiogenic switch', tipping the balance towards blood vessel growth (Bronckaers et al. 2014; Distler et al. 2003).

One of the main cell types in the angiogenic process are endothelial cells (ECs). As previously mentioned, these cells normally remain in a quiescent state, enclosed by a vascular basement membrane and mural cells such as pericytes and smooth muscle cells that provide support, protect the cells from the environment and prevent the cells from detaching (Potente et al. 2011). Extensive growth factor signalling, e.g. after a wound or inflammation, leads to endothelial activation and the transient development of specialised endothelial phenotypes (Phng and Gerhardt 2009). Together with vascular endothelial growth factor (VEGF), extensive Notch signalling enables the establishment of a well-coordinated pattern of tip and stalk cells (Potente et al. 2011; Phng and Gerhardt 2009). In response to pro-angiogenic signalling, tip cells will facilitate proteolytic breakdown of the vascular basement membrane by secretion of matrix metalloproteinases (MMPs) and subsequently lead the migrating front of endothelial cells by scanning the environment for angiogenic cues with their filopodia (Potente et al. 2011; Adams and Alitalo 2007). Stalk cells, on the other hand, will proliferate abundantly in order to extend the formed vessel sprout. The formation of intracellular vacuoles, which will fuse with vacuoles of adjoining ECs, will eventually lead to the development of a vessel lumen. Through the production of extracellular matrix (ECM) components, stalk cells also safeguard the integrity of the formed vessel sprout (Potente et al. 2011; Phng and Gerhardt 2009). Finally, a stable vascular network emerges by anastomosis of adjacent sprouts and the recruitment of mural cells. After perfusion, pro-angiogenic signalling will diminish and the ECs return to a resting phenotype (Potente et al. 2011).

3.2.3 Arteriogenesis

Arteriogenesis, i.e. the maturation and stabilisation of the nascent vascular structures, encompasses the active recruitment of pericytes and smooth muscle cells, the deposition of a supportive ECM and the tissue-specific specialisation of the vessel wall in order to ensure vascular function (Jain 2003).

During embryonic development, arteriovenous specification and endothelial differentiation, i.e. vessel specialisation, are not only determined by haemodynamic load but also comprise specific molecular interactions involving VEGF, Notch and members of the Eph receptor kinases and their ephrin ligand, which will eventually lead to a well-organised, tissue-specific network of arteries, veins and capillaries (Jain 2003; Swift and Weinstein 2009).

Similar to vasculogenesis and angiogenesis, vessel maturation is tightly regulated by different molecular signalling pathways. Transforming growth factor-beta (TGF-β), for example, is closely involved in the production of ECM as well as the induction and differentiation of mural cells. The recruitment of pericytes, on the other hand, is mediated by platelet-derived growth factor receptor-beta (PDGFR-β) signalling. Angiopoietin 1 and 2 (ANGPT1 and ANGPT2) also play a critical role in the process of arteriogenesis. Binding to their receptors, Tie1 and Tie2, promotes vessel stabilisation and enables leak resistance by tightening endothelial cell junctions. Interactions between ECs and mural cells are controlled by sphingosine-1-phosphate receptor signalling by causing changes in cytoskeleton organisation and cell adhesion (Jain 2003; Gaengel et al. 2009).

3.3 Blood and Lymph Vessels in the Dental Pulp

3.3.1 Tooth Development

During mammalian tooth development, strongly regulated reciprocal interactions take place between neural crest-derived mesenchymal tissues and ectodermally derived dental epithelium. Tooth morphogenesis and differentiation comprise different stages, with each exhibiting their own specific spatio-temporal events, eventually leading to tooth eruption (Jussila et al. 2013). Given the close relationship between the neurovascular supply of the tooth and tooth morphogenesis, mesenchymal invasion of both nerve fibres and blood vessels already occurs during the late cap stage and/or early bell stage (Jussila et al. 2013; Nait Lechguer et al. 2008). In addition, changes in vascular pressure presumably play a role in the timing and rate of tooth eruption, although definitive conclusions cannot be made at present (Burn-Murdoch 1990; Kjaer 2014; Wise and King 2008).

3.3.2 Vascular Anatomy of the Dental Pulp

The main vascular supply of the dental pulp originates from the maxillary artery, which branches off the external carotid artery. The maxillary artery flows into the dental artery, which enters the dental pulp through arterioles, forming the pulp microvasculature (Kim 1985). In terms of structural arrangement, the pulpal microcirculation is characterised by a strong hierarchical organisation: the arterioles spread throughout the central part of the dental pulp and eventually form a subodontoblastic capillary network (Kim 1985; Yu and Abbott 2007). This peripheral capillary plexus displays strong regional differences, ranging from a fishnet organisation in the roots to a dense network of hairpin-shaped capillaries in the pulp horn (Kim 1985). The blood vessels are mainly lined by a continuous layer of endothelium, except for the subodontoblastic capillaries which display endothelial fenestrations, reflecting the distinct metabolic demand in this region (Berggreen et al. 2010). The blood eventually drains into venules, which mainly comprise the central part of the pulp tissue and exit the tooth through the apical foramen (Kim 1985).

The pulpal microvasculature also displays certain specialised features, such as the presence of vascular shunts. These anastomoses are either arteriovenous, venous-venous or U-turn loops and presumably play an important role in the regulation of blood flow, given the direct connection between arterioles and venules which bypasses the aforementioned capillary plexus (Kim 1985; Yu and Abbott 2007).

Next to an extensive vascular network (Fig. 3.1b, c), dental pulp tissue also contains lymphatic vessels, which can be identified by their expression of VEGF receptor-3 (VEGFR-3) and lymphatic endothelial hyaluronan receptor-1 (LYVE-1) (Pimenta et al. 2003; Berggreen et al. 2009). These thin-walled vessels originate in the coronal region of the dental pulp and can be clearly distinguished from venules due to the absence of erythrocytes and the presence of wall discontinuities (Nanci 2008). Lymphatic vessels exit the dental pulp, either through large vessels in the apical foramen or through lateral canals in the radicular region (Berggreen et al. 2010; Nanci 2008).

3.3.3 Importance and Regulation of Dental Pulp Vasculature

As any vascular network, the main function of the pulpal microcirculation is to provide sufficient oxygen and nutrients to the tissue's residing cells as well as remove waste products. Studies have also described the relatively high interstitial tissue pressure within the dental pulp tissue, as compared to the vascular blood pressure. However, the constant tissue fluid volume within the pulp tissue indicates an important role for the dental pulp's microvascular network in the management of both the intraluminal vascular pressure and the pressure within the pulp tissue itself (Yu and Abbott 2007; Heyeraas 1989).

Given the low compliance of the dental pulp, the lack of a collateral blood supply and its important role in pressure and blood flow maintenance, strict regulation of the pulpal circulation is of utmost importance in order to safeguard the health of the dental pulp tissue (Yu and Abbott 2007). In physiological circumstances, vascular tone is regulated at different levels, i.e. through local, neurological and humoral mechanisms (Berggreen et al. 2010).

The dental pulp is a strongly innervated tissue, containing afferent sensory fibres, parasympathetic and sympathetic nerve fibres which are closely associated with the pulpal vascular system (Rodd and Boissonade 2003; Zhang et al. 1998; Caviedes-Bucheli et al. 2008). In addition to sympathetic vascular regulation, a wide array of neuropeptides released by sensory nerve fibres also actively modulates the pulp's vasculature, in particular through vasodilation. More specifically, substance P, calcitonin gene-related peptide (CGRP) and neurokinin A have been shown to cause long-lasting increases in pulpal blood flow upon tooth stimulation (Caviedes-Bucheli et al. 2008).

With regard to the local regulation of pulpal blood flow, different vasoactive agents have been shown to regulate vascular resistance according to the tissue's needs (reviewed in (Berggreen et al. 2010)). The production of NO, for example, has been detected in endothelial cells as well as odontoblasts and plays an important role in the regulation of vasodilation in a number of animal models (Berggreen et al. 2010; Berggreen and Heyeraas 1999; Toda et al. 2012). Endothelin-1 (EDN-1), on the other hand, has been shown to cause a dose-dependent reduction in pulpal blood flow both in vitro and in vivo (Yu et al. 2002). Aside from locally produced regulatory agents, pulpal blood flow can also be controlled at a humoral level, by vasoactive agents which reach the dental pulp through vascular transportation such as adrenaline, dopamine and angiotensin II (Berggreen et al. 2010).

3.4 Inflammation and Angiogenesis

As already mentioned, the dental pulp is a heavily innervated and vascularised tissue which serves many specialised physiological functions. Although its enclosure within the dentinal walls provides both mechanical support and protection, the pulp tissue is very vulnerable to insults such as trauma, caries and infections once the structural integrity of the pulp chamber is compromised. In case of acute inflammation, the resulting vasodilatation will cause an increase in pulp tissue pressure, given the low compliance of the tissue (Yu and Abbott 2007). Due to the resilient, gelatin-like ground substance of the dental pulp tissue, these pressure differences and the resulting cell death remain localised, except in the case of chronic inflammation which can lead to overall tissue necrosis (Yu and Abbott 2007; Heyeraas and Berggreen 1999). The severity of the inflammatory process can thus be considered as a determining factor for the onset of regeneration and repair, as research has shown that low-grade inflammation may induce angiogenesis and stem cell-mediated regeneration, while continuing inflammation leads to tissue destruction and molecular inhibition of regeneration (Cooper et al. 2010). In a rat model of apical periodontitis, for example, a gradual upregulation of VEGF isoforms and their receptors was detected in vascular ECs, inflammatory infiltrate, osteoclasts and stromal cells over a period of 21 days, which suggests extensive vascular and bone remodelling (Bletsa et al. 2012). Artese et al., on the other hand, reported a significant downregulation of both VEGF expression and microvessel density in human dental pulp tissues from patients suffering from irreversible pulpitis (Artese et al. 2002).

In addition to caries and infection, orthodontic tooth movement can also evoke an inflammatory response and thus affect pulp blood flow and angiogenesis (reviewed in (Javed et al. 2015)). Derringer et al., for example, observed an increased microvascular density in dental pulp tissue of teeth undergoing orthodontic force application for 2 weeks (Derringer et al. 1996). In accordance with these data, the same researchers reported the release of angiogenic growth factors, more specifically epidermal growth factor (EGF), bFGF, VEGF, TGF-β and PDGF, in response to orthodontic force (Derringer and Linden 2003, 2007). A number of studies also mentioned a transient change in pulp blood flow after prolonged exposure to orthodontic forces (reviewed in (Javed et al. 2015)).

As mentioned previously, neuropeptides play an important role in maintaining pulp homoeostasis through their regulation of pulpal blood flow. In addition to normal pulp physiology, neuropeptides also contribute to both neurogenic inflammation and regeneration and repair (Caviedes-Bucheli et al. 2008). In case of occlusal trauma, for example, the subsequent neurogenic inflammation and release of neuropeptides such as substance P promote angiogenesis, either by directly modulating endothelial cell behaviour or by stimulating paracrine mechanisms. The resulting increase in vascularity will promote mineralised tissue formation, both as a defence and repair mechanism (Caviedes-Bucheli et al. 2017). Neuropeptides can also modulate the inflammatory response and regulate angiogenesis through their interaction with dental pulp (stem) cells (Caviedes-Bucheli et al. 2008). An upregulation of CGRP in dental pulp tissue was observed after orthodontic force application, presumably leading to an increased angiogenic response within the dental pulp (Caviedes-Bucheli et al. 2011). Accordingly, El Karim et al. previously demonstrated an altered expression of angiogenic growth factors such as hepatocyte growth factor (HGF), EGF and placental growth factor, after in vitro exposure of dental pulp fibroblasts to different neuropeptides (El Karim et al. 2009).

3.5 The Promotion of Dental Pulp Angiogenesis: What are the Options?

3.5.1 Cell-Free Approaches

Angiogenesis requires a complicated interplay of numerous growth factors, cytokines and ECM components. Consequently, the first revascularisation strategies involved the application of angiogenic factors in biodegradable scaffolds. A wide variety of scaffolds have been tested in preclinical tooth regeneration studies or in vitro studies. Natural biomaterials include proteins such as collagen, fibrin and silk and polysaccharides such as chitosan, hyaluronic acid, alginate and agarose. Examples of synthetic biomaterials are organic polymers like polylactic acid (PLA) and poly(lactic-co-glycolic) acid (PLGA) or inorganic calcium phosphate materials such as hydroxyapatite (HA) and β-tricalcium phosphate (β-TCP) (reviewed in (Sharma et al. 2014)). These scaffolds are used as vehicles to deliver angiogenic growth factors, which do not only attract blood vessels but also induce stem cell homing. For instance, angiogenesis and tissue regeneration were augmented in subcutaneously implanted tooth slices treated with VEGF in immunodeficient mice

(Mullane et al. 2008). Collagen scaffolds loaded with FGF-2 successfully induced blood vessel formation and tissue regeneration in human roots implanted into the dorsum of rats (Suzuki et al. 2011). Combined delivery of bFGF, VEGF or PDGF with nerve growth factor (NGF) and bone morphogenetic protein-7 generated cellularised and vascularised tissues in real-size, native human teeth in mouse dorsum after 3 weeks of implantation (Kim et al. 2010).

Besides using single or combinations of recombinant proteins, natural cocktails of such factors can also be applied. Blood platelets, blood clots and consequently blood platelet concentrates such as platelet-rich plasma (PRP), platelet-rich fibrin (PRF) and leucocyte- and platelet-rich fibrin (L-PRF) contain a plethora of angiogenic factors including VEGF, FGF-2, thymidine phosphorylase and PDGF (Masoudi et al. 2016). A good example of the regenerative potential of blood platelets and their derivatives is the current practice in regenerative endodontics, which entails the induction of a blood clot by lacerating the periapical tissue. The blood clot serves as a scaffold for new ingrowing blood vessels but is also considered to attract stem cells from the apical papilla (SCAPs) towards the root canal. Blood platelet concentrates are cost-effective, contain a plethora of growth factors and can be autologously used. In a recent triple blind clinical trial, the use of PRP, PRF and induced bleeding in revascularisation of teeth with necrotic pulp and open apex was compared. PRP performed better than both other approaches with respect to periapical wound healing. All three treatments were comparable on grounds of root lengthening and lateral wall thickening (Shivashankar et al. 2017).

3.5.2 Stem Cell-Based Approaches for Pulp Revascularisation

As vascular access within the human tooth is localised at the apical foramen, the success of revascularisation and revitalisation approaches is largely determined by the size of this apical opening. In comparison to cell homing-based methods, which induce pulp revascularisation and healing in teeth with apical sizes ranging from 1.1 to 1.5 mm, stem cell-based approaches have been proven to successfully regenerate vascularised pulp tissue in pulpectomised canine teeth with apical foramen of 0.7 mm (Hilkens et al. 2015; Iohara et al. 2011). As stem cells do not only replace tissue but also produce of a broad range of (angiogenic) growth factors, these cells are widely studied in pulp revascularisation and regeneration.

During embryonic development as well as in the adult human body, several stem cell populations can be distinguished with each exhibiting their own characteristics. Given the elaborate ethical concerns associated with the isolation and use of embryonic stem cells, induced pluripotent stem cells (iPSCs) have proven to be valuable alternative source of pluripotent stem cells. In 2006, Takahashi et al. reported the creation of iPSCs through genetic reprogramming of somatic cells (Takahashi and Yamanaka 2006). Since then, extensive characterisation of these stem cells pointed out not only their elaborate differentiation potential but also their ability to promote angiogenesis in vitro and in vivo (reviewed in (Clayton et al. 2015)). Theoretically speaking, iPSCs can thus be considered as the stem cell type of choice in dental pulp revascularisation and regeneration. However, several disadvantages are associated with the use of these stem cells, such as differences in reprogramming efficiency, teratoma formation and activation of oncogenes associated with viral cell transformation (Malhotra 2016). Therefore, multipotent or adult stem cells, in particular mesenchymal stem cells (MSCs) and dental stem cells (DSCs), are assumed to be the most favourable cell type for application in regenerative dentistry.

3.5.2.1 Mesenchymal Stem Cells

In 1970, Friedenstein et al. reported the presence of so-called colony-forming unit fibroblasts, which were later on defined as MSCs (Friedenstein et al. 1970). Elaborate characterisation of these stem cells led to the establishment of minimal criteria, defined by the International Society for Cellular Therapy (ISCT), which these stem cells have to fulfil. More specifically, MSCs have to be adherent to plastic under standard culture conditions; they have to express cell surface markers CD73, CD90 and CD105 and lack the expression of CD14, CD34, CD45, CD79a and HLA-DR; and they display an in vitro trilineage differentiation capacity into adipogenic, chondrogenic and osteogenic cells (Dominici et al. 2006). Within the human body, MSCs can be found in a variety of different tissues, such as bone marrow, tendons, umbilical cord, adipose tissue and teeth, with bone marrow-derived MSCs (BM-MSCs) being one of the most widely studied and applied sources of MSCs (Arana et al. 2013; Bi et al. 2007; Huang et al. 2009; Kim et al. 2013).

In addition to an elaborate differentiation potential, BM-MSCs also display pronounced angiogenic properties. Secretome analysis identified the expression of a vast array of angiogenic growth factors, including but not limited to angiogenin, ANGPT1 and ANGPT2, FGF-2, HGF, insulin-like growth factor-1 (IGF-1), interleukin-8 (IL-8), monocyte chemotactic protein-1 (MCP-1), MMPs, TGF-β and VEGF (reviewed in (Bronckaers et al. 2014)). Besides the promotion of endothelial proliferation, migration and tubulogenesis in vitro (Estrada et al. 2009; Gruber et al. 2005; Potapova et al. 2007), BM-MSCs have also been shown to ameliorate angiogenesis in multiple animal models of peripheral artery disease, myocardial infarction and cerebral ischemia (reviewed in (Bronckaers et al. 2014)). With regard to their potential application in regenerative endodontics, BM-MSCs were reported to successfully generate pulp-like tissue in a rat pulpectomy model. However, the authors did not describe any signs of proper tissue vascularisation after transplantation (Ito et al. 2017). Zhang et al., on the other hand, demonstrated the regeneration of pulp-like tissue with a pronounced vascularisation after SDF-1-induced stem cell homing of systemically administered BM-MSCs (Zhang et al. 2015). Similar results were found after in situ transplantation of a CD31$^-$ side population of BM-MSCs in a canine model (Ishizaka et al. 2012). Despite their aforementioned high angiogenic potential, both the invasive and traumatic isolation procedures of BM-MSCs emphasise the need for an alternative source of MSCs (Holdsworth et al. 2003).

Adipose tissue-derived mesenchymal stem cells (AD-MSCs), for example, can be relatively easy isolated through liposuction. Similar to BM-MSCs, these stem cells also secrete several angiogenic growth factors, such as HGF, IGF-1, TGF-β and VEGF (Nakagami et al. 2005; Rehman et al. 2004). AD-MSCs were successfully applied in animal models of ischemic heart disease, wound healing and peripheral vascular disease (reviewed in (Zhao et al. 2017)). With regard to the use of AD-MSCs in dental pulp revascularisation and regeneration, a CD105$^+$ subpopulation of these stem cells was not able to form a significant amount of vascularised, pulp-like tissue in a canine pulpectomy model (Iohara et al. 2011). In contrast, Hung et al. described the successful regeneration of innervated and vascularised tooth implants by AD-MSCs and dental pulp stem cells (DPSCs). Potential differences in vascularisation rate of the newly formed tissue were not reported (Hung et al. 2011). When comparing the regenerative potential of CD31$^-$ side populations of DPSCs, BM-MSCs and AD-MSCs in a canine model with complete apical closure, Ishizaka et al. detected no significant differences between these stem cell populations with regard to their neovascularisation potential (Ishizaka et al. 2012). However, transplantation of a granulocyte colony-stimulating factor (G-CSF)-mobilised population of AD-MSCs led to the formation of a significantly lower volume of pulp-like tissue with significantly less angiogenesis in comparison to a similar population of DPSCs (Murakami et al. 2015)

3.5.2.2 Dental Stem Cells

Given their inherent capacity to repair and regenerate dental tissues, DSCs are one of the most widely studied stem cell populations for regenerative endodontic procedures. DPSCs, stem cells from human exfoliated deciduous teeth (SHEDs), SCAPs and dental follicle precursor cells (FSCs), in particular, have been successfully administered in different in vivo models of dental pulp regeneration (Hilkens et al. 2015; Ratajczak et al. 2016). According to the previously mentioned minimal criteria of the ISCT, DSCs are considered to be mesenchymal-like stem cells (Dominici et al. 2006; Huang et al. 2009). Over the past decade, an increasing amount of research has been performed regarding the ability of DSCs to promote angiogenesis in vitro and in vivo.

Angiogenic Properties of Dental Stem Cells

With regard to the angiogenic properties of DSCs, a number of studies have indicated their ability to secrete a broad range of angiogenic growth factors and stimulatory proteins such as angiogenin, ANGPT1 and ANGPT2, FGF-2, CSF, dipeptidyl peptidase IV, EDN-1, IGF-1, insulin-like growth factor-binding protein-3, IL-8, HGF, MMPs, MCP-1, PDGF, urokinase-type plasminogen activator and VEGF (reviewed in (Ratajczak et al. 2016)). Furthermore, the DSC secretome also contains a substantial amount of inhibitory proteins, more specifically endostatin, pentraxin-3, pigment epithelium-derived factor, plasminogen activator inhibitor-1, tissue inhibitor of matrix metalloproteinases and thrombospondin-1 (reviewed in (Ratajczak et al. 2016)).

Given their secretion of stimulatory as well as inhibitory proteins, the potential influence of DSCs on the behaviour of ECs has been widely investigated in different in vitro models (Ratajczak et al. 2016). With regard to endothelial proliferation, for example, our research group demonstrated no considerable impact of DPSCs, SCAPs or FSCs on the proliferation of human microvascular endothelial cells

(HMECs) (Hilkens et al. 2014). In contrast, hypoxia-preconditioned DPSCs were reported to cause a time-dependent augmentation of endothelial proliferation (Aranha et al. 2010), which confirmed earlier findings by Iohara et al., describing a pronounced increase in the proliferation and survival of human umbilical vein endothelial cells (HUVECs) caused by a $CD31^-/CD146^-$ subpopulation of DPSCs (Iohara et al. 2008). Next to endothelial proliferation, DPSCs and SCAPs have been proven to successfully induce endothelial migration towards a chemotactic gradient of proteins (Hilkens et al. 2014). DSCs are also able to promote endothelial tubulogenesis, as was shown in a variety of direct and indirect co-culture systems (Hilkens et al. 2014; Tran-Hung et al. 2006; Yuan et al. 2015; Dissanayaka et al. 2012; Janebodin et al. 2013). Regarding the potential influence of DSCs on the angiogenic process as a whole, our group and others identified a marked increase in the number of blood vessels after application of DPSCs or SCAPs in the chicken chorioallantoic membrane assay (Hilkens et al. 2014; Bronckaers et al. 2013; Woloszyk et al. 2016).

In addition to paracrine regulation of angiogenesis, MSCs are also understood to promote angiogenesis in a direct manner by differentiating into ECs (Sieveking and Ng 2009). With regard to DSCs, DPSCs, SCAPs and SHEDs in particular have been shown to successfully differentiate towards ECs (reviewed in (Ratajczak et al. 2016; About 2014)). DPSCs, for example, were reported to co-differentiate into endotheliocytes, following osteogenic differentiation of a sorted subpopulation (d'Aquino et al. 2007). Differentiated DPSCs were also able to form extensive capillary networks in vitro, as was shown by Marchionni and others (Barachini et al. 2014; Marchionni et al. 2009). Similar results were found for SHEDs, indicating a VEGF-induced upregulation of endothelial markers as well as capillary sprouting in vitro and in vivo (Bento et al. 2013; Cordeiro et al. 2008; Sakai et al. 2010; Zhang et al. 2016). Endothelial differentiation of SCAPs was recently reported by Bakopoulou et al., describing both the upregulation of endothelial markers and the development of capillaries in normoxic culture conditions. Ischemic preconditioning of the cells even led to the establishment of a more pronounced endothelial phenotype (Bakopoulou et al. 2015).

Dental Stem Cells in Dental Pulp Revascularisation and Regeneration

Over the past 15 years, a substantial amount of studies have been published concerning the potential application of DSCs in regenerative endodontic procedures. Both DPSCs and SCAPs have been proven to be a potent cell-based approach for the regeneration of vascularised, pulp-like tissue in a wide variety of in vivo models. Takeuchi et al., for example, reported the successful regeneration of dental pulp tissue after administration of a mobilised subpopulation of DSPCs in an ectopic root transplantation model. While there was no difference in vascularisation rate between the described cell homing-based approaches, the observed capillary density in the newly formed tissue was considerably higher after transplantation of DPSCs supported by a collagen gel (Takeuchi et al. 2015). Kuang et al. showed the formation of vascularised, pulp-like tissue containing a significantly higher number of blood vessels after transplantation of nanofibrous spongy microspheres containing hypoxia-primed DPSCs compared to DPSCs cultured under normoxic conditions

(Kuang et al. 2016). When combining DPSCs with VEGF in an ectopic root transplantation model, a notably higher amount of tissue was formed in comparison to root canals containing solely DPSCs. In terms of vascularisation, however, no significant differences between the experimental conditions were detected (Li et al. 2016). In situ transplantation of constructs containing either canine DPSCs and PRF or DPSCs alone led to a significant promotion of blood vessel formation in comparison to PRF particles alone (Chen et al. 2015). Another combined approach was used by Dissanayaka et al., describing the regeneration of vascularised pulp-like tissue after transplantation of a hydrogel containing DPSCs and HUVECs in an ectopic root transplantation model. This combined method led to more pronounced vascularisation in comparison to the root fragments containing DPSCs alone (Dissanayaka et al. 2015).

As previously described by Rombouts and others, the interaction between DSCs and their micro-environment is a crucial factor, not only in the engraftment of the transplanted cells but also in the regulation of their intrinsic behaviour such as the secretion of paracrine factors (Rombouts et al. 2017; Tran and Damaser 2015). Recent work from our group demonstrated the successful regeneration of vascularised, pulp-like tissue in 3D-printed, hydroxyapatite scaffolds. However, quantification of the vascularisation rate pointed out a significantly lower amount of blood vessels/mm² in the constructs containing DPSCs and/or SCAPs when compared to the negative control condition. These data, together with the observed formation of mineralised tissue within the stem cell constructs suggest a preferential osteogenic/odontogenic differentiation of DSCs rather than the expected promotion of angiogenesis within the applied time frame, which emphasises the determining role of the micro-environment at the time of transplantation partly determined by the experimental conditions such as the choice of scaffold material and duration of construct transplantation (Hilkens et al. 2017).

3.6 Conclusion and Future Perspectives

Over the past two decades, substantial advances have been made in unravelling the angiogenic process and in the application of pro-angiogenic proteins, blood platelet products and stem cells as approaches to induce blood vessel formation and subsequent dental pulp regeneration in animal models. In addition, recent innovations in tissue engineering, such as the use of bioprinted scaffolds, could play a promising role in regenerative dentistry. Athirasala et al., for example, recently developed printable alginate hydrogels with fractions of dentine matrix, which enhanced odontogenic differentiation of SCAPs encapsulated in these hydrogels (Athirasala et al. 2018). Nanotechnology, another promising scientific development, has made it possible to deliver proteins or drugs by means of vehicles such as agarose beads, collagen sponges, alginate gels and hydrogel microspheres, thereby allowing a slow and prolonged release of these substances into the micro-environment.

Despite the high potential of angiogenic approaches such as stem cells, 3D printing and recombinant proteins, more advances are needed before these therapies can enter the clinic. Cost-effectiveness, for example, as large-scale stem cell propagation, bioprinting or production of bioscaffolds, is currently non-existent or expensive. In addition, application of the aforementioned vascularisation approaches is labour intensive and still requires extensive monitoring. However, clinical translation remains complicated as multiple issues still need to be resolved, such as timing, dose and the presence of a suitable micro-environment/scaffold. The majority of the studies in the literature are based on subcutaneous implantation models in mice with healthy human teeth. These assays lack any signs of inflammation and bacterial infections and are often performed in immunocompromised animals. This is far removed from the clinical situation where pulp regeneration is mostly needed in pathological conditions such as necrosis, inflammation and apical periodontitis. Moreover, endodontic procedures entail the removal of the necrotic tissue and disinfection of the root canal which is potentially harmful for the biological tissues and their regenerative potential. Development of new animal models mimicking the clinical situations is thus needed to ascertain successful dentine-pulp regeneration with these procedures. In conclusion, despite the recent advances made in dental tissue engineering and the promotion of angiogenesis more specifically, there is still a long road ahead with regard to the application of effective revascularisation and regeneration treatment protocols in endodontics.

References

About I (2014) Pulp vascularization and its regulation by the microenvironment. In: Goldberg M (ed) The dental pulp: biology, pathology, and regenerative therapies. Springer, Berlin, pp 61–74

Adams RH, Alitalo K (2007) Molecular regulation of angiogenesis and lymphangiogenesis. Nat Rev Mol Cell Biol 8(6):464–478

Arana M et al (2013) Adipose tissue-derived mesenchymal stem cells: isolation, expansion, and characterization. Methods Mol Biol 1036:47–61

Aranha AM et al (2010) Hypoxia enhances the angiogenic potential of human dental pulp cells. J Endod 36(10):1633–1637

Artese L et al (2002) Vascular endothelial growth factor (VEGF) expression in healthy and inflamed human dental pulps. J Endod 28(1):20–23

Athirasala A et al (2018) A Dentin-derived hydrogel bioink for 3D printing of cell laden scaffolds for regenerative dentistry. Biofabrication 10:024101

Bakopoulou A et al (2015) Angiogenic potential and secretome of human apical papilla mesenchymal stem cells in various stress microenvironments. Stem Cells Dev 24(21):2496–2512

Barachini S et al (2014) Plasticity of human dental pulp stromal cells with bioengineering platforms: a versatile tool for regenerative medicine. Micron 67:155–168

Bento LW et al (2013) Endothelial differentiation of SHED requires MEK1/ERK signaling. J Dent Res 92(1):51–57

Berggreen E, Heyeraas KJ (1999) The role of sensory neuropeptides and nitric oxide on pulpal blood flow and tissue pressure in the ferret. J Dent Res 78(9):1535–1543

Berggreen E et al (2009) Characterization of the dental lymphatic system and identification of cells immunopositive to specific lymphatic markers. Eur J Oral Sci 117(1):34–42

Berggreen E, Bletsa A, Heyeraas KJ (2010) Circulation in normal and inflamed dental pulp. Endod Topics 17:2–11

Bi Y et al (2007) Identification of tendon stem/progenitor cells and the role of the extracellular matrix in their niche. Nat Med 13(10):1219–1227

Bletsa A, Virtej A, Berggreen E (2012) Vascular endothelial growth factors and receptors are up-regulated during development of apical periodontitis. J Endod 38(5):628–635

Bronckaers A et al (2013) Angiogenic properties of human dental pulp stem cells. PLoS One 8(8):e71104

Bronckaers A et al (2014) Mesenchymal stem/stromal cells as a pharmacological and therapeutic approach to accelerate angiogenesis. Pharmacol Ther 143(2):181–196

Burn-Murdoch R (1990) The role of the vasculature in tooth eruption. Eur J Orthod 12(1):101–108

Caviedes-Bucheli J et al (2008) Neuropeptides in dental pulp: the silent protagonists. J Endod 34(7):773–788

Caviedes-Bucheli J et al (2011) The effect of orthodontic forces on calcitonin gene-related peptide expression in human dental pulp. J Endod 37(7):934–937

Caviedes-Bucheli J et al (2017) Angiogenic mechanisms of human dental pulp and their relationship with substance P expression in response to occlusal trauma. Int Endod J 50(4):339–351

Chen YJ et al (2015) Potential dental pulp revascularization and odonto-/osteogenic capacity of a novel transplant combined with dental pulp stem cells and platelet-rich fibrin. Cell Tissue Res 361(2):439–455

Clayton ZE, Sadeghipour S, Patel S (2015) Generating induced pluripotent stem cell derived endothelial cells and induced endothelial cells for cardiovascular disease modelling and therapeutic angiogenesis. Int J Cardiol 197:116–122

Cooper PR et al (2010) Inflammation-regeneration interplay in the dentine-pulp complex. J Dent 38(9):687–697

Cordeiro MM et al (2008) Dental pulp tissue engineering with stem cells from exfoliated deciduous teeth. J Endod 34(8):962–969

d'Aquino R et al (2007) Human postnatal dental pulp cells co-differentiate into osteoblasts and endotheliocytes: a pivotal synergy leading to adult bone tissue formation. Cell Death Differ 14(6):1162–1171

Derringer KA, Linden RW (2003) Angiogenic growth factors released in human dental pulp following orthodontic force. Arch Oral Biol 48(4):285–291

Derringer K, Linden R (2007) Epidermal growth factor released in human dental pulp following orthodontic force. Eur J Orthod 29(1):67–71

Derringer KA, Jaggers DC, Linden RW (1996) Angiogenesis in human dental pulp following orthodontic tooth movement. J Dent Res 75(10):1761–1766

Dissanayaka WL et al (2012) Coculture of dental pulp stem cells with endothelial cells enhances osteo-/odontogenic and angiogenic potential in vitro. J Endod 38(4):454–463

Dissanayaka WL et al (2015) The interplay of dental pulp stem cells and endothelial cells in an injectable peptide hydrogel on angiogenesis and pulp regeneration in vivo. Tissue Eng Part A 21(3-4):550–563

Distler JH et al (2003) Angiogenic and angiostatic factors in the molecular control of angiogenesis. Q J Nucl Med 47(3):149–161

Dominici M et al (2006) Minimal criteria for defining multipotent mesenchymal stromal cells. The International Society for Cellular Therapy position statement. Cytotherapy 8(4):315–317

El Karim IA et al (2009) Neuropeptides regulate expression of angiogenic growth factors in human dental pulp fibroblasts. J Endod 35(6):829–833

Estrada R et al (2009) Secretome from mesenchymal stem cells induces angiogenesis via Cyr61. J Cell Physiol 219(3):563–571

Friedenstein AJ, Chailakhjan RK, Lalykina KS (1970) The development of fibroblast colonies in monolayer cultures of guinea-pig bone marrow and spleen cells. Cell Tissue Kinet 3(4):393–403

Gaengel K et al (2009) Endothelial-mural cell signaling in vascular development and angiogenesis. Arterioscler Thromb Vasc Biol 29(5):630–638

Gruber R et al (2005) Bone marrow stromal cells can provide a local environment that favors migration and formation of tubular structures of endothelial cells. Tissue Eng 11(5-6):896–903

Heyeraas KJ (1989) Pulpal hemodynamics and interstitial fluid pressure: balance of transmicrovascular fluid transport. J Endod 15(10):468–472

Heyeraas KJ, Berggreen E (1999) Interstitial fluid pressure in normal and inflamed pulp. Crit Rev Oral Biol Med 10(3):328–336

Hilkens P et al (2014) Pro-angiogenic impact of dental stem cells in vitro and in vivo. Stem Cell Res 12(3):778–790

Hilkens P et al (2015) Dental stem cells in pulp regeneration: near future or long road ahead? Stem Cells Dev 24(14):1610–1622

Hilkens P et al (2017) The angiogenic potential of DPSCs and SCAPs in an in vivo model of dental pulp regeneration. Stem Cells Int 2017:2582080

Holdsworth MT et al (2003) Pain and distress from bone marrow aspirations and lumbar punctures. Ann Pharmacother 37(1):17–22

Huang GT, Gronthos S, Shi S (2009) Mesenchymal stem cells derived from dental tissues vs. those from other sources: their biology and role in regenerative medicine. J Dent Res 88(9):792–806

Hung CN et al (2011) A comparison between adipose tissue and dental pulp as sources of MSCs for tooth regeneration. Biomaterials 32(29):6995–7005

Iohara K et al (2008) A novel stem cell source for vasculogenesis in ischemia: subfraction of side population cells from dental pulp. Stem Cells 26(9):2408–2418

Iohara K et al (2011) Complete pulp regeneration after pulpectomy by transplantation of CD105+ stem cells with stromal cell-derived factor-1. Tissue Eng Part A 17(15-16):1911–1920

Ishizaka R et al (2012) Regeneration of dental pulp following pulpectomy by fractionated stem/progenitor cells from bone marrow and adipose tissue. Biomaterials 33(7):2109–2118

Ito T et al (2017) Dental pulp tissue engineering of pulpotomized rat molars with bone marrow mesenchymal stem cells. Odontology 105:392

Jain RK (2003) Molecular regulation of vessel maturation. Nat Med 9(6):685–693

Janebodin K et al (2013) VEGFR2-dependent angiogenic capacity of pericyte-like dental pulp stem cells. J Dent Res 92(6):524–531

Javed F et al (2015) Influence of orthodontic forces on human dental pulp: a systematic review. Arch Oral Biol 60(2):347–356

Jussila M, Juuri E, Thesleff I (2013) Tooth morphogenesis and renewal. In: Huang GT, Thesleff I (eds) Stem cells in craniofacial development and regeneration. Blackwell-Wiley, Hoboken, NJ, pp 109–134

Kim S (1985) Microcirculation of the dental pulp in health and disease. J Endod 11(11):465–471

Kim JY et al (2010) Regeneration of dental-pulp-like tissue by chemotaxis-induced cell homing. Tissue Eng Part A 16(10):3023–3031

Kim DW et al (2013) Wharton's jelly-derived mesenchymal stem cells: phenotypic characterization and optimizing their therapeutic potential for clinical applications. Int J Mol Sci 14(6):11692–11712

Kjaer I (2014) Mechanism of human tooth eruption: review article including a new theory for future studies on the eruption process. Scientifica (Cairo) 2014:341905

Kuang R et al (2016) Nanofibrous spongy microspheres for the delivery of hypoxia-primed human dental pulp stem cells to regenerate vascularized dental pulp. Acta Biomater 33:225–234

Li X et al (2016) Pulp regeneration in a full-length human tooth root using a hierarchical nanofibrous microsphere system. Acta Biomater 35:57–67

Malhotra N (2016) Induced pluripotent stem (iPS) cells in dentistry: a review. Int J Stem Cells 9(2):176–185

Marchionni C et al (2009) Angiogenic potential of human dental pulp stromal (stem) cells. Int J Immunopathol Pharmacol 22(3):699–706

Masoudi E et al (2016) Platelet-rich blood derivatives for stem cell-based tissue engineering and regeneration. Curr Stem Cell Rep 2(1):33–42

Mullane EM et al (2008) Effects of VEGF and FGF2 on the revascularization of severed human dental pulps. J Dent Res 87(12):1144–1148

Murakami M et al (2015) Trophic effects and regenerative potential of mobilized mesenchymal stem cells from bone marrow and adipose tissue as alternative cell sources for pulp/dentin regeneration. Cell Transplant 24(9):1753–1765

Nait Lechguer A et al (2008) Vascularization of engineered teeth. J Dent Res 87(12):1138–1143

Nakagami H et al (2005) Novel autologous cell therapy in ischemic limb disease through growth factor secretion by cultured adipose tissue-derived stromal cells. Arterioscler Thromb Vasc Biol 25(12):2542–2547

Nanci A (2008) Dentin-pulp complex. In: Ten Cate's oral histology: development, structure, and function. Mosby Elsevier, St. Louis, MO, pp 191–238

Phng LK, Gerhardt H (2009) Angiogenesis: a team effort coordinated by notch. Dev Cell 16(2):196–208

Pimenta FJ, Sa AR, Gomez RS (2003) Lymphangiogenesis in human dental pulp. Int Endod J 36(12):853–856

Potapova IA et al (2007) Mesenchymal stem cells support migration, extracellular matrix invasion, proliferation, and survival of endothelial cells in vitro. Stem Cells 25(7):1761–1768

Potente M, Gerhardt H, Carmeliet P (2011) Basic and therapeutic aspects of angiogenesis. Cell 146(6):873–887

Ratajczak J et al (2016) The neurovascular properties of dental stem cells and their importance in dental tissue engineering. Stem Cells Int 2016:9762871

Rehman J et al (2004) Secretion of angiogenic and antiapoptotic factors by human adipose stromal cells. Circulation 109(10):1292–1298

Rodd HD, Boissonade FM (2003) Immunocytochemical investigation of neurovascular relationships in human tooth pulp. J Anat 202(2):195–203

Rombouts C et al (2017) Pulp vascularization during tooth development, regeneration, and therapy. J Dent Res 96(2):137–144

Sakai VT et al (2010) SHED differentiate into functional odontoblasts and endothelium. J Dent Res 89(8):791–796

Sharma S et al (2014) Biomaterials in tooth tissue engineering: a review. J Clin Diagn Res 8(1):309–315

Shivashankar VY et al (2017) Comparison of the effect of PRP, PRF and induced bleeding in the revascularization of teeth with necrotic pulp and open apex: a triple blind randomized clinical trial. J Clin Diagn Res 11(6):ZC34–ZC39

Sieveking DP, Ng MK (2009) Cell therapies for therapeutic angiogenesis: back to the bench. Vasc Med 14(2):153–166

Suzuki T et al (2011) Induced migration of dental pulp stem cells for in vivo pulp regeneration. J Dent Res 90(8):1013–1018

Swift MR, Weinstein BM (2009) Arterial-venous specification during development. Circ Res 104(5):576–588

Takahashi K, Yamanaka S (2006) Induction of pluripotent stem cells from mouse embryonic and adult fibroblast cultures by defined factors. Cell 126(4):663–676

Takeuchi N et al (2015) Similar in vitro effects and pulp regeneration in ectopic tooth transplantation by basic fibroblast growth factor and granulocyte-colony stimulating factor. Oral Dis 21(1):113–122

Toda N, Ayajiki K, Okamura T (2012) Neurogenic and endothelial nitric oxide regulates blood circulation in lingual and other oral tissues. J Cardiovasc Pharmacol 60(1):100–108

Tran C, Damaser MS (2015) Stem cells as drug delivery methods: application of stem cell secretome for regeneration. Adv Drug Deliv Rev 82-83:1–11

Tran-Hung L, Mathieu S, About I (2006) Role of human pulp fibroblasts in angiogenesis. J Dent Res 85(9):819–823

Wise GE, King GJ (2008) Mechanisms of tooth eruption and orthodontic tooth movement. J Dent Res 87(5):414–434

Woloszyk A et al (2016) Human dental pulp stem cells and gingival fibroblasts seeded into silk fibroin scaffolds have the same ability in attracting vessels. Front Physiol 7:140

Yu C, Abbott PV (2007) An overview of the dental pulp: its functions and responses to injury. Aust Dent J 52(1 Suppl):S4–S16

Yu CY et al (2002) An in vivo and in vitro comparison of the effects of vasoactive mediators on pulpal blood vessels in rat incisors. Arch Oral Biol 47(10):723–732

Yuan C et al (2015) Coculture of stem cells from apical papilla and human umbilical vein endothelial cell under hypoxia increases the formation of three-dimensional vessel-like structures in vitro. Tissue Eng Part A 21:1163

Zhang JQ, Nagata K, Iijima T (1998) Scanning electron microscopy and immunohistochemical observations of the vascular nerve plexuses in the dental pulp of rat incisor. Anat Rec 251(2):214–220

Zhang LX et al (2015) Systemic BMSC homing in the regeneration of pulp-like tissue and the enhancing effect of stromal cell-derived factor-1 on BMSC homing. Int J Clin Exp Pathol 8(9):10261–10271

Zhang Z et al (2016) Wnt/beta-catenin signaling determines the vasculogenic fate of post-natal mesenchymal stem cells. Stem Cells 34:576

Zhao L, Johnson T, Liu D (2017) Therapeutic angiogenesis of adipose-derived stem cells for ischemic diseases. Stem Cell Res Ther 8(1):125

Current and Future Views on Pulp Exposure Management and Epigenetic Influences

4

Henry F. Duncan and Yukako Yamauchi

4.1 Introduction

The pulp is protected in an unrestored tooth by an outer layer of enamel and dentine. This protection can be breached by trauma or carious processes rendering the dentine susceptible to microbial colonisation, which thereby stimulates an inflammatory response in the pulp. If the disease process is left untreated, the pulpitis will progressively increase in intensity ultimately resulting in pulp necrosis (Farges et al. 2015). If the irritating stimulus is removed prior to pulp necrosis and the tooth is adequately restored, then resolution of the inflamed pulp tissue is possible (Tronstad and Mjör 1972). The importance of retaining all or part the pulp has recently been highlighted as it is minimally invasive, less technically demanding and more biologically based compared with root canal treatment (Smith et al. 2016).

When managing a deep carious lesion, it is accepted that selective removal of the carious tissue and avoidance of pulpal exposure are the optimal treatment choice (Schwendicke et al. 2016); however, on occasions, the carious process has advanced to such an extent that pulpal exposure is unavoidable or clinical symptoms dictate that removal of part of the pulp is necessary to promote healing (Simon et al. 2013). Ascertaining the level of pulp inflammation, careful handling of the damaged pulp, the correct choice of capping material choice and subsequent restoration are all

H. F. Duncan (✉)
Division of Restorative Dentistry and Periodontology, Dublin Dental University Hospital, Dublin 2, Ireland

Division of Restorative Dentistry & Periodontology, Dublin Dental University Hospital, Trinity College Dublin, University of Dublin, Dublin 2, Ireland
e-mail: Hal.Duncan@dental.tcd.ie

Y. Yamauchi
Division of Restorative Dentistry & Periodontology, Dublin Dental University Hospital, Trinity College Dublin, University of Dublin, Dublin 2, Ireland

© Springer Nature Switzerland AG 2019
H. F. Duncan, P. R. Cooper (eds.), *Clinical Approaches in Endodontic Regeneration*,
https://doi.org/10.1007/978-3-319-96848-3_4

important aspects of the management of pulp exposure and are the focus of the first section of this chapter.

Current treatments, however, remain empirical and non-specific, and an improved understanding of the role of genetic and epigenetic factors in controlling cellular processes such as inflammation, mineralisation and repair is essential if we wish to develop new therapeutic solutions, as well as understand treatment failure. Epigenetic alterations, including DNA methylation and histone modification, have emerged as critical regulators of several cellular processes evident in the damaged pulp defence and repair response. The latter part of the chapter introduces these modifications from a clinical perspective explaining what they are, why they are important and what therapeutic opportunities they may present within vital pulp treatment (VPT).

4.2 Dentinogenesis and Pulp Repair after Exposure

The process of primary dentinogenesis begins during the late bell stage of tooth development, as the peripheral cells of the dental papilla undergo terminal differentiation into odontoblast cells (Ruch et al. 1995). Although the process has several similarities to osteogenesis, there are also differences as the odontoblast cell remains at the periphery of, and not encased in, the mineralised matrix as osteocytes are. By secreting an organic matrix, including collagen fibres, the odontoblast forms an outer mineralised shell of dentine but remains positioned at the interface between the pulp and dentine. The odontoblast's migration creates a trail as dentinal tubules, which generates a radial pattern throughout the dentine. The odontoblast process extends into the dentinal tubule and provides a history of the odontoblasts journey during primary dentinogenesis.

While the enamel-forming cells, ameloblasts, are only present during tooth development, odontoblasts can survive throughout the life of the tooth and continue to secrete secondary dentine, albeit at a greatly reduced rate compared with primary dentine formation. The secondary dentine is well organised, and its constant deposition leads to the natural physiological narrowing of the pulp chamber which is evident with increasing age (Morse 1991).

Dentine deposition is also induced locally in response to several stimuli including caries and trauma and as a result of restorative dental procedures, all of which can provoke inflammatory responses in the pulp, the nature and extent of which reflect the severity of the challenge (Mjör and Tronstad 1972). The deposition of tertiary dentine also alters depending on the severity of the stimuli with mild to moderate stimulation upregulating the matrix secretion of odontoblasts in a process called reactionary dentinogenesis (Lesot et al. 1994, Smith 2002), while more severe injury (e.g. pulp exposure) leads to odontoblast cell death and the recruitment of dental pulp stem/progenitor cells, which differentiate into odontoblast-like cells to form reparative dentine (Lesot et al. 1994) (Fig. 4.1). The formation of reparative dentine is under the influence of bioactive molecules released from the pulp and dentine matrix (Rutherford et al. 1993, Nakashima 1994, Cassidy et al. 1997, Smith and Lesot 2001). The source and nature of these progenitor cells are the

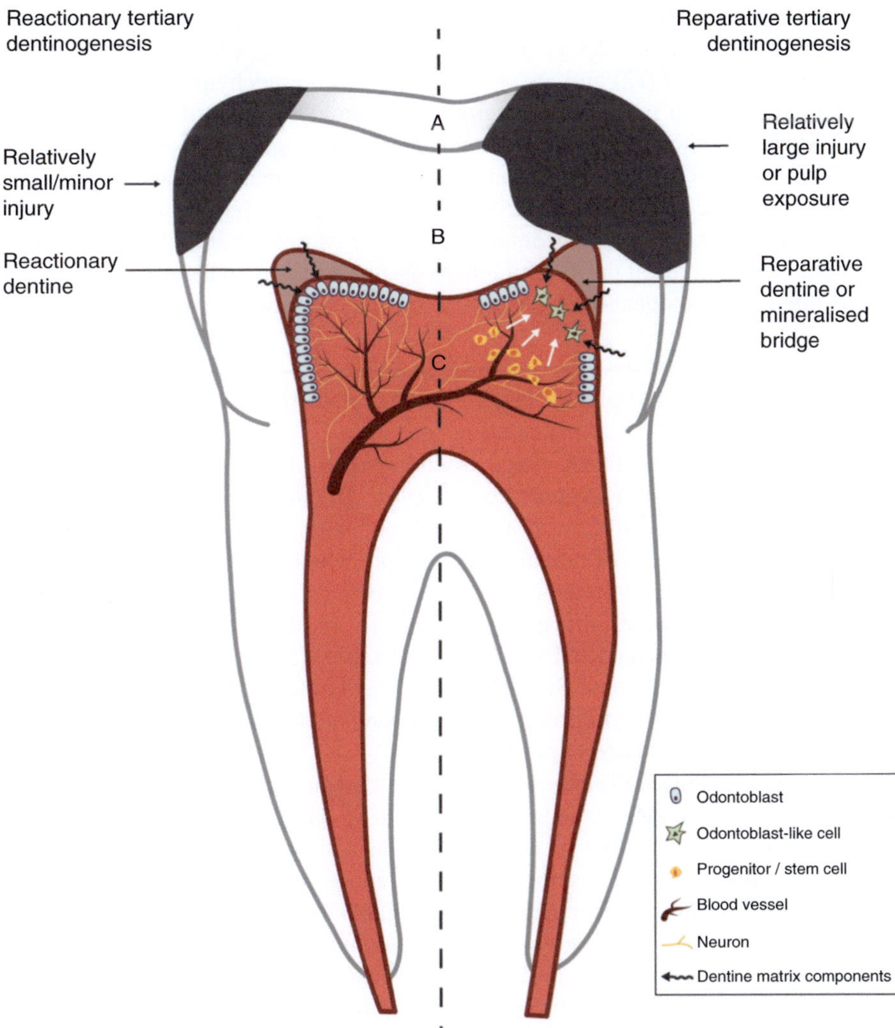

Fig. 4.1 Schematic illustration of the processes of tertiary dentine formation. Reactionary and reparative dentinogenesis processes differ in the source of the secreting cell. Reactionary dentine is formed by the existing primary odontoblast with a mild stimulus (e.g. early stage of carious disease) stimulating upregulation of existing odontoblast activity. During the reactionary dentinogenesis process, the odontoblasts recognise the bacterial products and released dentine matrix components (DMCs) diffusing through the dentine tubules, which increases cellular activity. Reparative dentine formation involves a more complex sequence of events in which a severe stimulus (e.g. increasing carious involvement of dentine) causes death of the primary odontoblasts, which are subsequently replaced following differentiation of progenitor or stem cells into odontoblast-like cells under the regulation of bioactive molecules (including DMCs). Although the nature of the cellular response is likely to be dependent upon the pulp environment, the mineralised tissue deposited at the pupal wound site will likely display a spectrum of dysplasia. (A) enamel; (B) dentine; (C) pulp

subject of considerable debate, being attributed to stem cell (SC) populations within the pulp (Smith and Lesot 2001), SCs migrating from outside the tooth (Feng et al. 2011, Frozoni et al. 2012) and also undifferentiated mesenchymal cells from cell-rich and central pulp perivascular regions (Fitzgerald et al. 1990, Machado et al. 2015). At present, there is no consensus regarding the progenitor population responsible for reparative dentine formation, although surface marker analysis generally confirms a mesenchymal origin (Simon and Smith 2014). Tertiary dentine formation occurs rapidly and in a less organised manner compared with primary dentine formation, and as a result the resulting hard tissue formation in the case of an exposure is often not homogeneous and lacks tubular continuity and structure.

4.3 Is Pulp Exposure a Negative Prognostic Factor?

Microbial irritation and microleakage around restorations are the dominant causes of pulpal inflammation (Kakehashi et al. 1965, Brännström and Nyborg 1973). Dentinal caries or defective restorations allow bacteria and their by-products to stimulate varying degrees of pulpal inflammation, which can be evident even when the carious process is only in the outer dentine (Brännström and Lind 1965). As the carious lesion approaches the pulp, the severity of the inflammatory response increases; however, it is reportedly only within the last 0.5 mm that the pulp becomes acutely inflamed (Reeves and Stanley 1966). This could account for the poor predictability of VPT with carious exposures (Mejàre and Cvek 1993), compared with traumatic, non-caries-related exposures.

If the pulp is traumatically exposed in an adult tooth, it is clear that VPT is a predictable procedure with a similar prognosis to pulpectomy and root canal treatment (Cvek 1978, Al-Hiyasat et al. 2006). If the pulp has been subject to a sustained bacterial onslaught by the caries process, the outcome of conservative vital pulp techniques is less certain with success rates ranging from less than 20% (Barthel et al. 2000, Bjørndal et al. 2017) to over 80% (Marques et al. 2015, Taha and Khazali 2017). The wide range of success quoted highlights the difficulties in comparing the results of individual pulp capping studies as the data is heterogeneous, with certain studies defining patient symptoms and pulpal diagnosis (Taha and Khazali 2017), while others include a mixed sample of both carious and traumatic exposures (Mente et al. 2014).

Certainly when managing caries in permanent teeth, it is generally accepted that clearing the margins of caries and creating a cleansable seal are essential. Interestingly, there has been less agreement over whether all carious dentine overlying the pulp should be removed (Ricketts et al. 2006, Marques et al. 2015). In a tooth with a deep carious lesion, which is considered to have a healthy pulp, selective caries removal is now recommended in preference to non-selective caries removal and the risk of pulp exposure (Bjørndal et al. 2010, 2017, Innes et al. 2016, Schwendicke et al. 2016). This caries management strategy for deep caries can be carried out in one visit as indirect pulp therapy or in two stages as a stepwise excavation technique (Schwendicke et al. 2016) (Fig. 4.2). Randomised controlled trials examining caries management strategies in permanent teeth are relatively rare; however, recently 5-year results of a previously published trial (Bjørndal et al. 2010)

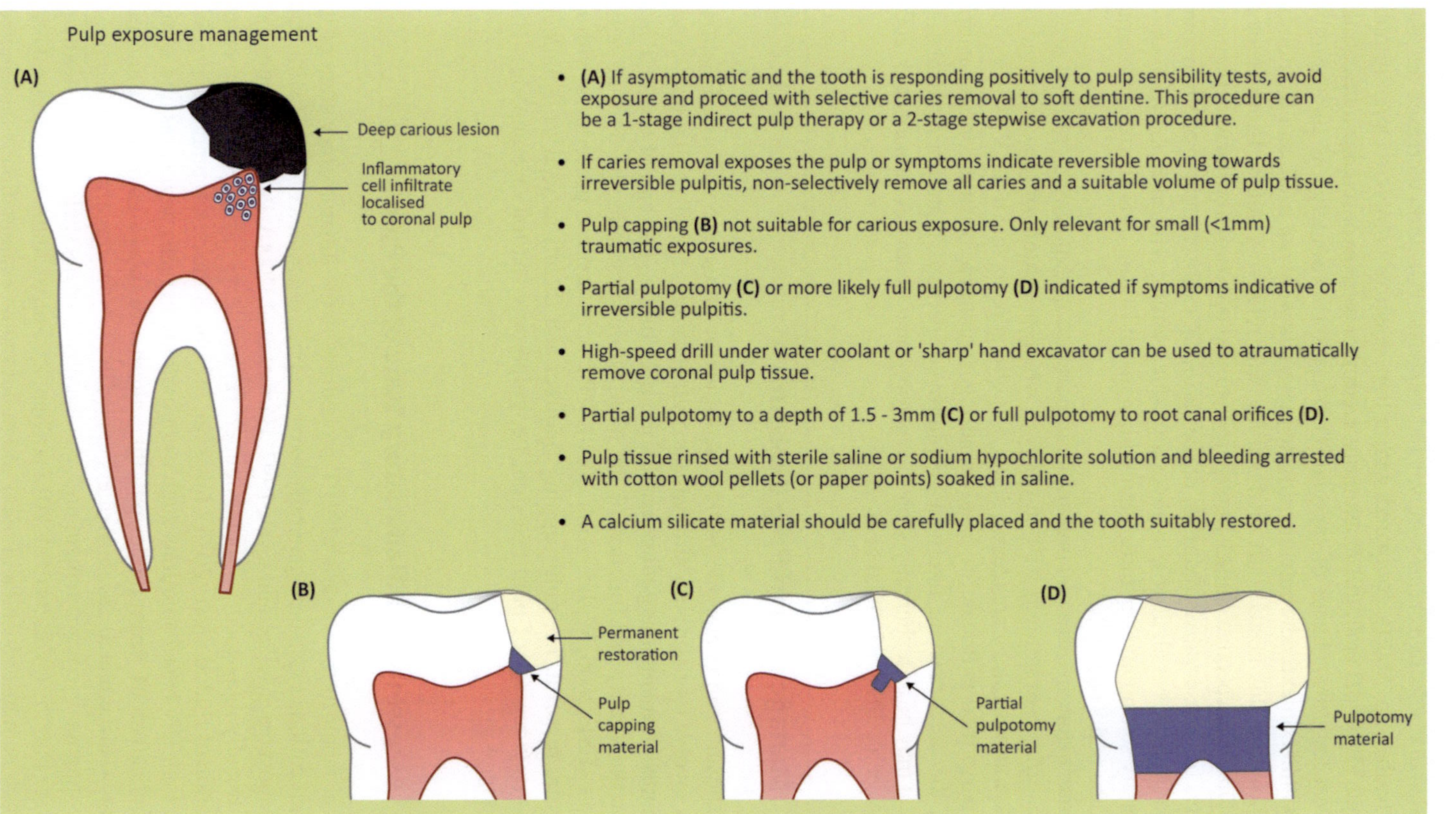

- **(A)** If asymptomatic and the tooth is responding positively to pulp sensibility tests, avoid exposure and proceed with selective caries removal to soft dentine. This procedure can be a 1-stage indirect pulp therapy or a 2-stage stepwise excavation procedure.

- If caries removal exposes the pulp or symptoms indicate reversible moving towards irreversible pulpitis, non-selectively remove all caries and a suitable volume of pulp tissue.

- Pulp capping **(B)** not suitable for carious exposure. Only relevant for small (<1mm) traumatic exposures.

- Partial pulpotomy **(C)** or more likely full pulpotomy **(D)** indicated if symptoms indicative of irreversible pulpitis.

- High-speed drill under water coolant or 'sharp' hand excavator can be used to atraumatically remove coronal pulp tissue.

- Partial pulpotomy to a depth of 1.5 - 3mm **(C)** or full pulpotomy to root canal orifices **(D)**.

- Pulp tissue rinsed with sterile saline or sodium hypochlorite solution and bleeding arrested with cotton wool pellets (or paper points) soaked in saline.

- A calcium silicate material should be carefully placed and the tooth suitably restored.

Fig. 4.2   Schematic illustration of the conservative management approach for deep caries and pulp exposure

concluded that selective caries removal and stepwise excavation increased the number of teeth with vitality compared with a non-selective complete caries removal technique (Bjørndal et al. 2017). Notably, teeth that were exposed during treatment had a very low (9%) chance of survival. This figure is extremely low and should be taken within context, new calcium silicate materials were not used, and the number of teeth within this nested part of the study was relatively small (Bjørndal et al. 2017). Other prospective studies have demonstrated opposing results with high success rates for conservative treatment of the cariously exposed pulp in an endodontic practice (Marques et al. 2015), in general practice setting (Hilton et al. 2013) and in a university setting investigating teeth with signs and symptoms of irreversible pulpitis (Taha and Khazali 2017).

In conclusion, in order to confirm the importance of exposure there is an urgent need for studies examining VPT in cases in which the extent of the caries and the pulpal symptomatology are clearly defined. It also appears that if the VPT is meticulously performed with careful tissue handling, magnification and correct material choice, the outcomes are likely to be improved, perhaps highlighting that these treatment may be as technically sensitive as root canal treatment (Bogen et al. 2008, Marques et al. 2015, Bjørndal et al. 2017).

4.4 Management of Pulp Exposure

Pulp exposure can occur due to trauma, caries or iatrogenic reasons. Treatment options involve tooth or pulp removal (i.e. pulpectomy) as well as vital pulp procedures aimed at maintaining all or part of the pulp tissue. The aim of the VPT is to preserve the vitality and function of the pulp, while stimulating hard tissue repair processes (ESE 2006, Witherspoon 2008). VPT encompasses procedures with no pulp tissue removal, i.e. pulp capping (indirect and direct) as well as techniques with varying degrees of pulp excision, i.e. pulpotomy (partial or complete) (ESE 2006) (Fig. 4.2).

4.4.1 Assessing the Inflammatory State of the Pulp

A critical factor in the success of VPT procedures is the inflammatory state of the pulp with carious exposures generally having a poor outcome compared with traumatic exposures (Mejàre and Cvek 1993, Barthel et al. 2000). Pulpal inflammation is traditionally classified as being either reversible or irreversible (American Association of Endodontists 2013); however, in light of the development of predictable biologically based solutions such as pulpotomy in teeth with signs and symptoms indicative of irreversible pulpitis, alternative classifications have been suggested (Hashem et al. 2015, Wolters et al. 2017). New classifications attempt to link the diagnosis to management and use diagnostic terms such as mild, moderate and severe pulpitis (Wolters et al. 2017) (Chap. 2). Pulpal status is determined after a thorough pain history and a clinical and radiographic examination, supplemented by specific tests, e.g. pulpal sensibility tests. Unfortunately, these methods based on clinical signs or symptoms are relatively crude only providing guidance and traditionally not understood to reflect the true histopathological status of the pulp (Garfunkel et al. 1973, Dummer et al. 1980). Notably, contradicting previous evidence, a recent publication demonstrated a strong correlation between histology and the signs and symptoms of reversible/irreversible pulpitis (Ricucci et al. 2014). This may be helpful as a lack of accuracy is problematic for clinicians as it is then difficult to forecast the likely prognosis of treatment preoperatively.

The symptoms of reversible pulpitis range from no complaint to a sharp pain sensation with hot/cold stimuli; usually, the pain resolves once the stimulus is removed. Spontaneous pain and sleep disturbance tend to indicate irreversible pulpitis (Dummer et al. 1980) with lingering pain after removal of the stimulus. However, relying too heavily on a patient's symptoms can mislead the clinician, as irreversible pulpitis may be symptomless in anywhere between 14% and 60% of cases (Seltzer et al. 1963, Michaelson and Holland 2002). Therefore, teeth treated by pulp capping or pulpotomy must be closely monitored (Fig. 4.3) to ensure continuing pulpal health.

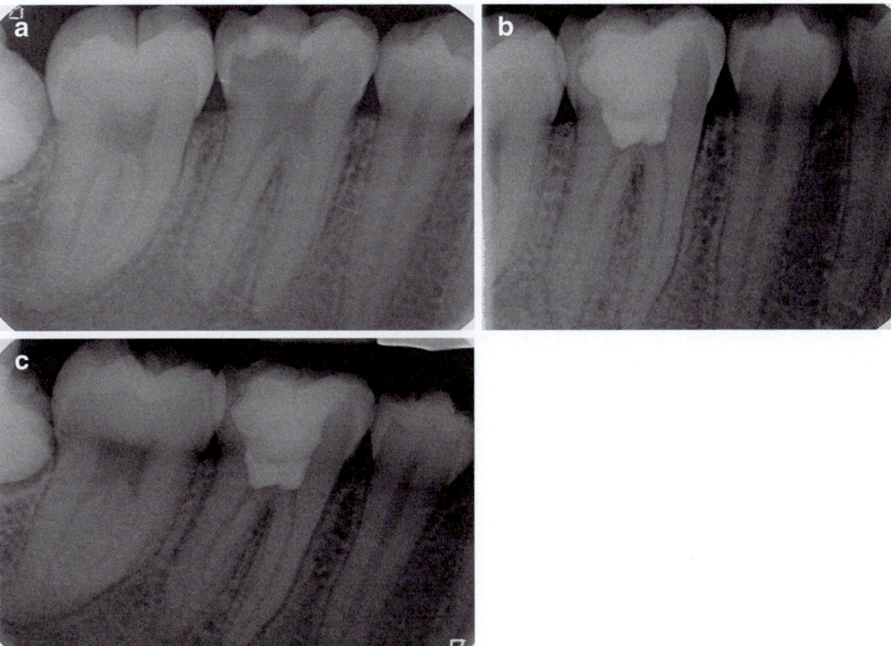

Fig. 4.3 (**a**) Radiograph of the lower right first molar demonstrated a large coronal radiolucency indicative of caries. There was no residual dentine visible between the carious front and the pulp. The patient reported pain for over a minute when drinking liquids. The tooth responded positively to pulp sensibility testing with a lingering response; however there was no apical radiolucency evident. (**b**) After gentle removal of the carious dentine, the pulp was exposed, and full coronal pulpotomy was carried out placing MTA before restoration. (**c**) When reviewed 6 months later, the tooth was not tender to percussion or palpation buccally. Radiographically there was no evidence of apical breakdown. Note that pulp sensibility testing is not predictable in these cases as it often gives a negative response

4.4.1.1 Pulpal Bleeding

A crude, but practical, indicator of the degree of pulpal inflammation may be assessment of the extent of bleeding after exposure (Matsuo et al. 1996). This has been studied in carious teeth and the bleeding placed into four categories; if the bleeding overflows at the pulp exposure site, but does not arrest within 30 s, the VPT procedure reportedly had a significantly poorer prognosis (Matsuo et al. 1996). Although seemingly logical, a difficulty in relying too strongly on pulpal bleeding as a diagnosis is that it will be influenced by local measures such as the type of local anaesthetic solution used, as well as whether the solution is administered as a block or infiltration (Pitt Ford et al. 1993, Odor et al. 1994).

4.4.1.2 Dental Pulp Tissue Management

The aim of conservative treatments of the exposed pulp is to preserve the vitality and function of the pulp tissue while stimulating hard tissue repair processes (ESE 2006, Witherspoon 2008). In general the removal of pulp tissue should be related to the patient's symptoms with traumatic exposures often requiring no pulp removal, while in carious exposures partial or full coronal pulpotomy is indicated (Figs. 4.2 and 4.3). The rationale for pulp tissue excision is that the inflammation and necrotic tissue is generally contained within the coronal pulp even in cases with signs and symptoms indicative of irreversible pulpitis (Ricucci et al. 2014). Notably, partial pulpotomy procedures in teeth with signs and symptoms of irreversible pulpitis have recently been shown to have good prognosis when 'capped' with the calcium silicate material and mineral trioxide aggregate (MTA) (Taha and Khazali 2017) but have a poor prognosis with calcium hydroxide (Bjørndal et al. 2017, Taha and Khazali 2017), while full pulpotomy procedures for carious exposures have been reported to have a greater than 80% outcome at 2 years (Simon et al. 2013, Qudeimat et al. 2017, Taha et al. 2017).

After exposure the pulpal wound should be cleansed of debris using sterile saline or sodium hypochlorite solution and the haemorrhage arrested by applying pressure using sterile paper points or cotton wool. Notably, although EDTA solution is the most effective solution for liberating dentine matrix components (Graham et al. 2006), it is best avoided due its tendency to stimulate renewed pulp bleeding. When the wound is dry, the chosen material should be carefully placed over the exposure, followed by a suitable permanent restoration.

4.4.2 Material Choice

Calcium hydroxide has been the material of choice for vital pulp procedures for many years (Zander and Glass 1949, Bjørndal et al. 2017); however, it possesses poor mechanical properties, an unspecific mechanism of action (Sangwan et al. 2013), does not seal well (Browne et al. 1983) and forms porous hard tissue repair over the pulp wound (Cox et al. 1996, Nair et al. 2008). An evolving understanding of pulp repair (Smith et al. 2016) and the introduction of calcium silicate materials including MTA and Biodentine have created new interest in VPT (Hilton et al. 2013,

Katge and Patil 2017). Notably, MTA has demonstrated superior histological (Aeinehchi et al. 2003, Nair et al. 2008) and clinical outcome compared with calcium hydroxide in VPT procedures (Hilton et al. 2013, Taha and Khazali 2017) and would now be considered the gold standard material for VPT applications (Chap. 6).

4.4.2.1 Role of Material

In general the successful healing of a pulpal exposure is not dependent on the material but on the pulpal reaction to the capping agent and the ability of the restoration to prevent bacterial microleakage (Tobias et al. 1982, Cox et al. 1985). That said, although pulpal repair is possible with a range of capping materials, the fundamental principles of an infection-free wound site, a relatively innocuous capping material and a high-quality hard tissue response remain (Bergenholtz 2005). Therefore, the predictability and potential success of pulp capping are influenced by the capping agent selected (Nair et al. 2008).

4.4.2.2 Timing of Permanent Restoration

After completion of a VPT procedure, it is important to restore the tooth immediately with a permanent restoration (Al-Hiyasat et al. 2006, Mente et al. 2010) rather than risk the breakdown on the early reparative process by encouraging bacterial microleakage around the temporary restoration (Bergenholtz et al. 1982). Glass ionomer (GI), resin-based composite (RBC) or amalgam restorations can generally be used alone or in combination; however, recently it was noted that bonding to calcium silicate materials was challenging with gaps between the GI and calcium silicate and breakdown of the bond between RBC and calcium silicate over time (Meraji and Camilleri 2017).

4.4.3 Clinical Questions

4.4.3.1 Is the Age of the Patient Relevant in the Treatment of Pulp Exposure?

Prospective studies analysing the histological response to VPT materials invariably involve young patients (Hörsted-Bindslev et al. 2003, Accorinte et al. 2008, Nair et al. 2008), as do clinical pulp capping outcome studies in carious teeth (Barrieshi-Nusair and Qudeimat 2006, Farsi et al. 2006, Taha et al. 2017). Younger patients, under the age of 20, are selected due to the greater blood supply, the potential for open root apices and increased cellularity of their pulps; it has been suggested that these characteristics should result in more predictable healing (Massler 1972). A recent prospective pulp capping study categorised the groups to above and below 40 years and concluded that treatment was less successful in older patients (Marques et al. 2015); however, another older study with a similar age range showed no difference (Matsuo et al. 1996). A recent prospective pulp capping study examining 229 teeth highlighted a trend indicating that calcium hydroxide did not perform as well as MTA in older patients; however, the result was not significant, and the authors proposed that a larger sample size would be required to properly test the hypothesis (Mente et al. 2014). In conclusion, there remains uncertainty, and as a result further adequately powered prospective clinical studies investigating patient age as a variable are required to ascertain if the promising new results (Taha et al. 2017) are applicable to the 'older' population.

4.4.3.2 Is the Size of the Exposure Important for Outcome?

In the case of traumatic exposures, the size of the exposed pulp does not appear to affect prognosis (Cvek 1978, Fuks et al. 1982). In carious teeth, it is logical to believe that the level of bacterial contamination and inflammation increases proportionally with size of the pulpal exposure; however, there is a paucity of evidence to support this (Zilbeman et al. 1989, Mejàre and Cvek 1993, Qudeimat et al. 2007). One randomised controlled trial comparing MTA and calcium hydroxide in carious exposures concluded that partial pulpotomy procedures were less successful if the exposure size was greater than 5 mm, although only relatively small numbers of teeth were included in the larger exposure groups (Chailertvanitkul et al. 2014). Perhaps a practical reason for small exposures performing better than large exposures is the difficulty in using hard-setting materials such as calcium hydroxide in larger deficits.

4.4.4   Gaps in Our Knowledge and Potential Solutions

Undoubtedly recent advances in the scientific understanding of pulp disease have improved the outcome of VPT procedures (Mente et al. 2014). However, current VPT procedures remain limited by an incomplete understanding of the intricate molecular processes which control the fate of dental pulp cells (DPCs) (Duncan et al. 2016a, b), an inability to accurately diagnose the pulp's inflammatory state (Chap. 1) and a reliance on capping materials whose action is non-specific (Ferracane et al. 2010). In order to find solutions, biological research should focus not only on the critical mediators of pulp disease and regeneration but also on the translational development of next-generation dental biomaterials aimed at tissue repair processes (Ferracane et al. 2010, Duncan et al. 2011). With a view to the future, the role of epigenetic influences on pulpal response and therapy has not been considered until recently; this will be the focus of the second section of this chapter.

4.5   Epigenetic Influences

Although every eukaryotic cell in an individual contains identical genetic material, phenotype and function vary depending on the cell's specific role. The control of cell fate is intricately orchestrated by complex molecular mechanisms (Portela and Esteller 2010), which enable certain genes to be expressed and others suppressed depending on cellular and tissue requirements (Horn and Peterson 2002). Transcription is largely regulated by chromatin conformation changes, a process regulated by epigenetic modifications. Epigenetics is defined as alterations which do not change the DNA sequence but affect chromatin conformation and subsequent regulation of gene expression (Barros and Offenbacher 2009, Arnsdorf et al. 2010).

Cellular genetic information is coded on DNA with approximately 146 base pairs of DNA tightly wound around a histone core; together this repeating unit is called a nucleosome (Luger 2003, Hake et al. 2004). Nucleosomes are assembled and repeatedly folded to form a higher-order structure, a process which enables the compaction of a significant volume of DNA (2 m in length) into the cell nucleus. This chromatin structure is dynamic, being constantly remodelled between a condensed and unfolded status, with these architectural alterations critical in modulating transcription. Generally, when the DNA is tightly wrapped around the core or the nucleosomes are densely packed, it is difficult for transcriptional factors to access binding sites on the DNA, which results in suppression of transcriptional activity. On the contrary a relaxed or open chromatin is considered transcriptionally active (Kleff et al. 1995, Margueron et al. 2005, Vaissière et al. 2008).

4.5.1 DNA Methylation

The principal types of epigenetic modifications are DNA methylation and histone modification (Nagase and Ghosh 2008, Vaissière et al. 2008) with DNA methylation being the only mechanism which directly interacts with the genome. In addition, gene expression can vary due to the function and interactions of RNA molecules themselves, and as a result increasing emphasis is being placed on the ability of non-coding RNA (ncRNA) transcripts, e.g. long ncRNAs (lncRNAs) and microRNAs (miRNAs), to modulate gene expression, and, thus, on ncRNAs role as epigenetic modifiers (Kelly et al. 2010).

DNA methylation generally occurs on cytosine residues at specific regions called CpG islands, which overlap gene promoter regions with methylation usually leading to repression of gene expression (Weber et al. 2007). Mechanistically, the methylation of the binding site on promoter region hinders the binding of transcriptional factors with DNA methylation patterns maintained by the cellular enzymes, DNA methyltransferases (DNMTs) (Jin and Robertson 2013).

4.5.2 Histone Modification

The post-translational modification of histone proteins in contrast to DNA methylation results in more labile or reversible epigenetic modification (Kelly et al. 2010). The histone core of the nucleosome structure consists of eight histones; however, the N-terminal histone tail is not incorporated in the structure and projects from the core. The tail is comprised of 20–30 amino acids, which can be modified by acetylation, methylation phosphorylation, ubiquitination and SUMOylation; however, the bulk of current research has focused on acetylation and methylation modifications (Zhang and Reinberg 2001). Histone methylation targets arginine and lysine residues on the histone tail (Zhang and Reinberg 2001) with the methylation of arginine a transcription activator, while methylation of lysine both induces and represses transcriptional activity. The process is complex with the gene expression changes dependent on the cell needs as well as the specific residue affected (Li et al. 2007). Lysine residues can also be acetylated, which leads to a promotion of gene expression, while deacetylation has a transcriptionally repressive effect (Taunton et al. 1996). Two groups of balancing enzymes, histone acetyltransferases (HATs) and histone deacetylases (HDACs), control the homeostatic balance of acetylation, and alterations in this balance modulate gene expression (Yang and Seto 2008). The mechanism for increased transcription has not been fully elucidated, but it is generally assumed that acetylation lowers histone affinity to the negatively charged DNA allowing greater accessibility for transcription factors (Clayton et al. 2006). Others have suggested that the range of histone tail (modifications) creates a pattern or code, and this 'histone code' recruits corresponding protein elements required for transcription (Turner 2007).

4.5.3 Non-coding RNA

NcRNAs are increasingly important epigenetic modifiers and include miRNAs and lncRNA. Gene expression involves a complex process of DNA transcription into mRNA, prior to mRNA translation into protein; however, in reality only a small portion of the genome is translated to protein (Lander et al. 2001, Kellis et al. 2014). The majority of the genome is transcribed as ncRNAs, which do not code for a protein, but play other roles (Mercer and Mattick 2013). NcRNA research has revealed a large variety of cellular functions, including ncRNA binding to complementary mRNA to induce degradation, which leads to an inhibition of gene expression as well as the direct interaction of miRNA with the process of DNA methylation or histone acetylation (Fabbri et al. 2007, Tao et al. 2015).

4.6 Dental Relevance of Epigenetic Modification

An evolving understanding of the intricacies of epigenetic modulation and transcriptional regulation/dysregulation highlights an important role for epigenetics in the pathogenesis of a range of human diseases (Kelly et al. 2010, You and Jones 2012). The importance of epigenetic influences in diseases such as cancer and mental and metabolic diseases has been demonstrated (Dugué et al. 2016, Cheng et al. 2017), and as a result significant effort has been directed towards developing epigenetic therapies targeted at methylation and acetylation processes (Egger et al. 2004, Wright 2013). Indeed, selected HDAC inhibitors (HDACis) have FDA approval for treating multiple myeloma (Grant et al. 2007). Recently an epigenetic role in pulp inflammation (Cardoso et al. 2010) and the development of potential epigenetic therapies in VPT (Duncan et al. 2011) and periodontal treatment have been reported (Huynh et al. 2017, Sehic et al. 2017).

Epigenetic regulation is also important in health with the epigenetic regulation of mineralisation processes in bone development and repair of particular relevance (Cantley et al. 2017). Bone has similarities to teeth both in the anatomic structure and the cellular composition (Karaoz et al. 2011, Isobe et al. 2015) including a resident population of mesenchymal stem cells able to differentiate into osteoblasts and other types of cells (Opsahl Vital et al. 2012). Runx2 is a transcriptional factor, which plays a pivotal role in osteoblast differentiation and bone formation, and there are clear indications of a strong association between HDACs with Runx2 (Schroeder et al. 2004, Jensen et al. 2007). Furthermore, other important epigenetic modifiers including miRNAs have been strongly linked to the control of osteoblast differentiation (Li et al. 2009) and odontogenic differentiation (Song et al. 2016).

4.6.1 Are Epigenetic Modifications Possible Therapeutic Targets in Dentistry?

In human DPCs, a range of HDAC enzymes are strongly expressed in odontoblasts (Klinz et al. 2012), while HDACis promote cell migration and mineralisation in rodent DPCs, increasing dentinogenesis-related proteins such as dentine matrix protein-1, bone morphogenic proteins and matrix metalloproteinases (Duncan et al. 2012, 2016a) (Fig. 4.4). In human DPCs, DNMT inhibition significantly enhances odontogenic differentiation (Zhang et al. 2015), while a correlation between miRNAs and odontoblast-like cell differentiation has been reported (Song et al. 2016). Similarly within periodontal tissues, both HDACs and ncRNAs have been demonstrated to be involved in the osteogenic differentiation processes in human periodontal ligament cells (Huynh et al. 2017, Qu et al. 2016).

4.6.2 Epigenetics and Pulp Exposure

In order for biologically based vital pulp procedures (e.g. direct pulp capping and partial pulpotomy) to be successful, there must be an environment conducive to repair. To enable effective repair and healing, inflammatory control (Chap. 7) as well as the promotion of mineralisation, angiogenesis (Chap. 4) and neurogenesis (Chap. 3) processes are all necessary (Grando Mattuella et al. 2007, Cooper et al. 2010). There is an opportunity for epigenetic-modifying agents targeting DNA methylation and histone acetylation to play a role in regenerative endodontics as they have previously been shown to be effective in reducing inflammation, promoting mineralisation and modulating regenerative processes in a range of cell types (Shanmugam and Sethi 2013, Gordon et al. 2015, Zhang et al. 2015). Notably, epigenetic modifications present attractive therapeutic targets firstly due to their association with disease and secondly as they are relatively easy to alter pharmacologically (Kelly et al. 2010, Gordon et al. 2015). Within dentistry, it has been postulated that the epigenetic reprogramming which accompanies the viral reprogramming of somatic cells to induced pluripotent SCs (iPSCs) (Takahashi and Yamanaka 2006,

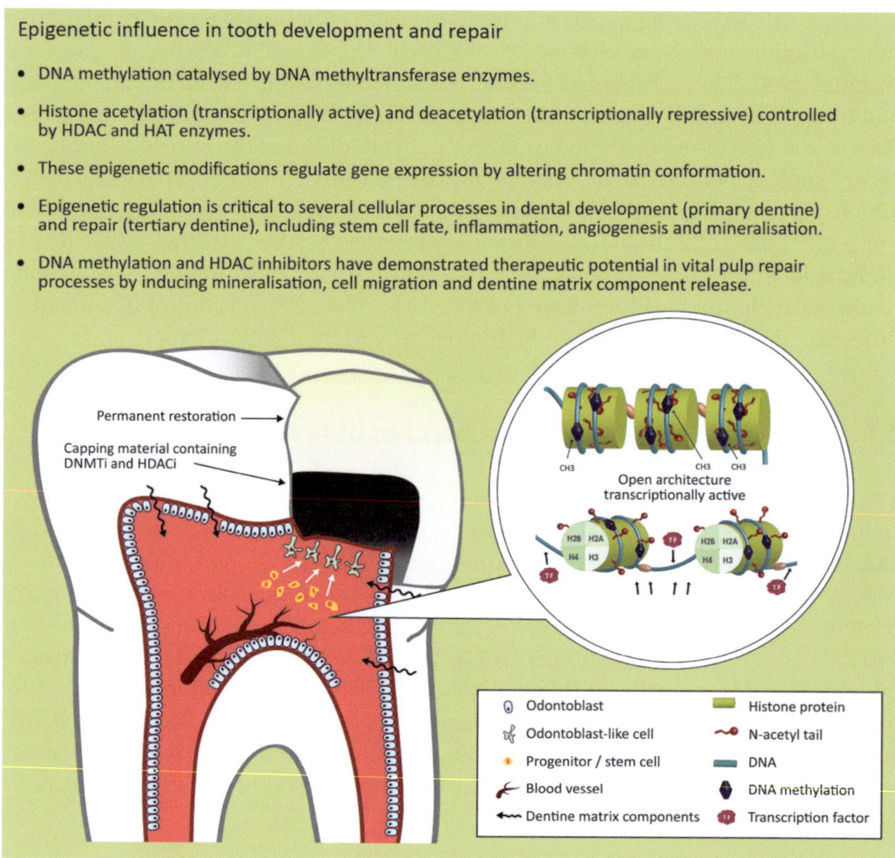

Fig. 4.4 Schematic illustration of the potential influence of epigenetic modifications in orchestrating development and repair within the dentine-pulp complex

Huangfu et al. 2008) might prove to be an important tool for wound healing or regeneration in periodontal tissues (Barros and Offenbacher 2009, 2014).

The enzymes that regulate epigenetic chromatin modifications, including methyltransferases, demethylases, HATs, and HDACs, are of particular therapeutic interest. HDACs have been demonstrated to be a particularly attractive target as they have been associated with the regulation of mineralisation and developmental cellular processes (Gordon et al. 2015) while also being readily inhibited pharmacologically (Richon et al. 1996). HDACi also represent exciting therapeutic candidates as their alterations of gene expression patterns modulate intracellular signalling, with subsequent effects on cell phenotype. The medical literature also reports that HDACi are associated with anti-inflammatory effects, pro-mineralisation, increased SC differentiation and overall improved regenerative responses (Leoni et al. 2002, Halili et al. 2009, Xu et al. 2009, Wang et al. 2010). Consequently, HDACi have the potential to enhance tertiary dentinogenesis by influencing the cellular and tissue processes critical to the success of VPT (Fig. 4.4). Furthermore, HDACi-induced modifications occur at low concentrations with minimal side effects, and therefore, they may offer the ability to develop an easily placed, inexpensive bio-inductive restorative material (Duncan et al. 2013).

> **Conclusions**
>
> Concerns over the destructive nature of dental treatment have led to the promotion of minimally invasive, biologically based dental restorative solutions. Within endodontics, this has resulted in a shift from root canal treatment (RCT) towards more conservative dental procedures aimed to protect the pulp and harness its natural regenerative capacity. Traditionally, VPT has been considered an unpredictable procedure, in part due to poor inflammatory control or low-quality mineralised tissue formation at the exposure site. New understanding of caries management, pulp inflammation, tissue handling and the introduction of calcium silicate cements have improved the outcome of VPT. Although the volume and quality of the repair are dependent on the dental material applied, currently available dental materials are limited by their cytotoxicity, non-specific action and poor reparative capacity. As a result there is a need for improved understanding and the development of better therapeutic solutions of the damaged pulp.
>
> Recently, the importance of epigenetic influence on the networks controlling dental pulp progenitor cell fate and differentiation has emerged. This involves acetylation, methylation, non-coding RNA expression and environmental signals. Further elucidation of individual epigenetic modifications is required to understand their influence on tooth development, pulp inflammation and odontogenic repair processes, prior to any proposed therapeutic clinical application. Potential future vital pulp therapies pharmacologically aimed at epigenetic or other cellular markers provide an opportunity for development of new dental restorative materials targeted at pulpal repair processes.

References

Accorinte ML, Holland R, Reis A et al (2008) Evaluation of mineral trioxide aggregate and calcium hydroxide as pulp-capping agents in human teeth. J Endod 1:1–6

Aeinehchi M, Eslami B, Ghanbariha M, Saffar AS (2003) Mineral trioxide aggregate (MTA) and calcium hydroxide as pulp-capping agents in human teeth: a preliminary report. Int Endod J 36:225–231

Al-Hiyasat AS, Barrieshi-Nusair KM, Al-Omari MA (2006) The radiographic outcomes of direct pulp-capping procedures performed by dental students: a retrospective study. J Am Dent Assoc 137:1699–1705

American Association of Endodontists (2013) Endodontic diagnosis. Accessed on 4 Jan 2018. https://www.aae.org

Arnsdorf EJ, Tummala P, Castillo AB, Zhang F, Jacobs CR (2010) The epigenetic mechanism of mechanically induced osteogenic differentiation. J Biomech 43:2881–2886

Barrieshi-Nusair KM, Qudeimat MA (2006) A prospective clinical study of mineral trioxide aggregate for partial pulpotomy in cariously exposed permanent teeth. J Endod 32:731–735

Barros SP, Offenbacher S (2009) Epigenetics: connecting environment and genotype to phenotype and disease. J Dent Res 88:400–408

Barros SP, Offenbacher S (2014) Modifiable risk factors in periodontal disease: epigenetic regulation of gene expression in the inflammatory response. Periodontol 2000 64:95–110

Barthel CR, Rosenkranz B, Leuenberg A, Roulet RF (2000) Pulp capping of carious exposures: treatment outcome after 5 and 10 years: a retrospective study. J Endod 26:525–528

Bergenholtz G, Cox CF, Loesche WJ, Syed SA (1982) Bacterial leakage around dental restorations: its effect on the dental pulp. J Oral Pathol 11:439–450

Bergenholtz G (2005) Advances since the paper by Zander and Glass (1949) on the pursuit of healing methods for pulpal exposures: historical perspectives. Oral Surg Oral Med Oral Pathol Oral Radiol Endod 100:S102–S108

Bjørndal L, Reit C, Bruun G et al (2010) Treatment of deep caries lesions in adults: randomized clinical trials comparing stepwise vs. direct complete excavation, and direct pulp capping vs. partial pulpotomy. Eur J Oral Sci 118:290–297

Bjørndal L, Fransson H, Bruun G et al (2017) Randomized clinical trials on deep carious lesions: 5-year follow-up. J Dent Res 96:747–753

Bogen G, Kim JS, Bakland LK (2008) Direct pulp capping with mineral trioxide aggregate: an observational study. J Am Dent Assoc 139:305–315

Brännström M, Lind PO (1965) Pulpal response to early dental caries. J Dent Res 144:1045–1050

Brännström M, Nyborg H (1973) Cavity treatment with a microbicidal fluoride solution: growth of bacteria and effect on the pulp. J Prosthet Dent 30:303–310

Browne RM, Tobias RS, Crombie IK, Plant CG (1983) Bacterial microleakage and pulpal inflammation in experimental cavities. Int Endod J 16:147–155

Cantley MD, Zannettino ACW, Bartold PM, Fairlie DP, Haynes DR (2017) Histone deacetylases (HDAC) in physiological and pathological bone remodelling. Bone 95:162–174

Cardoso FP, Viana MB, Sobrinho AP et al (2010) Methylation pattern of the IFN-gamma gene in human dental pulp. J Endod 36:642–646

Cassidy N, Fahey M, Prime SS, Smith AJ (1997) Comparative analysis of transforming growth factor-β isoforms 1-3 in human and rabbit dentine matrices. Arch Oral Biol 42:219–223

Chailertvanitkul P, Paphangkorakit J, Sooksantisakoonchai N et al (2014) Randomized control trial comparing calcium hydroxide and mineral trioxide aggregate for partial pulpotomies in cariously exposed pulps of permanent molars. Int Endod J 47:835–842

Cheng Z, Zheng L, Almeida FA (2017) Epigenetic reprogramming in metabolic disorders: nutritional factors and beyond. J Nutr Biochem 54:1–10

Clayton AL, Hazzalin CA, Mahadevan LC (2006) Enhanced histone acetylation and transcription: a dynamic perspective. Mol Cell 23:289–296

Cooper PR, Takahashi Y, Graham LW, Simon S, Imazato S, Smith AJ (2010) Inflammation-regeneration interplay in the dentine-pulp complex. J Dent 38:687–697

Cox CF, Bergenholtz G, Heys DR, Syed M, Fitzgerald M, Heys RJ (1985) Pulp capping of dental pulp mechanically exposed to oral microflora: a 1-2 year observation of wound healing in the monkey. J Oral Pathol 14:156–168

Cox CF, Sübay RK, Ostro E, Suzuki S, Suzuki SH (1996) Tunnel defects in dentin bridges: their formation following direct pulp capping. Oper Dent 21:4–11

Cvek M (1978) A clinical report on partial pulpotomy and capping with calcium hydroxide in permanent incisors with complicated crown fracture. J Endod 4:232–237

Dugué PA, Brinkman MT, Milne RL et al (2016) Genome-wide measures of DNA methylation in peripheral blood and the risk of urothelial cell carcinoma: a prospective nested case-control study. Br J Cancer 115:664–673

Dummer PM, Hicks R, Huws D (1980) Clinical signs and symptoms in pulp disease. Int Endod J 13:27–35

Duncan HF, Smith AJ, Fleming GJP, Cooper PR (2011) HDACi: cellular effects, opportunities for restorative dentistry. J Dent Res 90:1377–1388

Duncan HF, Smith AJ, Fleming GJ, Cooper PR (2012) Histone deacetylase inhibitors induced differentiation and accelerated mineralization of pulp-derived cells. J Endod 38:339–345

Duncan HF, Smith AJ, Fleming GJ, Cooper PR (2013) Histone deacetylase inhibitors epigenetically promote reparative events in primary dental pulp cells. Exp Cell Res 319:1534–1543

Duncan HF, Smith AJ, Fleming GJ, Partridge NC, Shimizu E, Moran GP, Cooper PR (2016a) The histone-deacetylase-inhibitor suberoylanilide hydroxamic acid promotes dental pulp repair mechanisms through modulation of matrix metalloproteinase-13 activity. J Cell Physiol 231:798–816

Duncan HF, Smith AJ, Fleming GJ, Cooper PR (2016b) Epigenetic modulation of dental pulp stem cells: implications for regenerative endodontics. Int Endod J 49:431–446

Egger G, Liang G, Aparicio A, Jones PA (2004) Epigenetics in human disease and prospects for epigenetic therapy. Nature 429:457–463

European Society of Endodontology (2006) Quality guidelines for endodontic treatment: consensus report of the European Society of Endodontology. Int Endod J 39:921–930

Fabbri M, Garzon R, Cimmino A et al (2007) MicroRNA-29 family reverts aberrant methylation in lung cancer by targeting DNA methyltransferases 3A and 3B. Proc Natl Acad Sci U S A 104:15805–15810

Farges JC, Alliot-Licht B, Renard E et al (2015) Dental pulp defence and repair mechanisms in dental caries. Mediators Inflamm 2015:230251

Farsi N, Alamoudi N, Balto K, Mushyat A (2006) Clinical assessment of mineral trioxide aggregate (MTA) as direct pulp capping in young permanent teeth. J Clin Pediatr Dent 31:72–76

Feng J, Mantesso A, De Bari C, Nishiyama A, Sharpe PT (2011) Dual origin of mesenchymal stem cells contributing to organ growth and repair. Proc Natl Acad Sci U S A 108:6503–6508

Ferracane JL, Cooper PR, Smith AJ (2010) Can interaction of materials with the dentin-pulp complex contribute to dentin regeneration? Odontology 98:2–14

Fitzgerald M, Chiego DJ Jr, Heys DR (1990) Autoradiographic analysis of odontoblast replacement following pulp exposure in primate teeth. Arch Oral Biol 35:707–715

Frozoni M, Zaia AA, Line SR, Mina M (2012) Analysis of the contribution of nonresident progenitor cells and hematopoietic cells to reparative dentinogenesis using parabiosis model in mice. J Endod 38:1214–1219

Fuks AB, Bielak S, Chosak A (1982) Clinical and radiographic assessment of direct pulp capping and pulpotomy in young permanent teeth. Pediatr Dent 4:240–244

Garfunkel A, Sela J, Ulmansky M (1973) Dental pulp pathosis: clinicopathologic correlations based on 109 cases. Oral Surg Oral Med Oral Pathol 35:110–117

Gordon JA, Stein JL, Westendorf JJ, van Wijnen AJ (2015) Chromatin modifiers and histone modifications in bone formation, regeneration, and therapeutic intervention for bone-related disease. Bone 81:739–745

Graham L, Cooper PR, Cassidy N, Nor JE, Sloan AJ, Smith AJ (2006) The effect of calcium hydroxide on solubilisation of bio-active dentine matrix. Biomaterials 27:2865–2873

Grando Mattuella L, Westphalen Bento L, de Figueiredo JA, Nör JE, de Araujo FB, Fossati AC (2007) Vascular endothelial growth factor and its relationship with the dental pulp. J Endod 33:524–530

Grant S, Easley C, Kirkpatrick P (2007) Vorinostat. Nat Rev Drug Discov 6:21–22

Hake SB, Xiao A, Allis CD (2004) Linking the epigenetic 'language' of covalent histone modifications to cancer. Br J Cancer 90:761–769

Halili MA, Andrews MR, Sweet MJ, Fairlie DP (2009) Histone deacetylase inhibitors in inflammatory disease. Curr Top Med Chem 9:309–319

Hashem D, Mannocci F, Patel S et al (2015) A clinical and radiographic assessment of the efficacy of calcium silicate indirect pulp capping: a randomized controlled clinical trial. J Dent Res 94:562–568

Hilton TJ, Ferracane JL, Mancl L, Northwest Practice-based Research Collaborative in Evidence-based Dentistry (NWP) (2013) Comparison of CaOH with MTA for direct pulp capping: a PBRN randomized clinical trial. J Dent Res 92:16S–22S

Horn PJ, Peterson CL (2002) Molecular biology. Chromatin higher order folding - wrapping up transcription. Science 297:1824–1827

Hörsted-Bindslev P, Vilkinis V, Sidlauskas A (2003) Direct capping of human pulps with a dentin bonding system or with calcium hydroxide cement. Oral Surg Oral Med Oral Pathol Oral Radiol Endod 96:591–600

Huangfu D, Maehr R, Guo W et al (2008) Induction of pluripotent stem cells by defined factors is greatly improved by small-molecule compounds. Nat Biotechnol 26:795–797

Huynh NC, Everts V, Salingcarnboriboon R, Ampornaramveth RS (2017) Histone deacetylases and their roles in mineralized tissue regeneration. Bone Rep 7:33–40

Innes NP, Frencken JE, Bjørndal L et al (2016) Managing carious lesions: consensus recommendations on terminology. Adv Dent Res 28:49–57

Isobe Y, Koyama N, Nakao K et al (2015) Comparison of human mesenchymal stem cells derived from bone marrow, synovial fluid, adult dental pulp, and exfoliated deciduous tooth pulp. Int J Oral Maxillofac Surg 45:124–131

Jensen ED, Nair AK, Westendorf JJ (2007) Histone deacetylase co-repressor complex control of Runx2 and bone formation. Crit Rev Eukaryot Gene Expr 17:187–196

Jin B, Robertson KD (2013) DNA methyltransferases (DNMTs), DNA damage repair, and cancer. Adv Exp Med Biol 754:3–29

Kakehashi S, Stanley HR, Fitzgerald RJ (1965) The effects of surgical exposures of dental pulps in germ-free and conventional laboratory rats. Oral Surg Oral Med Oral Pathol 20:340–349

Karaoz E, Demircan PC, Saglam O et al (2011) Human dental pulp stem cells demonstrate better neural and epithelial stem cell properties than bone marrow-derived mesenchymal stem cells. Histochem Cell Biol 136:455–473

Katge FA, Patil DP (2017) Comparative analysis of 2 calcium silicate-based cements (Biodentine and Mineral Trioxide Aggregate) as direct pulp-capping agent in young permanent molars: a split mouth study. J Endod 43:507–513

Kellis M, Wold B, Snyder MP et al (2014) Defining functional DNA elements in the human genome. Proc Natl Acad Sci U S A 111:6131–6138

Kelly TK, De Carvalho DD, Jones PA (2010) Epigenetic modifications as therapeutic targets. Nat Biotechnol 28:1069–1078

Kleff S, Andrulis ED, Anderson CW, Sternglanz R (1995) Identification of a gene encoding a yeast histone H4 acetyltransferase. J Biol Chem 270:24674–24677

Klinz FJ, Korkmaz Y, Bloch W, Raab WH, Addicks K (2012) Histone deacetylases 2 and 9 are coexpressed and nuclear localized in human molar odontoblasts in vivo. Histochem Cell Biol 137:697–702

Lander ES, Linton LM, Birren B et al (2001) Initial sequencing and analysis of the human genome. Nature 409:860–921

Leoni F, Zaliani A, Bertolini G et al (2002) The antitumor histone deacetylase inhibitor suberoylanilide hydroxamic acid exhibits antiinflammatory properties via suppression of cytokines. Proc Natl Acad Sci U S A 99:2995–3000

Lesot H, Smith AJ, Tziafas D, Begue-Kirn C, Cassidy N, Ruch JV (1994) Biologically active molecules and dental tissue repair: a comparative review of reactionary and reparative dentinogenesis with the induction of odontoblast differentiation in vitro. Cell Mat 4:199–218

Li B, Carey M, Workman JL (2007) The role of chromatin during transcription. Cell 128:707–719

Li Z, Hassan MQ, Jafferji M et al (2009) Biological functions of miR-29b contribute to positive regulation of osteoblast differentiation. J Biol Chem 284:15676–15684

Luger K (2003) Structure and dynamic behavior of nucleosomes. Curr Opin Genet Dev 13:127–135

Machado CV, Passos ST, Campos TM et al (2015) The dental pulp stem cell niche based on aldehyde dehydrogenase 1 expression. Int Endod J 49:755–763

Margueron R, Trojer P, Reinberg D (2005) The key to development: interpreting the histone code? Curr Opin Genet Dev 15:163–176

Marques MS, Wesselink PR, Shemesh H (2015) Outcome of direct pulp capping with mineral trioxide aggregate: a prospective study. J Endod 41:1026–1031

Massler M (1972) Therapy conductive to healing of the human pulp. Oral Surg Oral Med Oral Pathol 34:122–130

Matsuo T, Nakanishi T, Shimizu H (1996) A clinical study of direct pulp capping applied to carious-exposed pulps. J Endod 22:551–556

Mejàre I, Cvek M (1993) Partial pulpotomy in young permanent teeth with deep carious lesions. Endod Dent Traumatol 9:238–242

Mente J, Geletneky B, Ohle M et al (2010) Mineral trioxide aggregate or calcium hydroxide direct pulp capping: an analysis of the clinical treatment outcome. J Endod 36:806–813

Mente J, Hufnagel S, Leo M (2014) Treatment outcome of mineral trioxide aggregate or calcium hydroxide direct pulp capping: long-term results. J Endod 40:1746–1751

Meraji N, Camilleri J (2017) Bonding over dentin replacement materials. J Endod 43:1343–1349

Mercer TR, Mattick JS (2013) Structure and function of long noncoding RNAs in epigenetic regulation. Nat Struct Mol Biol 20:300–307

Michaelson PL, Holland GR (2002) Is pulpitis painful? Int Endod J 35:829–832

Mjör IA, Tronstad L (1972) Experimentally induced pulpitis. Oral Surg Oral Med Oral Pathol 34:102–108

Morse DR (1991) Age-related changes of the dental pulp complex and their relationship to systemic aging. Oral Surg Oral Med Oral Pathol 72:721–745

Nagase H, Ghosh S (2008) Epigenetics: differential DNA methylation in mammalian somatic tissues. FEBS J 275:1617–1623

Nair PNR, Duncan HF, Pitt Ford TR, Luder HU (2008) Histological, ultrastructural and quantitative investigations on the response of healthy human pulps to experimental capping with mineral trioxide aggregate: a randomized controlled trial. Int Endod J 41:128–150

Nakashima M (1994) Induction of dentin formation on canine amputated pulp by recombinant human bone morphogenetic proteins (BMP) -2 and -4. J Dent Res 73:1515–1522

Odor TM, Pitt Ford TR, McDonald F (1994) Effect of inferior alveolar nerve block anaesthesia on the lower teeth. Endod Dent Traumatol 10:144–148

Opsahl Vital S, Gaucher C et al (2012) Tooth dentin defects reflect genetic disorders affecting bone mineralization. Bone 50:989–997

Pitt Ford TR, Seare MA, McDonald F (1993) Action of adrenaline on the effect of dental local anaesthetic solutions. Endod Dent Traumatol 9:31–35

Portela A, Esteller M (2010) Epigenetic modifications and human disease. Nat Biotechnol 28:1057–1068

Qu Q, Fang F, Wu B et al (2016) Potential role of long non-coding RNA in osteogenic differentiation of human periodontal ligament stem cells. J Periodontol 87:127–137

Qudeimat MA, Barrieshi-Nusair KM, Owais AI (2007) Calcium hydroxide vs. mineral trioxide aggregates for partial pulpotomy of permanent molars with deep caries. Eur Arch Paediatr Dent 8:99–104

Qudeimat MA, Alyahya A, Hasan AA (2017) Mineral trioxide aggregate pulpotomy for permanent molars with clinical signs indicative of irreversible pulpitis: a preliminary study. Int Endod J 50:126–134

Reeves R, Stanley HR (1966) The relationship of bacterial penetration and pulpal pathosis in carious teeth. Oral Surg Oral Med Oral Pathol 22:59–65

Richon VM, Webb Y, Merger R et al (1996) Second generation hybrid polar compounds are potent inducers of transformed cell differentiation. Proc Natl Acad Sci U S A 93:5705–5708

Ricketts DN, Kidd EA, Innes N, Clarkson J (2006) Complete or ultraconservative removal of decayed tissue in unfilled teeth. Cochrane Database Syst Rev:CD003808

Ricucci D, Loghin S, Siqueira J Jr (2014) Correlation between clinical and histologic pulp diagnoses. J Endod 40:1932–1939

Ruch JV, Lesot H, Bègue-Kirn C (1995) Odontoblast differentiation. Int J Dev Biol 39:51–68

Rutherford RB, Wahle J, Tucker M, Rueger D, Charette M (1993) Induction of reparative dentine formation in monkeys by recombinant human osteogenic protein-1. Arch Oral Biol 38:571–576

Sangwan P, Sangwan A, Duhan J, Rohilla A (2013) Tertiary dentinogenesis with calcium hydroxide: a review of proposed mechanisms. Int Endod J 46:3–19

Schwendicke F, Frencken JE, Bjørndal L et al (2016) Managing carious lesions: consensus recommendations on carious tissue removal. Adv Dent Res 28:58–67

Schroeder TM, Kahler RA, Li X, Westendorf JJ (2004) Histone deacetylase 3 interacts with Runx2 to repress the osteocalcin promoter and regulate osteoblast differentiation. J Biol Chem 279:41998–42007

Sehic A, Tulek A, Khuu C, Nirvani M, Sand LP, Utheim TP (2017) Regulatory roles of microRNAs in human dental tissues. Gene 596:9–18

Seltzer S, Bender IB, Ziontz M (1963) The dynamics of pulpal inflammation: correlations between diagnostic data and actual histologic findings in the pulp. Oral Surg Oral Med Oral Pathol 16:871–876

Shanmugam MK, Sethi G (2013) Role of epigenetics in inflammation-associated diseases. Subcell Biochem 61:627–657

Simon S, Smith AJ (2014) Regenerative endodontics. Br Dent J 216:E13

Simon S, Perard M, Zanini M et al (2013) Should pulp chamber pulpotomy be seen as a permanent treatment? Some preliminary thoughts. Int Endod J 46:79–87

Smith AJ (2002) Pulp responses to caries and dental repair. Caries Res 36:223–232

Smith AJ, Lesot H (2001) Induction and regulation of crown dentinogenesis: embryonic events as a template for dental tissue repair? Crit Rev Oral Biol Med 12:425–437

Smith AJ, Duncan HF, Diogenes A, Simon S, Cooper PR (2016) Exploiting the bioactive properties of the dentin-pulp complex in regenerative endodontics. J Endod 42:47–56

Song Z, Chen LL, Wang RF et al (2016) MicroRNA-135b inhibits odontoblast-like differentiation of human dental pulp cells by regulating Smad5 and Smad4. Int Endod J 50:685–693

Taha NA, Khazali MA (2017) Partial pulpotomy in mature permanent teeth with clinical signs indicative of irreversible pulpitis: a randomized clinical trial. J Endod 43:1417–1421

Taha NA, Ahmad MB, Ghanim A (2017) Assessment of mineral trioxide aggregate pulpotomy in mature permanent teeth with carious exposures. Int Endod J 50:117–125

Takahashi K, Yamanaka S (2006) Induction of pluripotent stem cells from mouse embryonic and adult fibroblast cultures by defined factors. Cell 126:663–676

Tao H, Yang JJ, Shi KH (2015) Non-coding RNAs as direct and indirect modulators of epigenetic mechanism regulation of cardiac fibrosis. Expert Opin Ther Targets 19:707–716

Taunton J, Hassig CA, Schreiber SL (1996) A mammalian histone deacetylase related to the yeast transcriptional regulator Rpd3p. Science 272:408–411

Tobias RS, Plant CG, Browne RM (1982) Reduction in pulpal inflammation beneath surface-sealed silicates. Int Endod J 15:173–180

Tronstad L, Mjör IA (1972) Capping of the inflamed pulp. Oral Surg Oral Med Oral Pathol 34:477–485

Turner BM (2007) Defining an epigenetic code. Nat Cell Biol 9:2–6

Vaissière T, Sawan C, Herceg Z (2008) Epigenetic interplay between histone modifications and DNA methylation in gene silencing. Mutat Res 659:40–48

Wang G, Badylak SF, Heber-Katz E, Braunhut SJ, Gudas LJ (2010) The effects of DNA methyltransferase inhibitors and histone deacetylase inhibitors on digit regeneration in mice. Regen Med 5:201–220

Weber M, Hellmann I, Stadler MB et al (2007) Distribution, silencing potential and evolutionary impact of promoter DNA methylation in the human genome. Nat Genet 39:457–466

Witherspoon DE (2008) Vital pulp therapy with new materials: new directions and treatment perspectives-permanent Teeth. J Endod 34:S25–S28

Wolters WJ, Duncan HF, Tomson PL, Karim IE, McKenna G, Dorri M, Stangvaltaite L, van der Sluis LWM (2017) Minimally invasive endodontics: a new diagnostic system for assessing pulpitis and subsequent treatment needs. Int Endod J 50:825–829

Wright J (2013) Epigenetics: reversible tags. Nature 498:S10–S11

You JS, Jones PA (2012) Cancer genetics and epigenetics: two sides of the same coin? Cancer Cell 22:9–20

Xu Y, Hammerick KE, James AW et al (2009) Inhibition of histone deacetylase activity in reduced oxygen environment enhances the osteogenesis of mouse adipose-derived stromal cells. Tissue Eng Part A 15:3697–3707

Yang XJ, Seto E (2008) The Rpd3/Hda1 family of lysine deacetylases: from bacteria and yeast to mice and men. Nat Rev Mol Cell Biol 9:206–218

Zander HA, Glass RL (1949) The healing of phenolized pulp exposures. Oral Surg Oral Med Oral Pathol 2:803–810Y

Zhang Y, Reinberg D (2001) Transcription regulation by histone methylation: interplay between different covalent modifications of the core histone tails. Genes Dev 15:2243–2360

Zhang D, Li Q, Rao L, Yi B, Xu Q (2015) Effect of 5-Aza-2'-deoxycytidine on odontogenic differentiation of human dental pulp cells. J Endod 41:640–645

Zilbeman U, Mass E, Sarnat E (1989) Partial pulpotomy in carious permanent molars. Am J Dent 2:147–150

Current and Future Views on Biomaterial Use in Regenerative Endodontics

5

Eliseu A. Münchow and Marco C. Bottino

5.1 Introduction

Dental pulp plays a vital role in tooth development as it harbours progenitor/stem cells (DPSCs) that proliferate and differentiate into dentine-secreting odontoblasts (Gronthos et al. 2002). Dental trauma and the bacterial infection (caries) of dental pulp lead to inflammation, and if left untreated, pulpal necrosis and apical periodontitis will eventually develop (Albuquerque et al. 2014a; Galler 2016). While trauma is more commonly associated with an accidental injury (Andreasen and Kahler 2015), caries may depend on several variables, especially those related to poor oral hygiene and sugar intake (Selwitz et al. 2007).

Traumatic dental injuries have recently become a public health problem worldwide (Zaleckiene et al. 2014); they are more prevalent in the permanent than the primary dentition and occur in earlier stages of life, i.e. before age 20 (Glendor 2009). Concerning caries, data from the latest National Health and Nutrition Examination Survey (Dye et al. 2015) revealed ~21% of children aging 6–11 years and ~58% of adolescents aging 12–19 years have experienced dental caries in their permanent dentition. When properly managed, tooth decay is a reversible condition; however, if neglected, caries may induce inflammatory reactions at the pulp, leading to tissue necrosis and, ultimately, root canal therapy (Larsen and Fiehn 2017).

In the United States, over 15 million patients undergo root canal therapy each year (American Association of Endodontics 2016), resulting in a major socioeconomic burden. Traditional root canal treatment remains the standard of care for

E. A. Münchow
Department of Dentistry, Health Science Institute, Federal University of Juiz de Fora, Governador Valadares, MG, Brazil

M. C. Bottino (✉)
Department of Cariology, Restorative Sciences, and Endodontics, University of Michigan School of Dentistry, Ann Arbor, MI, USA
e-mail: mbottino@umich.edu

© Springer Nature Switzerland AG 2019
H. F. Duncan, P. R. Cooper (eds.), *Clinical Approaches in Endodontic Regeneration*,
https://doi.org/10.1007/978-3-319-96848-3_5

mature, fully developed teeth with pulpal necrosis, and it involves the chemome-chanical debridement and sealing of the canal system with an inert rubber-like material (Huang 2011). However, immature permanent teeth present a very unique anatomy, i.e. wide open root apex and thin root dentinal walls (Albuquerque et al. 2014a; Galler 2016; Diogenes et al. 2014). Given the wide open root apex, which halts the possibility of achieving an apical seal and thin dentinal walls, performing traditional root canal therapy on necrotic immature teeth is not advisable (Albuquerque et al. 2014a; Galler 2016; Diogenes et al. 2014). Thus, apexification using either calcium hydroxide ($Ca(OH)_2$) or mineral trioxide aggregate (MTA) has been used to induce apical closure (Cvek 1972, 1973; Damle et al. 2012). Although apexification supports apical closure, it neither promotes root development nor restores the immunologic competence of pulp (Jeeruphan et al. 2012; Wang et al. 2010). Additionally, apexification eliminates any further chance for complete root development (e.g. dentinal wall thickening and apical maturation), thus increasing the chance of future root fracture (Cvek 1992; Diogenes et al. 2016).

Regeneration of the pulp-dentine complex holds the promise of extending the function of the natural dentition, particularly in cases where traumatic injuries to permanent immature teeth halt root maturation and full development (Albuquerque et al. 2014a, b; Diogenes et al. 2014, 2016). The clinically available regenerative strategy, namely, evoked bleeding (EB), employs intracanal medications, including triple (TAP, ciprofloxacin, metronidazole and minocycline) and double (DAP, minocycline-free) highly concentrated antibiotic pastes or $Ca(OH)_2$. Following proper disinfection, the intentional laceration of periapical tissue is performed to provoke bleeding allowing intracanal delivery of apical stem cells and formation of a fibrin-based scaffold which induces tissue regeneration (Albuquerque et al. 2014a; Galler 2016; Diogenes et al. 2014, 2013). It is worth noting that this form of medi-cation was introduced into the clinics without precise information as to the thera-peutic dose to be used, which would retain its antimicrobial effect while minimising its toxicity on host tissues and cells. There is a compelling level of data indicating that both intracanal medicaments and chemical irrigants can negatively affect the survival and function of dental stem cells (Albuquerque et al. 2014a; Galler 2016; Diogenes et al. 2014). Meanwhile, the blood clot-derived fibrin scaffold might not be the most ideal matrix to act as a scaffold. Thus, the purpose of this chapter is to discuss the latest discoveries on biocompatible strategies of root canal disinfection and the use of biomaterials (scaffolds), stem cells and growth factors in dental pulp tissue regeneration.

5.2 The Role of Disinfection in Regenerative Endodontics

In regenerative endodontics, both root canal disinfection and blood clot formation (i.e. fibrin-based scaffold) have been shown to play a critical role in new tissue for-mation and overall root maturation and development. Despite these promising results, the biological outcome of the therapy is rather unpredictable (Diogenes et al. 2013; Banchs and Trope 2004; Bose et al. 2009; Cehreli et al. 2011; Iwaya et al. 2001; Petrino et al. 2010). Bone healing and root development do not necessarily confirm the formation of tissue that closely resembles the pulp-dentine complex within root canals. In fact, the histological examination of tissue formed inside the root canals of teeth treated with regenerative procedures reveals apposition of a cementum-like tissue, which is responsible for canal narrowing and an increase in length (Gomes-Filho et al. 2013; Martin et al. 2013). Additionally, the ingrowth of a connective tissue similar to the periodontal ligament, along with a bone-like tissue, was identified inside root canals (Diogenes et al. 2013; Lin et al. 2013; Becerra et al. 2014). Unpredictability of the histologic results could relate to many factors (Albuquerque et al. 2014a; Galler 2016; Diogenes et al. 2014, 2013). It has previously been understood that inflammation derived from TAP remnants (da Silva et al. 2010) or from the healing process itself (Wang et al. 2010) could impair the formation of new pulp tissue. More recently, the effect of residual bacteria on the outcome of pulp regeneration was confirmed in vivo (Verma et al. 2017), thus showing a strong association with inflammation. In that study, residual bacteria were found to be mostly located in the coronal part of the canal, far from the inflammation zone and regenerated tissues located at the apical region. The authors stated that, at the coronal part of the canal, bacteria have the ability to grow faster than at the apical part, where vital tissues are present and the host response is strongly available to control infection. Interestingly, a study by Vishwanat et al. (Vishwanat et al. 2017) demonstrated that residual biofilm arrested within the intracanal space may promote osteoblastic versus dentinogenic gene expression of stem cells from the apical papilla (SCAP), preventing the formation of new dentine-like tissue. For those reasons, true pulp regeneration remains a clinical challenge, especially due to the presence of residual bacteria/biofilm within the root canal system. Therefore, antimicrobial strategies that assure a strong disinfection capacity without jeopardising the environment, such as enabling stem cell differentiation, are still needed.

5.2.1 An Overview of Conventional Antimicrobial Therapy

Originally, the first antimicrobial agent used in regenerative endodontic protocols was the so-called triple antibiotic paste (TAP) (Hoshino et al. 1996). Its mixture is efficient against a wide range of oral pathogens that are important in polymicrobial infection naturally found in necrotic teeth. Several studies have confirmed the positive effects of TAP in disinfecting the root canal system (Banchs and Trope 2004; Albuquerque et al. 2015a), although it may not eliminate all cultivable bacteria. In the study by Windley et al. (Windley 3rd et al. 2005), TAP was able to eliminate approximately 75% of the total amount of pathogens. It can be assumed that infected teeth are more resistant to disinfection when compared to soft tissues due to the presence of dentinal tubules. Indeed, bacteria may form planktonic and biofilm cultures, limiting complete action of antimicrobial agents (Diogenes and Hargreaves 2017). Consequently, residual bacteria may stay entrapped within the depth of the dentinal tubules, surviving the disinfection protocol. Even though TAP is broadly used worldwide, some case reports have revealed that this triple mixture may stain the tooth, provoking strong discolouration and unpleasing aesthetic issues (Albuquerque et al. 2015a; Kahler and Rossi-Fedele 2016; Porter et al. 2016). This is a consequence of the minocycline component, and in order to eliminate this staining side effect, minocycline has been replaced by nonstaining antibiotics, including but not limited to amoxicillin/clavulanic acid (Nosrat et al. 2013), clarithromycin/fosfomycin (Mandras et al. 2013) and cefaclor (Ruparel et al. 2012). Antimicrobial pastes containing only two antibiotics have been proposed, as in the case of double antibiotic paste (DAP) comprised of ciprofloxacin and metronidazole (Iwaya et al. 2001). Notwithstanding, bacteria elimination is usually greater when TAP is used, compared to DAP (Latham et al. 2016).

In spite of their antimicrobial effects or discolouration potential, antibiotic pastes used in regenerative endodontics are known to pose a critical risk to regeneration, since the high concentration of antibiotics is potentially toxic to DPSCs and SCAP (Galler et al. 2015; Althumairy et al. 2014; Martin et al. 2014). Additionally, it has been demonstrated that TAP may inhibit the release of growth factors from dentine (Galler et al. 2015), thus potentially affecting the regenerative process. One attempt has been made to reduce the final cytotoxicity of antibiotic pastes, i.e. reducing the concentration of medicaments. According to the study by Latham et al. (Latham et al. 2016), which compared the antimicrobial and cytotoxic potential of TAP and DAP at different antibiotic concentrations (e.g. 0.1, 1 and 10 mg/mL), the less concentrated pastes, though being non-toxic to stem cells, were not potent enough to eliminate bacteria, thus allowing a greater number of viable bacteria in the dentinal tubules when compared to the more concentrated formulations. On the other hand, pastes containing 10 mg/mL of antibiotics were effective in reducing the level of viable bacteria, but they were also associated with greater cytotoxicity. In a similar study by Ruparel et al. (Ruparel et al. 2012), the authors tested the effects of TAP and DAP at concentrations of 0.01, 0.1, 1, 10 and 100 mg/mL; they found that concentrations below 1 mg/mL had no detectable effect on stem cell survival (nearly 100% cell survival), whereas concentrations of 1, 10 and 100 mg/mL resulted in approximately 58%, 8% and 1.3% of stem cell survival, respectively. Thus, an impasse exists between the maximum disinfection potential and minimal cytotoxic effects of conventional TAP and DAP pastes. To that end, alternative antimicrobial strategies have been proposed, which will be the focus of the next section.

5.2.2 Nanofibrous Intracanal Drug Delivery Systems

In recent years, electrospinning or electrostatic spinning, a textile technology, has been employed to fabricate antibiotic-containing polymer-based nanofibers for drug delivery applications in dentistry (Albuquerque et al. 2014a; Bottino et al. 2012, 2013). The theory behind the use of antibiotic-containing nanofibers as a three-dimensional (3D) tubular drug delivery construct (Albuquerque et al. 2014a; Porter et al. 2016; Bottino et al. 2015) that can be placed inside the root canal system of necrotic teeth (Fig. 5.1) is based on the fact that the addition of low antibiotic

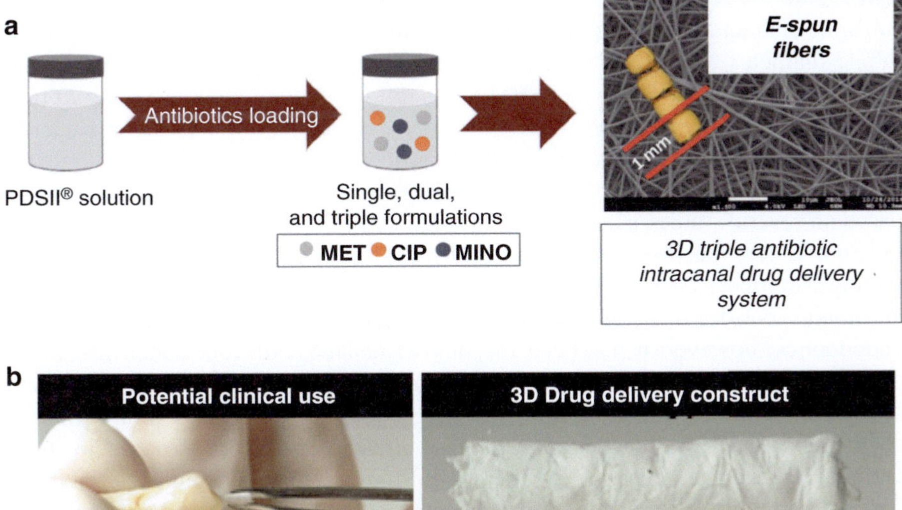

Fig. 5.1 (**a**) Synthesis of triple antibiotic-eluting nanofibers. Polymer solubilisation in hexafluoro-2-propanol. Single, dual or triple antibiotic incorporation (MET, CIP and MINO) into the solution before electrospinning. Representative scanning electron micrograph (SEM) of triple antibiotic-containing fibres and 3D constructs (in yellow, superimposed on the SEM image). Image obtained from reference (Palasuk et al. 2014), with permission. (**b**) Potential clinical use of the recently developed 3D patient-specific drug delivery construct. Image obtained from reference (Bottino et al. 2017), with permission

concentrations and the slow drug release provided by these nanofibrous constructs will eradicate infection and thus create a bacteria-free environment favourable to tissue regeneration (Albuquerque et al. 2014a, 2015a, b, 2016; Porter et al. 2016; Bottino et al. 2013; Palasuk et al. 2014; Kamocki et al. 2015a, b).

In electrospinning, a polymer solution/melt containing the desired concentration of antibiotics is prepared in order to produce nanofibers (Albuquerque et al. 2014a; Bottino et al. 2012, 2013). The chosen polymer solution can be incorporated with one or a combination of antibiotics, making it possible to fabricate fibres with a narrow or wide spectrum of action (e.g. ciprofloxacin [CIP], metronidazole [MET] and minocycline [MINO], among others) that have been shown to inhibit the growth of endodontic pathogens (Bottino et al. 2013; Palasuk et al. 2014; Kamocki et al. 2015a, b). In a recent study, CIP-containing polymer nanofibers were tested against *Enterococcus faecalis* (*Ef*) biofilms developed on human root fragments (Albuquerque et al. 2015b). An *Ef* suspension was inoculated on dentine specimens for 5 days to enable biofilm formation which were then exposed (direct contact) to CIP-containing (5 and 25 wt.%CIP) nanofibers. A thick biofilm mass was observed using scanning electron microscopy (SEM) along the whole root segment, with a remarkable concentration of bacteria on the middle third, likely due to intrinsic substrate characteristics (e.g. uniform distribution of dentinal tubules and a similar tubule diameter) (Wang et al. 2012). Antimicrobial assays involving the use of colony-forming units (CFU) and SEM methodologies found that this young *Ef* biofilm was susceptible to 25 wt.%CIP nanofibers, demonstrating maximum bacterial biofilm elimination (Albuquerque et al. 2015b).

In an attempt to improve the antimicrobial effects of these unique nanofibers and based on several studies using TAP as the standard of care in regenerative endodontics, our group was the first to develop triple (MET, CIP and MINO) antibiotic-eluting nanofibers (Albuquerque et al. 2015a). The chosen bacteria, *Actinomyces naeslundii*, consisted of uncommon bacterial species used for in vitro studies in endodontics; however, it has been recently associated with root canal infections, particularly in cases of undeveloped traumatised teeth (Nagata et al. 2014). *A. naeslundii* was cultured on dentine specimens for 7 days to allow for biofilm formation on the surface and inside dentinal tubules. Infected specimens exposed to triple antibiotic-eluting nanofibers (i.e., TAP scaffold) revealed significant bacterial death based on confocal laser scanning microscopy (CLSM) data when using the Live/ Dead Cell assay (Fig. 5.2) (Albuquerque et al. 2015a).

Noteworthy, the aforementioned studies focused on facultative anaerobic bacteria; however, root canal colonisation, mainly in primary infections, is often composed of strict anaerobic species (Gomes et al. 2004). Therefore, recent research (Albuquerque et al. 2016) used *Porphyromonas gingivalis* to induce a 7-day biofilm on human dentine through the careful limitation of environmental conditions. The established *P. gingivalis* biofilm was also susceptible to triple antibiotic-eluting nanofibers (Albuquerque et al. 2016).

Further research related to the fabrication of antibiotic-eluting fibres has focused on improving the staining limitation discussed previously. One study in particular (Porter et al. 2016) tested the effects of different TAP pastes and triple antibiotic-eluting nanofibers formulated with either minocycline or doxycycline on dentine colour changes. The authors observed that nanofibers containing minocycline or doxycycline produced similar colour changes when compared to their respective TAP systems, although the doxycycline-treated groups presented less discolouration than those treated using conventional minocycline. A different study by Karczewski et al. (Karczewski et al. 2018) intended to replace minocycline with clindamycin, i.e. another potent antibiotic with a wide spectrum of action, testing the antimicrobial properties, cell compatibility and dentine discoloration. The authors demonstrated that these modified antibiotic-eluting nanofibers may present remarkable antimicrobial effects, a cell-friendly behaviour (biocompatibility) and a stain-free property (Fig. 5.3), since no discoloration was seen. Not less important, clindamycin has demonstrated in vitro proangiogenic activity (Radomska-Lesniewska et al. 2010), which may be considered a critical step to the recreation of the dentine-pulp complex, since angiogenesis is essential for oxygen and nutrient transport to regenerated cells (Saghiri et al. 2015). Conversely, MINO was revealed to negatively affect angiogenesis by decreasing vascular endothelial growth factor secretion and suppressing neovasculogenesis of endothelial cells (Li et al. 2014). In

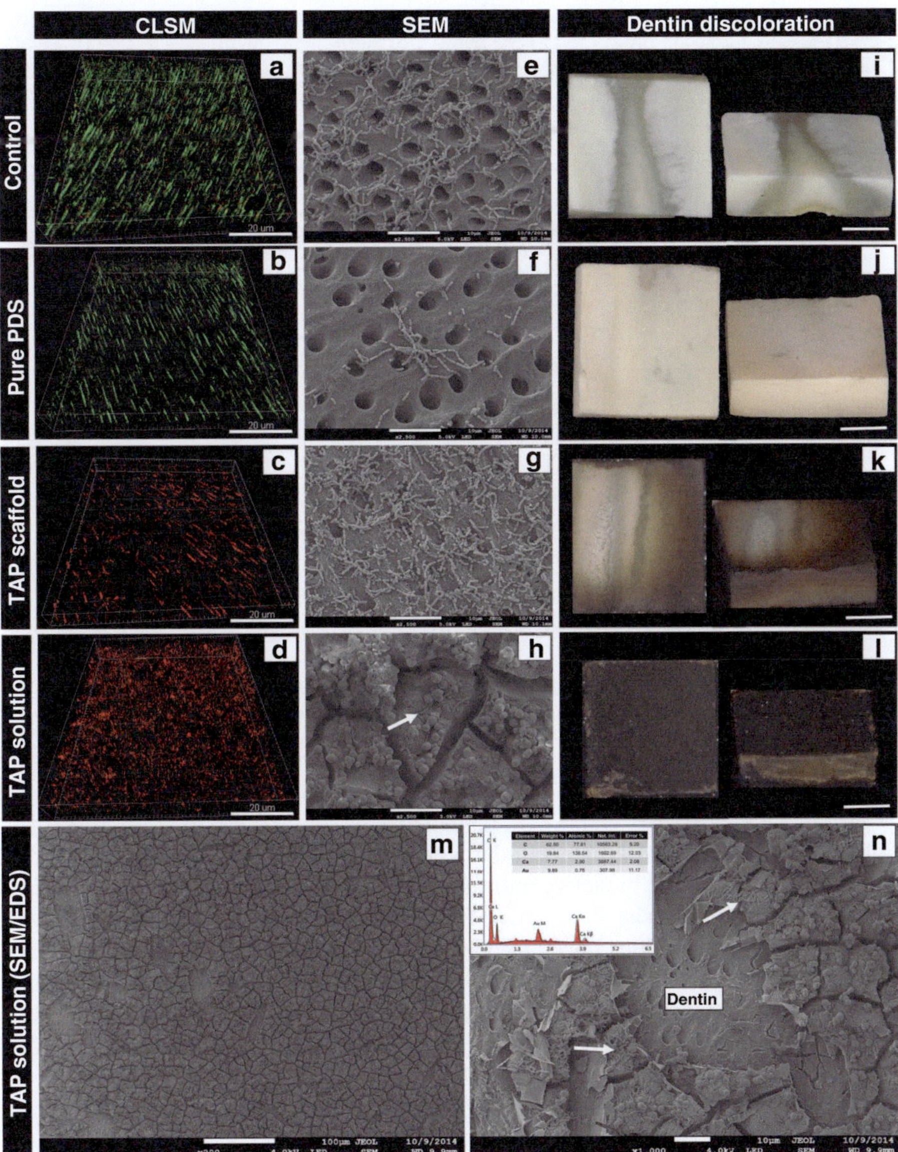

Fig. 5.2 CLSM images were collected in sequential illumination mode by using 488 and 552 nm laser lines. Fluorescent emission was collected in two HyD spectral detectors with filter range set up to 500–550 and 590–655 nm for green (SYTO9) and red dye (PI), respectively. CLSM macro-photographs of 7-day *A. naeslundii* biofilm (negative control) growth inside dentinal tubules (**a**), infected dentine treated with pure PDS (**b**), TAP scaffold (**c**) and TAP solution (**d**) for 3 days. SEM images of *A. naeslundii* biofilm on the dentine surface (negative control) (**e**) treated by pure PDS (**f**), TAP scaffold (**g**) and TAP solution (**h**). Dentine discolouration images of negative control (**i**), pure PDS (**j**), TAP scaffold (**k**) and TAP solution (**l**) groups. Representative SEM images (original magnification, ×200 and ×1000) of TAP solution-treated dentine showing calcium-enriched (Ca) insoluble agglomerates attached to the dentine surface (**m**) and covering dentinal tubules (**n**) as demonstrated by energy-dispersive X-ray spectroscopy (EDS) analyses (inset EDS image **n**); *A. naeslundii* can be seen on the surface of this insoluble complex (white arrows) (**n** and **h**). Image obtained from reference (Albuquerque et al. 2015a), with permission

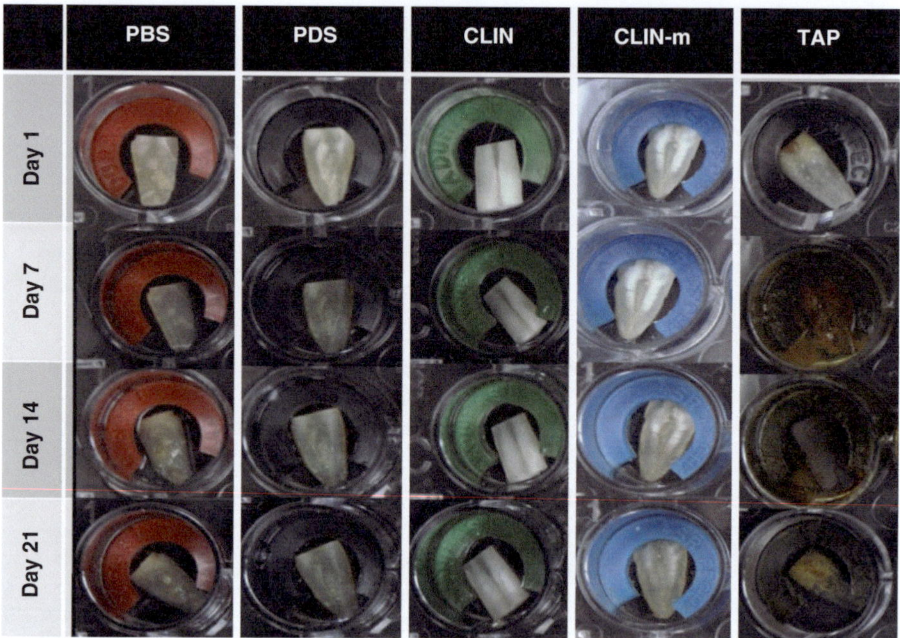

Fig. 5.3 Representative macrophotographs showing human dentine colour stability/change after 1, 7, 14 and 21 days of exposure to control (PBS), antibiotic-free (PDS), CLIN and CLIN-m nanofibers and triple antibiotic paste (TAP). Image obtained from reference (Karczewski et al. 2018), with permission

light of this, replacing MINO by clindamycin into TAP formulations would contribute to the use of a more bioactive antimicrobial agent and perhaps to improved cell survival and angiogenesis.

Collectively, our studies have provided abundant background information to not only test the antimicrobial efficacy of these nanofibers on multispecies biofilms in vitro but to also explore their clinical efficacy using preclinical animal models of periapical disease (Fig. 5.4).

5.2.3 Alternative Antimicrobial Strategies

Other strategies, in lieu of using antibiotic-eluting nanofibers, have also demonstrated important root canal disinfection. For example, the 2010 study by Sousa et al. (Sousa et al. 2010) prepared novel amoxicillin-loaded microspheres constituted of poly(D-L-lactide-co-glycolide) and zein (i.e. a class of prolamine protein), showing effective antimicrobial activity against *Ef*. The authors also demonstrated that, by varying the content of zein, the release of amoxicillin could be modulated to a level where it could achieve a more effective intracanal dressing, thus improving the disinfection potential of the microspheres. Another strategy showing

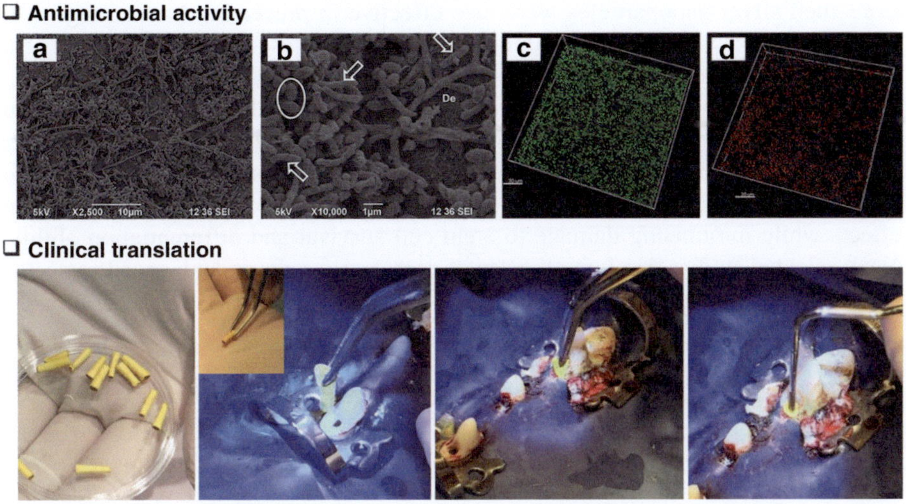

□ **Antimicrobial activity**

□ **Clinical translation**

Fig. 5.4 Antimicrobial activity of triple antibiotic-eluting nanofibers against a 7-day dual-species (*Actinomyces naeslundii* and *Enterococcus faecalis*) biofilm formed on dentine specimens. (**a**) Lower-magnification SEM image showing a homogeneous distribution of the two bacterial cells. (**b**) Higher-magnification SEM image revealing the rod-shaped *A. naeslundii* (arrows) and cocci-shaped *E. faecalis* (circle) bacterial cells over the dentine (De) surface. Confocal laser scanning micrographs of (**c**) 7-day dual-species biofilm growth on dentine (live bacteria = green) and (**d**) confocal image showing the elimination of most of the bacteria (dead bacteria = red) by the formulated triple antibiotic-eluting nanofibers. Scale bars = 30 µm. Clinical translation: placement of 3D tubular triple antibiotic-eluting construct into the root canal of a periapical lesion dog model, to act as a localised intracanal drug delivery system. Image obtained from reference (Bottino et al. 2017), with permission

effective antibiofilm properties against *Ef* is the use of photo-triggered drug delivery system made of nano-graphene oxide and indocyanine green (i.e. a cyanine dye generally used in medical diagnoses with known antimicrobial properties upon photoactivation), as shown in the study by Akbari et al. (Akbari et al. 2017). Besides being effective against *Ef* biofilm, indocyanine green-loaded nano-graphene oxide was prepared using much lower concentrations of active indocyanine green, compared to how this molecule is conventionally used, thus presenting less cytotoxic behaviour and less potential for causing tooth staining.

A recent strategy considered effective against oral biofilms relates to the use of silver nanoparticles in the form of core-shell compounds applied as an irrigant solution during the disinfection step (Ertem et al. 2017). Silver is already known for its broad-spectrum antibacterial activities, although silver nanoparticles may possess a tendency toward particle aggregation under ambient conditions, leading to a significant reduction in their antimicrobial effects. To overcome this limitation, the authors of that study proposed the following method to increase nanoparticles' stabilisation: using a porous silica shell to encapsulate the silver nanoparticles. As a result, for the first time, this proof-of-concept study demonstrated the long-term antimicrobial potential of the nanoparticle-based approach for endodontic infection treatment.

Core-shell silver nanoparticles were also effective in preventing biofilm regrowth when combined with suitable cleaning compounds and less cytotoxic than classical antimicrobial agents.

The foregoing strategies have proven to be effective in the control of intracanal infection, and perhaps they may be the focus of regenerative studies for the proper disinfection of immature permanent teeth with pulp necrosis. Taken together, future insights in this field need to be designed in an attempt to maximise the antimicrobial effects while minimising damage to stem cell survival and differentiation ability. Next, selected studies involving the use of dental stem cells and advanced scaffolds for dental pulp regeneration are discussed.

5.3 Regenerative Strategies for Dental Pulp Regeneration

Besides a more cell-friendly disinfection strategy, a number of developments in tissue engineering, primarily related to the synthesis of scaffolds, have provided the foundational knowledge for reliable and predictable regeneration of the pulp-dentine complex. According to the American Society for Testing Materials (ASTM—F2150), a scaffold is defined as "the support, delivery vehicle, or matrix for facilitating the migration, binding, or transport of cells or bioactive molecules used to replace, repair, or regenerate tissues". It should precisely replicate the features of the native extracellular matrix (ECM) at the nanoscale to regulate cell function and encourage and regulate specific events at the cellular and tissue levels (Bunyaratavej and Wang 2001; Owens and Yukna 2001). Moreover, scaffolds should be synthesised from biocompatible and biodegradable material(s) to avoid immune responses. A myriad of polymers, both synthetic, e.g. poly[lactic] acid (PLA), and natural (e.g. collagen), have been used in gas foaming, as well as salt leaching techniques, to obtain macroporous scaffolds. Meanwhile, nanofibrous scaffolds have been processed via electrospinning, self-assembly and phase separation (Albuquerque et al. 2014a).

In electrospinning, polymer nanofibers are obtained by the creation and elongation of an electrified jet (Albuquerque et al. 2014a). Various polymer solutions can be used and modified through mixing with other chemical reagents, polymers, nanoparticles, growth factors (GFs) and cells to generate unique nanofibers (Albuquerque et al. 2014a). Meanwhile, molecular self-assembly has been used to fabricate nanofibrous scaffolds through spontaneous molecular arrangement via non-covalent interactions (Albuquerque et al. 2014a). This technique allows recapitulation of collagen's supramolecule formation and enhances cell adhesion (Albuquerque et al. 2014a). Moreover, these unique nanofibers present major clinical advantages as they are assembled in solution and result in gels that are biocompatible and can be used for stem cell transplantation (Albuquerque et al. 2014a). However, this technique has limitations in terms of controlling pore size/shape within the scaffold and in producing sufficient mechanical properties (Albuquerque et al. 2014a). Accordingly, an alternative method, commonly referred to as thermally induced phase separation, has been incorporated in the fabrication of macro-/

micropore networks within 3D nanofibrous scaffolds (Albuquerque et al. 2014a). Taken together, recent advances in the field of biomaterials have allowed researchers to obtain scaffolds that can be easily injected in the desired site to aid in stem cell transplantation or to serve as delivery vehicles for bioactive factors. Some of the latest developments include the testing of innovative scaffolds/stem cell constructs in conjunction with therapeutic agents, and these are presented next as evidence of the translational potential of tissue engineering in regenerative endodontics. Of note, the next section has been divided into cell-free and cell transplantation approaches. In brief, the former approach comprises a cell-free strategy in which no exogenous cells are used/transplanted into the root canal system to propagate cell proliferation, whereas the latter approach induces regenerative outcomes by transplanting stem cells into the desired site.

5.3.1   Cell-Free Approaches

Cell-homing approaches to engineer dental pulp are based on the recruitment of resident stem cells by endogenous, dentine-derived growth factors, which induce cell migration into a custom-made scaffold, as well as proliferation and differentiation of the cells (Galler and Widbiller 2017). The utilisation of exogenous bioactive molecules that can be adsorbed, tethered or encapsulated into scaffolds to attract stem/progenitor cells adjacent to the root apices of endodontically treated teeth has demonstrated great clinical prospects. A recent report (Kim et al. 2010) highlighted the regeneration of dental-pulp-like tissue based solely on the intracanal delivery of fibroblast growth factor (FGF2) and/or vascular endothelial growth factor (VEGF) without stem cell transplantation. A recellularised and revascularised connective tissue integrated with the native dentinal wall in root canals was observed following in vivo implantation of endodontically treated human teeth in mouse dorsum for 3 weeks. In addition, combined delivery of a cocktail of GFs (FGF2, VEGF and platelet-derived growth factor [PDGF]) with a basal set of nerve growth factor (NGF) and bone morphogenetic protein 7 (BMP-7) led to the formation of tissues with patent vessels and new dentine regeneration (Kim et al. 2010). Several recent studies have begun to demonstrate that the release of specific biomolecules (e.g. TGF-β1, FGF-2, BMP-2, PDGF and VEGF) by certain irrigants and medicaments can favour the activity and proliferation of host stem cells, thereby incorporating the concept of a cell-homing mechanism in which the medium becomes a more welcoming environment for cell sustainability.

The identification of biomolecules, including but not limited to GFs and matrix molecules sequestered within dentine and dental pulp, affords a unique opportunity to make these signalling cues available in the regenerative process after a biocompatible disinfection approach. It has been proposed that the liberation of these biomolecules by certain irrigants and medicaments can potentially circumvent the use of non-human exogenous biomolecules (Widbiller et al. 2018). For a conditioning agent, it is extremely desirable to present a demineralising effect on dentine inorganic content, which would favour the release of any GFs or matrix proteins that are naturally archived within the dentine substrate. For instance, EDTA (ethylenediaminetetraacetic acid) is mostly used as an irrigant in endodontic therapy, and according to a recent study by Galler et al. (Galler et al. 2016), EDTA was capable of inducing substantial release of GFs when kept in direct contact with dentine for 10 min; conversely, irrigation using sodium hypochlorite was not able to induce the release of any bioactive molecule from dentine. Notably, conditioning of dentine surfaces with EDTA has shown to result in chemotactic effects on dental pulp cells, promoting cell adhesion and differentiation into pulp-like cells (Galler et al. 2016). A representative illustration of clinically viable cell-homing approach is depicted in Fig. 5.5.

5.3.2 Cell Transplantation Strategies

Cell-based/transplantation approaches use exogenous scaffolds and/or stem cells as the starting point to produce regenerated tissue after transplantation into the desired site (Albuquerque et al. 2014a). The basis for the cell transplantation approach is not new in dentistry; it was first presented by Mooney et al. in 1996 (Mooney et al. 1996). Subsequently, DPSCs have been transplanted and combined into inorganic compounds to form dentine-like structures in mice (Gronthos et al. 2000) or to increase dentine-pulp regeneration within the root canals of mini dogs when combined with platelet-rich plasma (Zhu et al. 2013). Other stem cell lineages (e.g. stem cells obtained from human exfoliated deciduous teeth [SHEDs] or SCAPs) were also effective in the regeneration of dentine-pulp tissues (Cordeiro et al. 2008; Huang et al. 2013, 2010). Nonetheless, the latest developments in this field include testing innovative scaffolds/stem cell constructs in conjunction with therapeutic agents, and these are presented next as evidence of the translational potential of tissue engineering in regenerative endodontics.

Fig. 5.5 Schematic illustrating a clinically viable protocol of a cell-homing approach to engineer dental pulp in immature permanent teeth with pulp necrosis (**a**), and the sequence of events/stages associated to the cell-homing approach that may occur into the root canal system under regeneration (**b**). In (**a**), disinfection of the root canal system is paramount to allow bacteria elimination, followed by dentine conditioning using EDTA solution for up to 10 min, which contributes for endogenous growth factor (GF) release; next, rinsing with saline solution is performed under ultrasonic activation, allowing the collection of GFs. The GF-containing solution will be then mixed with the liquid components of a scaffold material, forming a GF-laden scaffold/hydrogel, which will be injected into the root canal system, with subsequent polymerisation (e.g. usually photopolymerisation due to the presence of photoinitiators composing the scaffold material). Restoration with bioactive materials is advisable in order to maintain the pulpal space sealed. Lastly, followups including clinical and radiographic examination must be performed until complete regeneration of the dentine-pulp complex. In (**b**), the presence of GFs into the custom-made GF-laden scaffold induces chemotaxis (i.e. stem cell migration from the root apex), being the first stage in the cell-homing approach. After chemotaxis, the cells begin to proliferate within the GF-laden scaffold, increasing in number (second stage). In the sequence, cells attach to the inner root-dentine surface (third stage), allowing cell differentiation into pulp-like cells (fourth stage)

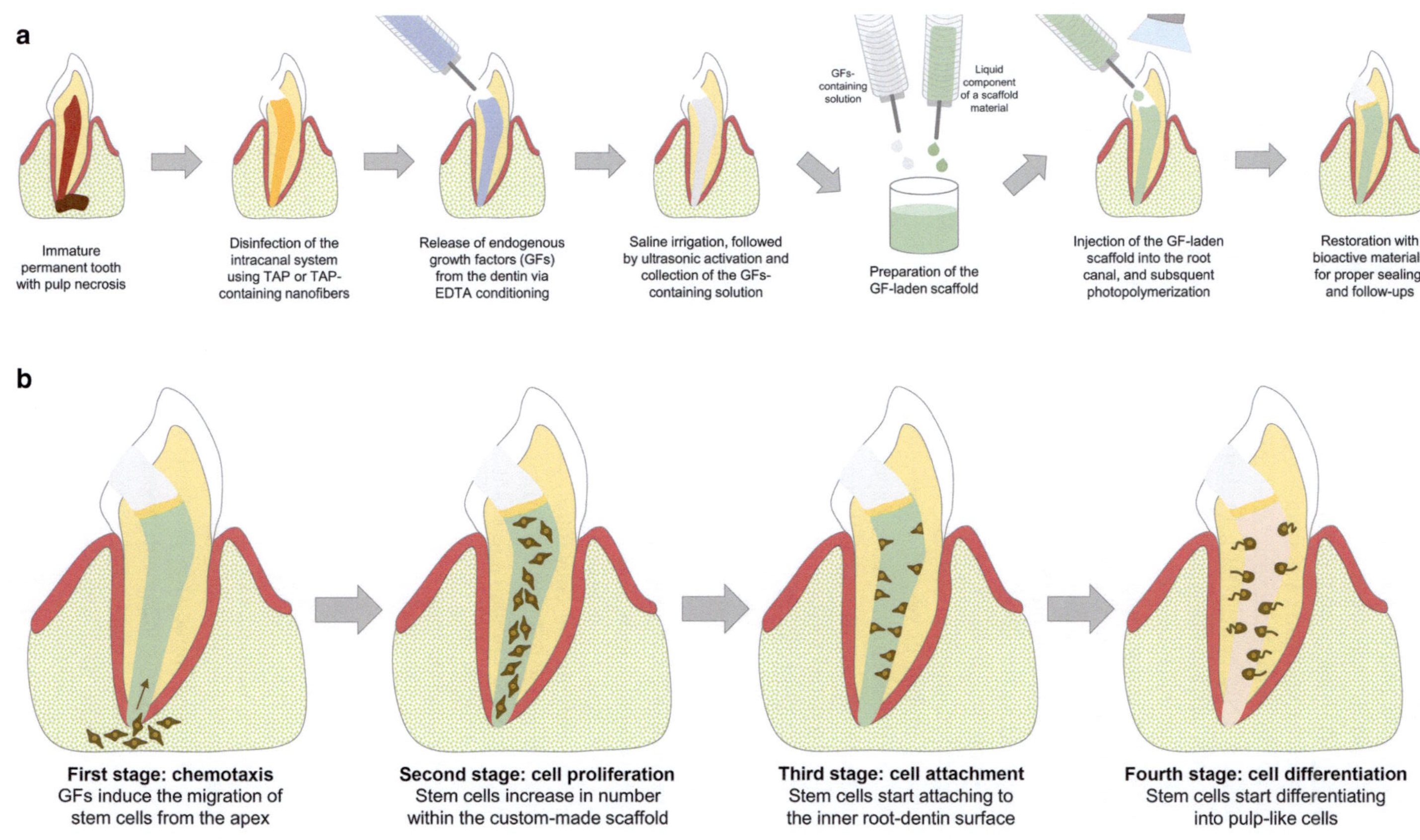
a
Immature permanent tooth with pulp necrosis
Disinfection of the intracanal system using TAP or TAP-containing nanofibers
Release of endogenous growth factors (GFs) from the dentin via EDTA conditioning
Saline irrigation, followed by ultrasonic activation and collection of the GFs-containing solution
GFs-containing solution
Liquid component of a scaffold material
Preparation of the GF-laden scaffold
Injection of the GF-laden scaffold into the root canal, and subsquent photopolymerization
Restoration with bioactive materials for proper sealing, and follow-ups
b
First stage: chemotaxis
GFs induce the migration of stem cells from the apex
Second stage: cell proliferation
Stem cells increase in number within the custom-made scaffold
Third stage: cell attachment
Stem cells start attaching to the inner root-dentin surface
Fourth stage: cell differentiation
Stem cells start differentiating into pulp-like cells

Nanostructured, self-assembling microspheres have also been used to deliver DPSCs into the pulpal space, as demonstrated elsewhere (Kuang et al. 2015, 2016). Indeed, a novel, star-shaped block copolymer constituted of poly(L-lactic acid)-block-poly-(L-lysine) and capable of self-assembling into nanofibrous spongy microspheres (NF-SMS) was synthesised, supporting DPSC proliferation and DSPP expression in vitro. Nanostructured microspheres have also been investigated for GF delivery (Niu et al. 2016). In that study, a microsphere platform was used to concurrently release fluocinolone acetonide (FA) to suppress inflammation, as well as BMP-2 to enhance odontogenic differentiation of DPSCs. A constant linear release of FA and a rapid BMP-2 release were observed in in vitro systems that reduced inflammation on DPSCs and enhanced differentiation.

Gelatin methacryloyl-based (GelMA) hydrogel was recently investigated for dental pulp regeneration (Khayat et al. 2017). GelMA is composed of denatured collagen and retains RGD (i.e. arginine-glycine-aspartic acid) adhesive domains and presents sensitivity to MMPs (i.e. metalloproteinases), thus enhancing cell binding and matrix degradation. In that study (Khayat et al. 2017), human DPSCs and human umbilical vein endothelial cells (HUVECs) were encapsulated in 5% GelMA and used to fabricate experimental constructs that were injected into human tooth root segments; acellular GelMA constructs and empty root segments were also prepared to serve as control groups. All constructs/root segments were cultured in osteogenic media for 13 days, followed by subcutaneous implantation in mouse dorsum for 4 or 8 weeks. The authors observed that the cellular GelMA construct allowed formation of highly cellularised and vascularised hDPSC/HUVEC-derived pulp-like tissue in the root segments and facilitated cell attachment to the tooth root inner dentine surface, formation of cellular extensions into the dentine tubules as well as elaboration of reparative dentine matrix. Overall, the GelMA hydrogel was also considered suitable for cell encapsulation and is easily tunable by varying the concentrations of GelMA and photoinitiators and, more recently, by using light-visible irradiation (Monteiro et al. 2018), which would pertain to a more clinically relevant setting (Fig. 5.6), since dental curing lights operating in the visible range are more frequent in the dental practice and may produce less deleterious effects on DNA and cellular function (Kappes et al. 2006). Figure 5.6 illustrates the potential clinical translation of the proposed strategy.

A particularly interesting study by Athirasala et al. (Athirasala et al. 2017) tested the effects of a tunable cell-laden GelMA hydrogel on the fabrication of an engineered pre-vascularised dental pulp-like tissue construct using a root canal model. In that study (Athirasala et al. 2017), the authors used root fragments of human premolars to obtain two root halves, which were properly sterilised using UV light and standardised immersion protocol. The two halves were then reattached and secured by wrapping them with laboratory film (Parafilm M); and EDTA conditioning was performed in order to expose the bioactive molecules sequestered within the dentine. The next step was to fabricate the microchannels of the engineered pulp-dentine complex; to that end, sacrificial agarose was used to synthesise 500 μm-thick fibres via a 3D printing-inspired method recently proposed (Bertassoni

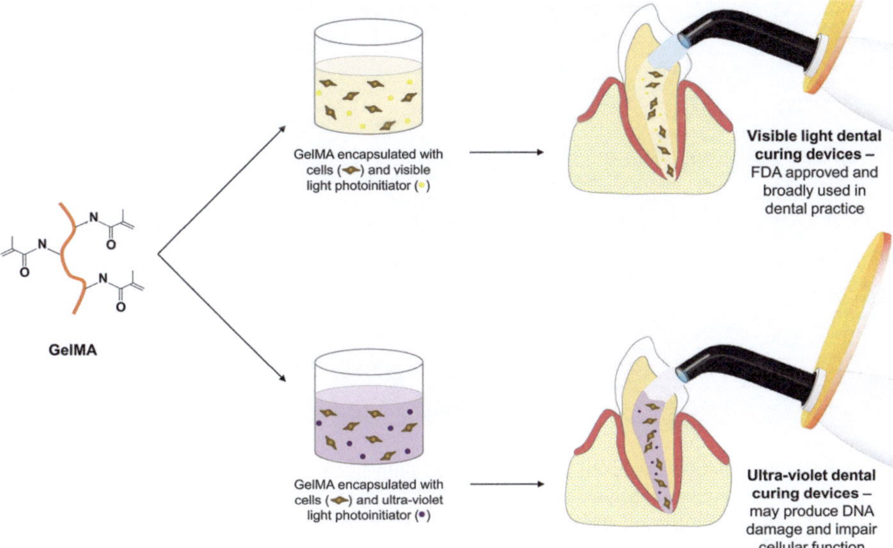

Fig. 5.6 Schematic showing a novel strategy to engineer pre-vascularised, cell-laden hydrogel pulp-like tissue constructs in full-length root canals in vitro by sequential GelMA polymerisation using visible light. First, GelMA macromer is synthesised by mixing gelatin with methacrylic anhydride, followed by lithium phenyl-2,4,6-trimethylbenzoylphosphinate (LAP) photoinitiator incorporation and consequent cell encapsulation, which is performed by suspending cells in the GelMA hydrogel. The resulting cell-laden hydrogel construct is then placed into the intracanal space, followed by photopolymerisation using a dental curing light unit. Image adapted with permission from reference (Monteiro et al. 2018)

et al. 2014a), followed by manually positioning pre-solidified sacrificial fibres inside the tooth, which was fulfilled with GelMA hydrogel. After photopolymerisation of the GelMA hydrogel, the final step of this root canal model consisted of complete aspiration/removal of the agarose fibres using a light vacuum and glass pipette (Bertassoni et al. 2014b). With fabrication of the tunable cell-laden GelMA hydrogel, diverse cells were seeded into the fabricated microchannels, and the tissue construct was cultured in standardised culture medium. In this study by Athirasala et al. (Athirasala et al. 2017), the authors demonstrated a novel and effective strategy to engineer pre-vascularised pulp-like tissue constructs using tunable cell-laden GelMA hydrogels (Fig. 5.7), showing optimal spreading and proliferation of cells near the dentine walls and important formation of endothelial monolayers with active angiogenic sprouts in fabricated microchannels after 7 days in culture, as shown in Fig. 5.8.

Overall, both pulp regeneration strategies discussed show promising applications in the field. Nevertheless, it is important to consider that the cell-homing approach involves the use of resident stem cells (i.e. derived from the patient) and non-complex mechanisms of pulp regeneration, thus representing a cost-effective method of inducing tissue regeneration, whereas the cell transplantation approach may involve

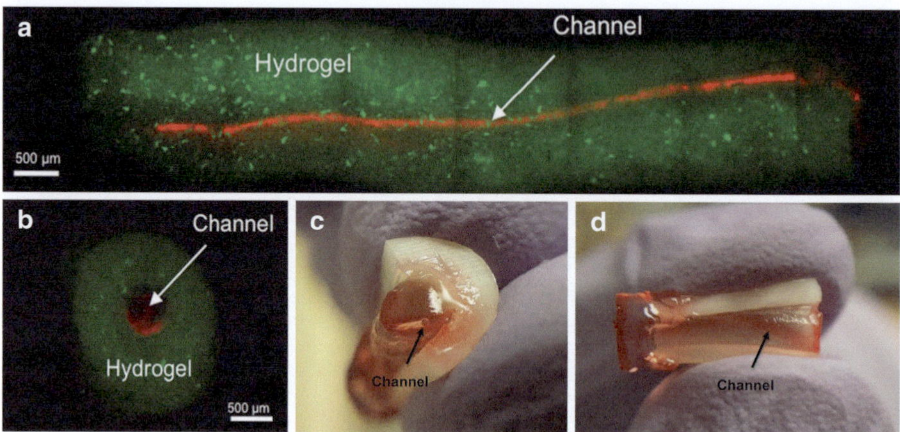

Fig. 5.7 Representative images of pre-vascularised pulp-like tissue construct, showing longitudinal (**a**) and cross-sectional (**b**) views of the GelMA hydrogels loaded with green fluorescent microparticles and the fabricated microchannel loaded with red fluorescent microparticle solution. Images of GelMA hydrogels from occlusal (**c**) and longitudinal (**d**) perspectives. Images obtained from reference (Athirasala et al. 2017), with permission

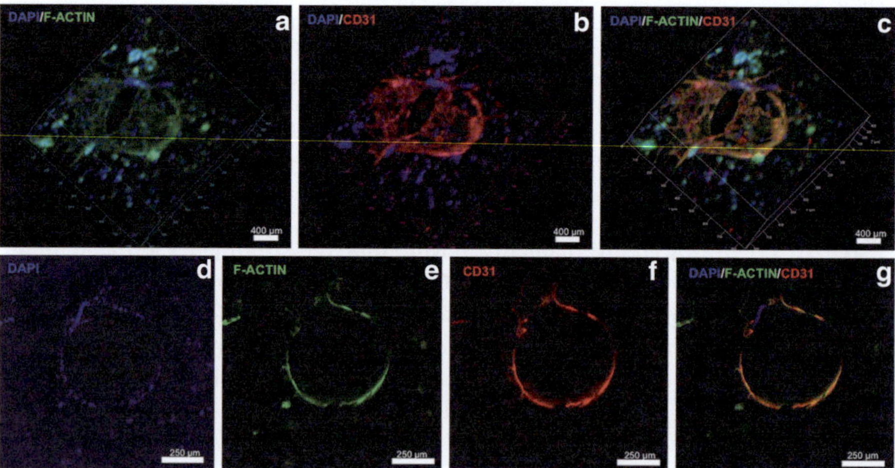

Fig. 5.8 Confocal images demonstrating the presence of endothelialised microchannels in the GelMA hydrogel, cultured in a full-length dental pulp-like tissue construct. Images (**a–c**) represent the 3D rendering, and images (**d–g**) indicate the cross-sectional slices of confocal images, showing endothelial colony-forming cell monolayer formation and angiogenic sprouts in the engineered constructs on day 7 (cells were stained with DAPI [blue], actin [green] and CD31 [red]). Images obtained from reference (Athirasala et al. 2017), with permission

a combination of exogenous stem cells and scaffolds/hydrogels/microspheres, which are usually expensive and complex/time-consuming to fabricate. This may limit clinical application of the cell transplantation approach compared with the cell-homing approach.

5.4   Conclusions and Future Outlook

Over the past decade, in spite of significant advancement and amendments of the EB technique, accumulating evidence regarding the key aspects deemed to negatively affect clinical outcome (e.g. the cytotoxic behaviour of antibiotic pastes and sodium hypochlorite irrigation), only one report has shown true pulp-like tissue formation. As a result, numerous research groups have been working intensively on tissue engineering-based strategies for regenerative endodontics. Noteworthy, preclinical (animal model) demonstration (Iohara et al. 2011; Ishizaka et al. 2012; Nakashima and Iohara 2011) of pulp regeneration by DPSCs has suggested that clinically effective human pulp regeneration (Nakashima et al. 2017) is now closer to application than it has ever been.

Concerning the major outcomes achieved over the past few years, we can list the following: (1) DPSCs revealed higher angiogenic and neurogenic potential compared with bone marrow-derived or adipose-derived mesenchymal stem cells; (2) complete pulp regeneration has been shown upon autologous transplantation of DPSC cells into the pulpectomised root canals of dogs; and (3) complete pulp regeneration with coronal dentine formation in the pulpectomised root canal of dogs was observed, showing reduced number of inflammatory cells, decreased cell death and major increase in neurite outgrowth. Other preclinical results also exist, and they generally confirm the efficacy and safety of stem cell transplantation mechanisms, aiding the initiation of a clinical trial with the consent of the Japanese Ministry of Health, Labour and Welfare (Nakashima et al. 2017). Besides the positive outcomes observed in several reports, and based on current knowledge, a key aspect for clinical success refers to the development of a biocompatible disinfection approach. Our group has focused on the design and synthesis of 3D patient-specific cytocompatible antibiotic-eluting nanofibers for intracanal drug delivery. In vivo preclinical (animal) studies are currently being conducted to validate these results. Next, the development of a regenerative strategy using advanced scaffolds, loaded or not with stem cells and/or growth factors to stimulate pulp and dentine regeneration after attaining a bacteria-free niche, is warranted to establish novel therapeutics to treat teeth with necrotic pulp.

Acknowledgements M.C.B. acknowledges funding from the NIH/NIDCR (Grants K08DE023552 and R01DE026578). The content is solely the responsibility of the authors and does not necessarily represent the official views of the National Institutes of Health.

References

Akbari T, Pourhajibagher M, Hosseini F, Chiniforush N, Gholibegloo E, Khoobi M, Shahabi S, Bahador A (2017) The effect of indocyanine green loaded on a novel nano-graphene oxide for high performance of photodynamic therapy against Enterococcus faecalis. Photodiagnosis Photodyn Ther 20:148–153

Albuquerque MT, Valera MC, Nakashima M, Nor JE, Bottino MC (2014a) Tissue-engineering-based strategies for regenerative endodontics. J Dent Res 93:1222–1231

Albuquerque MT, Junqueira JC, Coelho MB, de Carvalho CA, Valera MC (2014b) Novel in vitro methodology for induction of Enterococcus faecalis biofilm on apical resorption areas. Indian J Dent Res 25:535–538

Albuquerque MT, Ryan SJ, Munchow EA, Kamocka MM, Gregory RL, Valera MC, Bottino MC (2015a) Antimicrobial effects of novel triple antibiotic paste-mimic scaffolds on Actinomyces naeslundii biofilm. J Endod 41:1337–1343

Albuquerque MT, Valera MC, Moreira CS, Bresciani E, de Melo RM, Bottino MC (2015b) Effects of ciprofloxacin-containing scaffolds on enterococcus faecalis biofilms. J Endod 41:710–714

Albuquerque MT, Evans JD, Gregory RL, Valera MC, Bottino MC (2016) Antibacterial TAP-mimic electrospun polymer scaffold: effects on P. gingivalis-infected dentin biofilm. Clin Oral Investig 20:387–393

Althumairy RI, Teixeira FB, Diogenes A (2014) Effect of dentin conditioning with intracanal medicaments on survival of stem cells of apical papilla. J Endod 40:521–525

American Association of Endodontics (2016). Accessed on 2 May 2016. http://www.aae.org

Andreasen FM, Kahler B (2015) Diagnosis of acute dental trauma: the importance of standardized documentation: a review. Dent Traumatol 31:340–349

Athirasala A, Lins F, Tahayeri A, Hinds M, Smith AJ, Sedgley C, Ferracane J, Bertassoni LE (2017) A novel strategy to engineer pre-vascularized full-length dental pulp-like tissue constructs. Sci Rep 7:3323

Banchs F, Trope M (2004) Revascularization of immature permanent teeth with apical periodontitis: new treatment protocol? J Endod 30:196–200

Becerra P, Ricucci D, Loghin S, Gibbs JL, Lin LM (2014) Histologic study of a human immature permanent premolar with chronic apical abscess after revascularization/revitalization. J Endod 40:133–139

Bertassoni LE, Cardoso JC, Manoharan V, Cristino AL, Bhise NS, Araujo WA, Zorlutuna P, Vrana NE, Ghaemmaghami AM, Dokmeci MR, Khademhosseini A (2014a) Direct-write bioprinting of cell-laden methacrylated gelatin hydrogels. Biofabrication 6:024105

Bertassoni LE, Cecconi M, Manoharan V, Nikkhah M, Hjortnaes J, Cristino AL, Barabaschi G, Demarchi D, Dokmeci MR, Yang Y, Khademhosseini A (2014b) Hydrogel bioprinted microchannel networks for vascularization of tissue engineering constructs. Lab Chip 14:2202–2211

Bose R, Nummikoski P, Hargreaves K (2009) A retrospective evaluation of radiographic outcomes in immature teeth with necrotic root canal systems treated with regenerative endodontic procedures. J Endod 35:1343–1349

Bottino MC, Thomas V, Schmidt G, Vohra YK, Chu TM, Kowolik MJ, Janowski GM (2012) Recent advances in the development of GTR/GBR membranes for periodontal regeneration--a materials perspective. Dent Mater 28:703–721

Bottino MC, Kamocki K, Yassen GH, Platt JA, Vail MM, Ehrlich Y, Spolnik KJ, Gregory RL (2013) Bioactive nanofibrous scaffolds for regenerative endodontics. J Dent Res 92:963–969

Bottino MC, Yassen GH, Platt JA, Labban N, Windsor LJ, Spolnik KJ, Bressiani AH (2015) A novel three-dimensional scaffold for regenerative endodontics: materials and biological characterizations. J Tissue Eng Regen Med 9:E116–E123

Bottino MC, Pankajakshan D, Nör JE (2017) Advanced scaffolds for dental pulp and periodontal regeneration. Dent Clin N Am 61:689–711

Bunyaratavej P, Wang HL (2001) Collagen membranes: a review. J Periodontol 72:215–229

Cehreli ZC, Isbitiren B, Sara S, Erbas G (2011) Regenerative endodontic treatment (revascularization) of immature necrotic molars medicated with calcium hydroxide: a case series. J Endod 37:1327–1330

Cordeiro MM, Dong Z, Kaneko T, Zhang Z, Miyazawa M, Shi S, Smith AJ, Nor JE (2008) Dental pulp tissue engineering with stem cells from exfoliated deciduous teeth. J Endod 34:962–969

Cvek M (1972) Treatment of non-vital permanent incisors with calcium hydroxide. I. Follow-up of periapical repair and apical closure of immature roots. Odontol Revy 23:27–44

Cvek M (1973) Treatment of non-vital permanent incisors with calcium hydroxide. II. Effect on external root resorption in luxated teeth compared with effect of root filling with guttapucha. A follow-up. Odontol Revy 24:343–354

Cvek M (1992) Prognosis of luxated non-vital maxillary incisors treated with calcium hydroxide and filled with gutta-percha. A retrospective clinical study. Endod Dent Traumatol 8:45–55

Damle SG, Bhattal H, Loomba A (2012) Apexification of anterior teeth: a comparative evaluation of mineral trioxide aggregate and calcium hydroxide paste. J Clin Pediatr Dent 36:263–268

Diogenes A, Hargreaves KM (2017) Microbial modulation of stem cells and future directions in regenerative endodontics. J Endod 43:S95–S101

Diogenes A, Henry MA, Teixeira FB, Hargreaves KM (2013) An update on clinical regenerative endodontics. Endod Topics 28:2–23

Diogenes AR, Ruparel NB, Teixeira FB, Hargreaves KM (2014) Translational science in disinfection for regenerative endodontics. J Endod 40:S52–S57

Diogenes A, Ruparel NB, Shiloah Y, Hargreaves KM (2016) Regenerative endodontics: a way forward. J Am Dent Assoc 147:372–380

Dye B, Thornton-Evans G, Li X, Iafolla T (2015) Dental caries and tooth loss in adults in the United States, 2011-2012. NCHS Data Brief 197:1

Ertem E, Gutt B, Zuber F, Allegri S, Le Ouay B, Mefti S, Formentin K, Stellacci F, Ren Q (2017) Core-shell silver nanoparticles in endodontic disinfection solutions enable long-term antimicrobial effect on oral biofilms. ACS Appl Mater Interfaces 9:34762–34772

Galler KM (2016) Clinical procedures for revitalization: current knowledge and considerations. Int Endod J 49:926–936

Galler KM, Widbiller M (2017) Perspectives for cell-homing approaches to engineer dental pulp. J Endod 43:S40–S45

Galler KM, Buchalla W, Hiller KA, Federlin M, Eidt A, Schiefersteiner M, Schmalz G (2015) Influence of root canal disinfectants on growth factor release from dentin. J Endod 41:363–368

Galler KM, Widbiller M, Buchalla W, Eidt A, Hiller KA, Hoffer PC, Schmalz G (2016) EDTA conditioning of dentine promotes adhesion, migration and differentiation of dental pulp stem cells. Int Endod J 49:581–590

Glendor U (2009) Aetiology and risk factors related to traumatic dental injuries--a review of the literature. Dent Traumatol 25:19–31

Gomes BP, Pinheiro ET, Gade-Neto CR, Sousa EL, Ferraz CC, Zaia AA, Teixeira FB, Souza-Filho FJ (2004) Microbiological examination of infected dental root canals. Oral Microbiol Immunol 19:71–76

Gomes-Filho JE, Duarte PC, Ervolino E, Mogami Bomfim SR, Xavier Abimussi CJ, Mota da Silva Santos L, Lodi CS, Penha De Oliveira SH, Dezan E Jr, Cintra LT (2013) Histologic characterization of engineered tissues in the canal space of closed-apex teeth with apical periodontitis. J Endod 39:1549–1556

Gronthos S, Mankani M, Brahim J, Robey PG, Shi S (2000) Postnatal human dental pulp stem cells (DPSCs) in vitro and in vivo. Proc Natl Acad Sci U S A 97:13625–13630

Gronthos S, Brahim J, Li W, Fisher LW, Cherman N, Boyde A, DenBesten P, Robey PG, Shi S (2002) Stem cell properties of human dental pulp stem cells. J Dent Res 81:531–535

Hoshino E, Kurihara-Ando N, Sato I, Uematsu H, Sato M, Kota K, Iwaku M (1996) In-vitro antibacterial susceptibility of bacteria taken from infected root dentine to a mixture of ciprofloxacin, metronidazole and minocycline. Int Endod J 29:125–130

Huang GT (2011) Dental pulp and dentin tissue engineering and regeneration: advancement and challenge. Front Biosci 3:788–800

Huang GT, Yamaza T, Shea LD, Djouad F, Kuhn NZ, Tuan RS, Shi S (2010) Stem/progenitor cell-mediated de novo regeneration of dental pulp with newly deposited continuous layer of dentin in an in vivo model. Tissue Eng Part A 16:605–615

Huang GT, Al-Habib M, Gauthier P (2013) Challenges of stem cell-based pulp and dentin regeneration: a clinical perspective. Endod Topics 28:51–60

Iohara K, Imabayashi K, Ishizaka R, Watanabe A, Nabekura J, Ito M, Matsushita K, Nakamura H, Nakashima M (2011) Complete pulp regeneration after pulpectomy by transplantation of CD105+ stem cells with stromal cell-derived factor-1. Tissue Eng Part A 17:1911–1920

Ishizaka R, Iohara K, Murakami M, Fukuta O, Nakashima M (2012) Regeneration of dental pulp following pulpectomy by fractionated stem/progenitor cells from bone marrow and adipose tissue. Biomaterials 33:2109–2118

Iwaya SI, Ikawa M, Kubota M (2001) Revascularization of an immature permanent tooth with apical periodontitis and sinus tract. Dent Traumatol 17:185–187

Jeeruphan T, Jantarat J, Yanpiset K, Suwannapan L, Khewsawai P, Hargreaves KM (2012) Mahidol study 1: comparison of radiographic and survival outcomes of immature teeth treated with either regenerative endodontic or apexification methods: a retrospective study. J Endod 38:1330–1336

Kahler B, Rossi-Fedele G (2016) A review of tooth discoloration after regenerative endodontic therapy. J Endod 42:563–569

Kamocki K, Nor JE, Bottino MC (2015a) Effects of ciprofloxacin-containing antimicrobial scaffolds on dental pulp stem cell viability-In vitro studies. Arch Oral Biol 60:1131–1137

Kamocki K, Nor JE, Bottino MC (2015b) Dental pulp stem cell responses to novel antibiotic-containing scaffolds for regenerative endodontics. Int Endod J 48:1147–1156

Kappes UP, Luo D, Potter M, Schulmeister K, Runger TM (2006) Short- and long-wave UV light (UVB and UVA) induce similar mutations in human skin cells. J Invest Dermatol 126:667–675

Karczewski A, Feitosa SA, Hamer EI, Pankajakshan D, Gregory RL, Spolnik KJ, Bottino MC (2018) Clindamycin-modified triple antibiotic nanofibers: a stain-free antimicrobial intracanal drug delivery system. J Endod 44:155–162

Khayat A, Monteiro N, Smith EE, Pagni S, Zhang W, Khademhosseini A, Yelick PC (2017) GelMA-encapsulated hDPSCs and HUVECs for dental pulp regeneration. J Dent Res 96:192–199

Kim JY, Xin X, Moioli EK, Chung J, Lee CH, Chen M, Fu SY, Koch PD, Mao JJ (2010) Regeneration of dental-pulp-like tissue by chemotaxis-induced cell homing. Tissue Eng Part A 16:3023–3031

Kuang R, Zhang Z, Jin X, Hu J, Gupte MJ, Ni L, Ma PX (2015) Nanofibrous spongy microspheres enhance odontogenic differentiation of human dental pulp stem cells. Adv Healthc Mater 4:1993–2000

Kuang R, Zhang Z, Jin X, Hu J, Shi S, Ni L, Ma PX (2016) Nanofibrous spongy microspheres for the delivery of hypoxia-primed human dental pulp stem cells to regenerate vascularized dental pulp. Acta Biomater 33:225–234

Larsen T, Fiehn NE (2017) Dental biofilm infections - an update. Acta Pathol Microbiol Immunol Scand 125:376–384

Latham J, Fong H, Jewett A, Johnson JD, Paranjpe A (2016) Disinfection efficacy of current regenerative endodontic protocols in simulated necrotic immature permanent teeth. J Endod 42:1218–1225

Li CH, Liao PL, Yang YT, Huang SH, Lin CH, Cheng YW, Kang JJ (2014) Minocycline accelerates hypoxia-inducible factor-1 alpha degradation and inhibits hypoxia-induced neovasculogenesis through prolyl hydroxylase, von Hippel-Lindau-dependent pathway. Arch Toxicol 88:659–671

Lin J, Shen Y, Haapasalo M (2013) A comparative study of biofilm removal with hand, rotary nickel-titanium, and self-adjusting file instrumentation using a novel in vitro biofilm model. J Endod 39:658–663

Mandras N, Roana J, Allizond V, Pasqualini D, Crosasso P, Burlando M, Banche G, Denisova T, Berutti E, Cuffini AM (2013) Antibacterial efficacy and drug-induced tooth discolouration of antibiotic combinations for endodontic regenerative procedures. Int J Immunopathol Pharmacol 26:557–563

Martin G, Ricucci D, Gibbs JL, Lin LM (2013) Histological findings of revascularized/revitalized immature permanent molar with apical periodontitis using platelet-rich plasma. J Endod 39:138–144

Martin DE, De Almeida JF, Henry MA, Khaing ZZ, Schmidt CE, Teixeira FB, Diogenes A (2014) Concentration-dependent effect of sodium hypochlorite on stem cells of apical papilla survival and differentiation. J Endod 40:51–55

Monteiro N, Thrivikraman G, Athirasala A, Tahayeri A, Franca CM, Ferracane JL, Bertassoni LE (2018) Photopolymerization of cell-laden gelatin methacryloyl hydrogels using a dental curing light for regenerative dentistry. Dent Mater 34:389

Mooney DJ, Powell C, Piana J, Rutherford B (1996) Engineering dental pulp-like tissue in vitro. Biotechnol Prog 12:865–868

Nagata JY, Soares AJ, Souza-Filho FJ, Zaia AA, Ferraz CC, Almeida JF, Gomes BP (2014) Microbial evaluation of traumatized teeth treated with triple antibiotic paste or calcium hydroxide with 2% chlorhexidine gel in pulp revascularization. J Endod 40:778–783

Nakashima M, Iohara K (2011) Regeneration of dental pulp by stem cells. Adv Dent Res 23:313–319

Nakashima M, Iohara K, Murakami M, Nakamura H, Sato Y, Ariji Y, Matsushita K (2017) Pulp regeneration by transplantation of dental pulp stem cells in pulpitis: a pilot clinical study. Stem Cell Res Ther 8:61

Niu X, Liu Z, Hu J, Rambhia KJ, Fan Y, Ma PX (2016) Microspheres assembled from chitosan-graft-poly(lactic acid) micelle-like core-shell nanospheres for distinctly controlled release of hydrophobic and hydrophilic biomolecules. Macromol Biosci 16:1039–1047

Nosrat A, Li KL, Vir K, Hicks ML, Fouad AF (2013) Is pulp regeneration necessary for root maturation? J Endod 39:1291–1295

Owens KW, Yukna RA (2001) Collagen membrane resorption in dogs: a comparative study. Implant Dent 10:49–58

Palasuk J, Kamocki K, Hippenmeyer L, Platt JA, Spolnik KJ, Gregory RL, Bottino MC (2014) Bimix antimicrobial scaffolds for regenerative endodontics. J Endod 40:1879–1884

Petrino JA, Boda KK, Shambarger S, Bowles WR, McClanahan SB (2010) Challenges in regenerative endodontics: a case series. J Endod 36:536–541

Porter ML, Munchow EA, Albuquerque MT, Spolnik KJ, Hara AT, Bottino MC (2016) Effects of novel 3-dimensional antibiotic-containing electrospun scaffolds on dentin discoloration. J Endod 42:106–112

Radomska-Lesniewska DM, Skopinska-Rozwska E, Malejczyk J (2010) The effect of clindamycin and lincomycin on angiogenic activity of human blood mononuclear cells. C Eur J Immunol 35:217–222

Ruparel NB, Teixeira FB, Ferraz CC, Diogenes A (2012) Direct effect of intracanal medicaments on survival of stem cells of the apical papilla. J Endod 38:1372–1375

Saghiri MA, Asatourian A, Sorenson CM, Sheibani N (2015) Role of angiogenesis in endodontics: contributions of stem cells and proangiogenic and antiangiogenic factors to dental pulp regeneration. J Endod 41:797–803

Selwitz RH, Ismail AI, Pitts NB (2007) Dental caries. Lancet 369:51–59

da Silva LA, Nelson-Filho P, da Silva RA, Flores DS, Heilborn C, Johnson JD, Cohenca N (2010) Revascularization and periapical repair after endodontic treatment using apical negative pressure irrigation versus conventional irrigation plus triantibiotic intracanal dressing in dogs' teeth with apical periodontitis. Oral Surg Oral Med Oral Pathol Oral Radiol Endod 109:779–787

Sousa FF, Luzardo-Alvarez A, Perez-Estevez A, Seoane-Prado R, Blanco-Mendez J (2010) Development of a novel AMX-loaded PLGA/zein microsphere for root canal disinfection. Biomed Mater 5:055008

Verma P, Nosrat A, Kim JR, Price JB, Wang P, Bair E, Xu HH, Fouad AF (2017) Effect of residual bacteria on the outcome of pulp regeneration in vivo. J Dent Res 96:100–106

Vishwanat L, Duong R, Takimoto K, Phillips L, Espitia CO, Diogenes A, Ruparel SB, Kolodrubetz D, Ruparel NB (2017) Effect of bacterial biofilm on the osteogenic differentiation of stem cells of apical papilla. J Endod 43:916–922

Wang X, Thibodeau B, Trope M, Lin LM, Huang GT (2010) Histologic characterization of regenerated tissues in canal space after the revitalization/revascularization procedure of immature dog teeth with apical periodontitis. J Endod 36:56–63

Wang Z, Shen Y, Haapasalo M (2012) Effectiveness of endodontic disinfecting solutions against young and old Enterococcus faecalis biofilms in dentin canals. J Endod 38:1376–1379

Widbiller M, Eidt A, Lindner SR, Hiller KA, Schweikl H, Buchalla W, Galler KM (2018) Dentine matrix proteins: isolation and effects on human pulp cells. Int Endod J 51:e278

Windley W 3rd, Teixeira F, Levin L, Sigurdsson A, Trope M (2005) Disinfection of immature teeth with a triple antibiotic paste. J Endod 31:439–443

Zaleckiene V, Peciuliene V, Brukiene V, Drukteinis S (2014) Traumatic dental injuries: etiology, prevalence and possible outcomes. Stomatologija 16:7–14

Zhu W, Zhu X, Huang GT, Cheung GS, Dissanayaka WL, Zhang C (2013) Regeneration of dental pulp tissue in immature teeth with apical periodontitis using platelet-rich plasma and dental pulp cells. Int Endod J 46:962–970

Current Understanding and Future Applications in Dentine-Pulp Complex Inflammation and Repair

6

Paul Roy Cooper, Jean-Christophe Farges, and Brigitte Alliot-Licht

6.1 Introduction

Erupted teeth are covered by symbiotic microbial communities organised in biofilms, mainly composed of Gram-positive saprophytic bacteria. These biofilms adhere to the enamel surface and are normally harmless to the tooth; however, increased bacterial metabolic activity in response to a sugar-rich environment results in the release of acids that progressively demineralise the enamel (Hamilton 2000; Farges et al. 2009). A carious lesion thus develops which is characterised by the formation of a cavity within which "cariogenic" bacteria grow and release additional acids deepening the lesion. The dentine subsequently becomes affected and demineralised by this activity of microorganisms, such as *Streptococci*, *Lactobacilli* and *Actinomyces*, that predominate the local Gram-positive microflora (Love and Jenkinson 2002). Proliferating intra-dentinal bacteria release by-products which diffuse down the dentinal tubules and towards the peripheral pulp. Concomitantly

P. R. Cooper (✉)
Oral Biology, School of Dentistry, College of Medical and Dental Sciences,
University of Birmingham, Birmingham, UK
e-mail: p.r.cooper@bham.ac.uk

J.-C. Farges
Institut de Biologie et Chimie des Protéines, Laboratoire de Biologie Tissulaire et Ingénierie thérapeutique, UMR 5305 CNRS/Université Lyon 1, Lyon, France

Université Lyon 1, Faculté d'Odontologie, Université de Lyon, Lyon, France

Service de Consultations et de Traitements Dentaires, Hospices Civils de Lyon, Lyon, France

B. Alliot-Licht
Centre de Recherche en Transplantation et Immunologie UMR 1064, INSERM,
Université de Nantes, Nantes, France

Faculté d'Odontologie, Université de Nantes, Nantes, France

Service Odontologie Conservatrice et Pédiatrique, CHU Nantes, Nantes, France

© Springer Nature Switzerland AG 2019
H. F. Duncan, P. R. Cooper (eds.), *Clinical Approaches in Endodontic Regeneration*,
https://doi.org/10.1007/978-3-319-96848-3_6

the demineralisation of the dentine matrix, due to the acidic environment, releases the bioactive molecules archived within it (Cooper et al. 2011). The recognition of the bacterial components initially by the odontoblasts at the pulp periphery is the trigger for local protective events including the production, by pulp cells, of antibacterial, immune, inflammatory and dentinogenic molecules. This activity aims to both limit the bacterial infection and block its progression to the pulp by the formation of tertiary dentine at the pulp-dentine interface. If the bacterial invasion remains unchecked, however, irreversible pulpitis will occur which will ultimately lead to pulp necrosis and infection within the tooth root canal system. Invading microorganisms will then disseminate into the periapical regions and trigger periapical disease (Love and Jenkinson 2002; Heyeraas and Berggreen 1999). These series of events result in important dental and supporting tissue damage, and ultimately the tooth may be lost following periodontal tissue destruction. If the early-stage dentine infection is clinically removed by the practitioner, the pulp inflammation should subside (Hahn and Liewehr 2007a) and tissue healing with tertiary dentine formation can occur (Lesot et al. 1994). The newly formed dentine will protect the pulp from further infection as well as from any restorative filling material placed. From a clinical standpoint, it is reasonable to speculate that the induction of tertiary dentine, by distancing the pulp from the affected dentine, will help protect the pulp, promote healing and maintain pulp vitality, thereby enhancing tooth longevity. The identification of the molecular and cellular mediators, which dampen the immune/inflammatory response, while stimulating tertiary dentine formation, and which may promote a return to pulp tissue homeostasis and health following bacterial infection resolution, has therapeutic potential (Farges et al. 2009, 2013; Cooper et al. 2014; Gaudin et al. 2015). Subsequently studies are underway aimed at obtaining a better understanding of the events that initiate and control the pulp's antibacterial-, immune- and dentinogenic-mediated defences to enable the development of novel treatments.

6.2 Early Stages of the Dentine-Pulp Complex's Host Defence Response

Due to their location and cellular processes penetrating into the dentinal tubules, odontoblasts are the first cells within the tooth to be encountered by the molecular components released by the invading pathogens (Durand et al. 2006; Veerayutthwilai et al. 2007). Pathogen recognition occurs via the detection of bacterial structures termed pathogen-associated molecular patterns (PAMPs), and these are sensed by a limited number of so-called pattern recognition receptors (PRRs). A key class of PRRs is the Toll-like receptor (TLR) family, which is essential for triggering the effector phase of the innate immune response (Fig. 6.1) (Beutler 2009; Kawai and Akira 2010; Kumar et al. 2011). TLR-2 and TLR-4 detect the Gram-positive and Gram-negative cell membrane components lipoteichoic acid (LTA) and lipopolysaccharide (LPS), respectively. They have been shown to be present on odontoblasts from healthy pulp, indicating the tissue is equipped to initially recognise early

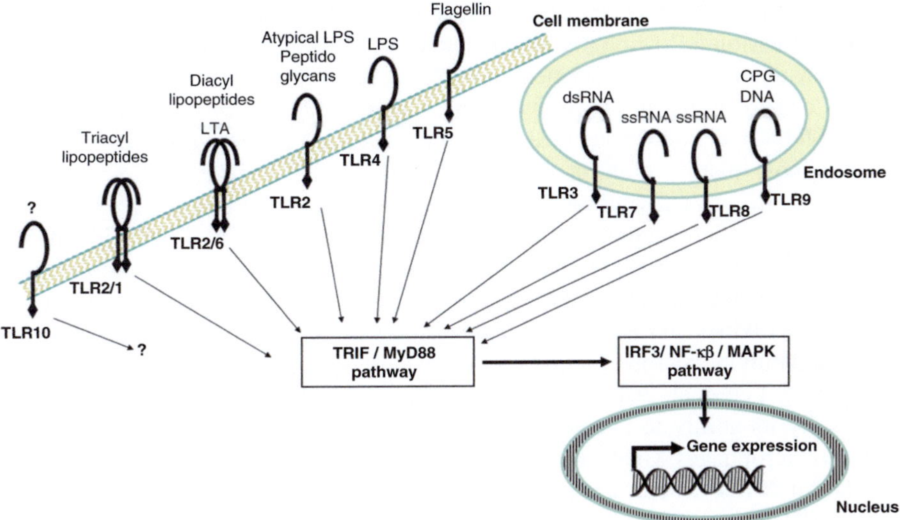

Fig. 6.1 Overview of Toll-like receptor (TLR) signalling pathways which sense bacterial components (examples indicated above each TLR). Pathogen recognition receptors (PRRs) are present on cells present in the dentine-pulp complex (as described in the main text body), and their binding of microbial components results in transcriptional activation of pro-inflammatory and dental repair-associated genes. TLRs comprise two components and form homo- or heterodimers which are located on the outer cell membrane or on endosomal membranes. The binding of the bacterial components initially results in activation of downstream intracellular signalling molecules including TRIF and MyD88. Activation of these molecules results in further IRF, NF-κB and MAPK signalling activation which culminates in nuclear translocation and transcription factor activation. The cytoplasmic PRRs of NOD (nucleotide-binding oligomerization domain)-1 (Gram positive) and NOD-2 (Gram negative) have also been reported as being present in dental cells, and they transduce signals via NF-κB, NALP3 (NACHT, LRR and pyrin domain-containing protein 3) and caspase-1 signalling. ? = the ligand and downstream signalling from TLR10 are not yet known. Abbreviations: IRF = IFN regulatory factor; MAPK = mitogen-activated protein kinase; MyD88 = myeloid differentiation primary response gene 88; NF-κB = nuclear factor-κB; TRIF = Toll/IL-1R (TIR) domain-containing adaptor protein inducing IFN-β

dentine infection (Veerayutthwilai et al. 2007; Jiang et al. 2006). TLR2 is reportedly upregulated in odontoblasts beneath caries lesions (Farges et al. 2009), indicating that these cells can adapt and potentially increase their sensitivity for pathogen recognition.

TLR activation results in upregulation of innate immune responses manifested by local release of antimicrobial agents and pro-inflammatory cytokines and chemokines which recruit and activate immune/inflammatory cells (Viola and Luster 2008; Turner et al. 2014). Notably, odontoblasts have been shown to express several antimicrobial agents, such as beta-defensins (BDs) and nitric oxide (NO). The BD family comprise of cationic, broad-spectrum antimicrobial peptides that elicit their killing mechanisms by forming channel-like micropores that disrupt membrane integrity and induce leakage of the microbial cell content (Pazgier et al. 2006; Sørensen et al. 2008; Semple and Dorin 2012; Mansour et al. 2014). In general

BD-1 is constitutively expressed, whereas BD-2, BD-3 and BD-4 are induced in tissue expression following microbial contact with the host. Several in vitro studies have now reported BD involvement in pulpal defence during caries. BD-2 has been shown to exert antibacterial activity against *Streptococcus mutans* and *Lactobacillus casei* (Shiba et al. 2003; Song et al. 2009; Lee and Baek 2012), while BD-3 is active against more mature biofilms containing *Actinomyces naeslundii*, *Lactobacillus salivarius*, *Streptococcus mutans* and *Enterococcus fæcalis* (Lee et al. 2013a). BD-2 can also feedback by autocrine and paracrine mechanisms to amplify the inflammatory response and can upregulate interleukin (IL)-6 and IL-8 in odontoblast-like cells in vitro (Dommisch et al. 2007). A positive feedback mechanism may exist between cytokines and BD-2 as its expression can be stimulated by the cytokines IL-1α and tumour necrosis factor (TNF)-α in cultured human dental pulp cells (Kim et al. 2010; Lee et al. 2011). The pro-inflammatory effects of BD-2 are also highlighted by its ability to chemoattract immature antigen-presenting dendritic cells (DCs), macrophages, CD4+ memory T cells and natural killer (NK) cells (Semple and Dorin 2012). Studies using a tooth organ culture model have shown that odontoblast BD-2 gene expression was not affected by TLR2 activation; however, BD-1 and BD-3 transcript levels were downregulated (Veerayutthwilai et al. 2007). Interestingly BD-2 gene expression was elevated following TLR4 activation. In vivo studies have also shown that odontoblasts in healthy tissue express BD-1 and BD-2 (Dommisch et al. 2005; Paris et al. 2009). Combined, these data indicate that BDs are differentially expressed in the pulp tissue and that there is a low level of constitutive expression of BDs by odontoblasts and other cells within the pulp protecting the tissue from infection. There is, however, a degree of controversy regarding expression levels of BDs in inflamed dental pulp. Initially BD-1 and BD-2 were reported to be decreased in irreversible pulpitis (Dommisch et al. 2007); however, more recent work has shown increases in BD-1 and BD-4 (but not BD-2 and BD-3) in pulp tissue at a similar stage of disease (Paris et al. 2009). Clearly further studies are required to better understand the role and regulation of BDs in dentine-pulp complex health and disease.

Reactive nitrogen species (RNS), such as NO, are potent antibacterial molecules. They are highly diffusible free radicals generated by the oxidative action of NO synthases, of which there are three isoforms, NOS1 (neuronal NOS), NOS2 (inducible NOS) and NOS3 (endothelial NOS), which produces NO from L-arginine. NOS1 and NOS3 are constitutively expressed in most healthy tissues; however, NOS2 can be induced following microbial challenge. NOS2 is mostly involved in host defence due to the relatively high micromolar range amounts of NO that it can generate over long time periods (hours to days) (Nathan 1992; Nussler and Billiar 1993; MacMicking et al. 1997; Coleman 2001; Guzik et al. 2003; Arthur and Ley 2013; Bogdan 2015). Notably, NOS2 was only detected at relatively low levels in healthy human pulp but was significantly upregulated in inflamed pulps (Law et al. 1999; Di Nardo Di Maio et al. 2004). Interestingly in an experimental rat incisor pulp model of inflammation, NOS2 activation also promoted an increase in neutrophil and macrophage influx (Kawanishi et al. 2004; Kawashima et al. 2005). This process may be mediated by the chemoattractant,

IL-8, as NO is known to stimulate its production in human pulp cells. Recent studies have also indicated that human odontoblasts constitutively release NO which might provide an important defence mechanism against *Streptococcus mutans*, and in inflamed tissue, its release is further mediated by NOS2 activation to combat the later stages of disease (Korkmaz et al. 2011; Min et al. 2008; Silva-Mendez et al. 1999; Farges et al. 2015).

Numerous in vitro studies have demonstrated the ability of odontoblasts to produce inflammatory cytokines and chemokines when exposed to PAMPs (Durand et al. 2006; Veerayutthwilai et al. 2007). Indeed odontoblast-like cells in vitro have been shown to be responsive to LTA via TLR2 detection resulting in upregulation of TLR2 itself as well as the nucleotide-binding oligomerization domain-containing protein 2 (NOD2), a cytosolic pattern recognition receptor (PRR). This exposure activated NF-κB and p38 mitogen-activated protein kinase (MAPK) signalling pathways (Fig. 6.1), inhibited dentinogenesis and promoted the production of several pro-inflammatory chemokines, including CCL2, CXCL1, CXCL2, CXCL8 (IL-8) and CXCL10 (Farges et al. 2009, 2011; Durand et al. 2006; Staquet et al. 2008; Keller et al. 2010, 2011). This chemokine "storm" will lead to chemoattraction and activation of a range of immune cells within the pulp. During the early stages of caries, immature DCs are initially attracted and accumulate at strategic sites beneath the lesion in readiness to capture foreign antigens. Subsequently there is also a progressive and sequential accumulation of T cells/lymphocytes, macrophages, neutrophils and B cells/lymphocytes in the pulp as the lesion and bacterial infection increase (Hahn and Liewehr 2007a; Farges et al. 2003; Jontell et al. 1998). Others have shown that the pleiotropic cytokine, IL-6, regulates many aspects of the local immune responses and is strongly upregulated by odontoblasts in vitro following TLR2 exposure (Farges et al. 2011; Hunter and Jones 2015; Nibali et al. 2012). IL-6 is critical to the differentiation of T helper (Th) 17 cells, while IL-6 inhibits regulatory T-cell (Treg) differentiation. Notably the main function of Tregs is to restrain excessive effector T-cell responses. IL-6 has also been shown to be important in promoting the secretion of acute-phase proteins such as LPS-binding protein (LBP) (Turner et al. 2014) as well as increasing vascular permeability to facilitate immune cell movement. It is therefore conceivable that odontoblast-derived IL-6 may modulate several functions in the infected pulp including oedema formation in response to bacterial infection.

IL-10 is a modulatory cytokine previously shown to be upregulated in bacterial infected pulps, and it has also been shown to be upregulated in odontoblast-like cells in vitro upon TLR2 engagement (Farges et al. 2011; Lee et al. 2012). IL-10 acts as an immunosuppressive cytokine, and for example, is able to decrease the production of the pro-inflammatory cytokines IL-6 and IL-8 (Li and Flavell 2008) and inhibit the Th1 and Th2 immune responses while promoting Treg differentiation (Saraiva and O'Garra 2010; Kaji et al. 2010). Subsequently it has been proposed that, as odontoblasts express this molecule, they therefore have the ability to molecularly limit local tissue inflammatory intensity (Farges et al. 2011).

Recent work studying the role of LBP has shown that this acute-phase protein attenuates pro-inflammatory cytokine production by preventing the binding to host cells of several bacterial cell wall components including LPS, LTA, lipopeptides and peptidoglycan (Lee et al. 2012). In vitro, LBP has been shown to be upregulated in TLR2-activated odontoblast-like cells (Carrouel et al. 2013) and is also elevated in bacteria-challenged inflamed pulps. Potentially this molecule might decrease the effects of bacterial components, thereby also enabling modulation of the local dental immune response.

In summary, several studies demonstrate that odontoblasts are able to detect microorganisms and then respond to defend the tooth using their antibacterial arsenal (e.g. BDs, NO) and by signalling (e.g. chemokines, cytokines) to alert immune cells to combat the infection. This response is analogous to that found in other bodily tissues which become infected.

6.3 Immune Cell Responses in the Pulp

Clinically the removal of the tooth's decayed and infected hard tissues aims to lead to decreased pulpal inflammation, tissue healing and homeostatic recovery. Similar to other peripheral tissues, the healthy dental pulp is known to contain sentinel immune cells, including macrophages, DCs and T cells which undertake immuno-surveillance (Farges et al. 2003; Jontell et al. 1998; Mangkornkarn et al. 1991; Izumi et al. 1995). Recent work has shown that leukocytes comprise ~1% of the total cell population in non-erupted healthy human third molar pulps (Gaudin et al. 2015). Following infection these numbers significantly increase due to chemoattraction from the circulatory system. Neutrophils are recruited in high numbers to the infected pulp, where they aim to combat the bacteria via intra- and extracellular killing mechanisms. In addition there is an increase in monocyte numbers which differentiate into macrophages (Cooper et al. 2011, 2014, 2010; Hahn and Liewehr 2007a, b; Jontell et al. 1998; Okiji et al. 1997). Bacterial phagocytosis by the macrophages activates T cells which trigger an adaptive immune response in association with DCs. Immature DCs are also attracted for bacterial antigen capture by odontoblast-derived chemokines (Hahn and Liewehr 2007a; Durand et al. 2006; Staquet et al. 2008; Jontell et al. 1998). Antigen uptake activates the maturation of DCs which then express a range of cytokines that regulate both the innate and adaptive immune responses. The latter is activated following DC migration to regional lymph nodes where they present antigens to and activate naive CD4+ T cells. The activated naive CD4+ T cells subsequently differentiate into effector CD4+ T helper cells (including Th1, Th2 or Th17 subsets) or induced regulatory T cells (Tregs) (Onoe et al. 2007). Recent analysis of T-cell populations in healthy human dental pulp has indicated that cytotoxic CD8+ T cells represent ~21% of total leukocytes and CD4+ T cells represent ~11%, with DCs ~4% of the leukocyte population (Gaudin et al. 2015). There is a progressive and sequential accumulation of CD4+ and CD8+ T cells as pulpal disease progresses (Cooper et al. 2011; Jontell et al. 1998; Okiji et al. 1997). Our knowledge of the mechanisms that regulate Th1, Th2 or Th17 responses in the pulp is essential to better understand pulp pathogenesis; however, currently data is minimal. Interestingly a recent study has proposed that the control of IL-6 activity by MMP-3 could decrease Th2 and Th17 responses which may enable pulp regenerative events (Eba et al. 2012). NK cells have recently been identified in rat molar and incisor pulps, and they have also been shown to contribute to ~2.5% of the leukocyte population in healthy human pulps (Gaudin et al. 2015; Kawashima et al. 2006; Renard et al. 2016). Natural killer T (NKT) cells have also been detected in healthy rat pulp (Eba et al. 2012), and these cells play a major developmental role in Th1 versus Th2 immune responses (Kawashima et al. 2006). B cells are also reportedly present in healthy pulp tissue with their numbers significantly increasing during disease progression (Cooper et al. 2011; Gaudin et al. 2015; Hahn and Liewehr 2007b; Renard et al. 2016).

It is important to limit damage to the pulp that can occur collaterally by the complex immune cell mechanisms which are attempting to eliminate the microbial infection. Regulatory immune cells, such as Tol-DCs, may play a major role in this process (Tanoue et al. 2010; Banchereau and Steinman 1998). Notably they induce central and peripheral tolerance through different cellular and molecular mechanisms including T-cell depletion or anergy, induced Treg differentiation from naive CD4+ T cells and production of a variety of immunomodulatory mediators such as PD-L1, PD-L2, heme oxygenase-1 (HO-1), HLA-G, galectin-1, DC-SIGN, IL-10, TGF-β, indoleamine 2,3-dioxygenase (IDO), IL-27 and NO (Morelli and Thomson 2007; Li and Shi 2015). Tregs express molecules that inhibit or suppress the effector T-cell and Th cell responses. Interestingly, Tregs were identified in healthy human dental pulp (Gaudin et al. 2015), and a relatively large numbers of Tregs have recently been reported in severely inflamed human pulps (Bruno et al. 2010). Furthermore within healthy human pulp, there is also now evidence for the presence of a specific subset of immunoregulatory DCs which express HO-1 and protect cells against inflammatory and oxidative stress (Gaudin et al. 2015; Bruno et al. 2010). In addition myeloid-derived suppressor cells (MDSCs) which regulate immune responses have also been identified in healthy pulp (Gabrilovich and Nagaraj 2009; Dugast et al. 2008; Drujont et al. 2014). Notably the heterogeneous population of MDSCs can be expanded by exposure to bacterial components, such as LPS, and these regulate alloreactive T cells via HO-1 and IL-10 secretion (De Wilde et al. 2009). In an experimental rat incisor pulp model of reversible inflammation induced by LPS, an accumulation of an MDSC-enriched population and an increase of the expression of HO-1 and IL-10 were observed (Renard et al. 2016).

The healthy dental pulp is well equipped to detect and subsequently mount an efficient and effective immune response against invading bacteria. The range of resident leukocytes is much broader in healthy pulp than previously understood, and the immune and inflammatory response to the invading pathogens is complex. As the disease progresses, a range of immune cells are recruited from the circulatory system and these mature to reinforce the tissue's defence potential. Further work to better understand the pulp's cellular inflammatory response is warranted to enable development of novel immuno-therapeutics which could be exploited by the dental practitioner.

6.4   Interplay Between Pulp Inflammation and Healing

The immune and healing/repair responses within the tooth tissue are intimately associated. Indeed if possible, the tooth initially upregulates its dentinogenic responses to "wall off" any invading bacteria; if this first line of defence is overwhelmed however, the host's classical immune-inflammatory response is invoked to combat the bacterial invasion. Postnatal repair mechanisms within the dentine-pulp complex are well described and resemble tooth developmental processes in which progenitor cells in the dental papilla are molecularly signalled to differentiation into odontoblasts. During primary dentinogenesis, these newly formed odontoblasts secrete predentine which matures into dentine. In this cyclical process of dentine deposition, the mature odontoblasts continue to communicate with the dentine via their cellular processes which extend into the tubules. Subsequently bioactive molecules secreted by the odontoblast become fossilised within the dentine during its development (Jernvall and Thesleff 2000). The release of these dentine entombed signalling molecules later in life results in cellular events which modulate tooth tissue repair.

Primary dentinogenesis is reported to occur at a rate of ~4 µm/day of dentine deposition, while secondary dentinogenesis (which occurs throughout life after tooth root formation) decreases to a rate of ~0.4 µm/day (Nanci 2003). Tertiary dentinogenesis results in new dentine formation which distances and protects the surviving pulp from potential invading bacteria and is the tooth's natural wound healing response. Two distinct tertiary dentinogenic processes have been described (Fig. 6.2). Following relatively mild dental injury such as during early-stage caries, the primary odontoblasts become reactivated and secrete a reactionary dentine which has tubular continuity with the primary and secondary dentine. A greater injurious challenge, however, such as that occurring during a rapidly progressing carious lesion, results in primary odontoblast cell death beneath the lesion (Bjørndal 2008; Bjørndal and Darvann 1999). This cell death is potentially a result of bacterial toxins, components released from the demineralised dentine and/or local release of high levels of proinflammatory mediators. If, however, local conditions become conducive, for example, if the infection is clinically controlled or becomes arrested, stem/progenitor cells either within the pulp or ones more distant from it are recruited to the site of injury and differentiate into odontoblast-like cells. The tertiary dentine formed by these cells occurs at a similar rate of deposition to that of primary dentinogenesis, and clinically this can result in dentine bridge formation (Smith et al. 1995).

These two tertiary dentinogenic processes differ in their complexity. Reactionary dentinogenesis is comparatively simple and requires only upregulation of existing odontoblast activity, whereas reparative dentinogenesis involves several processes including progenitor cell homing, proliferation, differentiation and upregulation of dentine synthesis (Fig. 6.2) (Fitzgerald et al. 1990; Magloire et al. 1996). The source of the signalling molecules necessary for both these processes is derived from the bacterial acid demineralised dentine substrate (Smith et al. 1995, 2012; Simon et al. 2011). This molecular release due to the hard tissue breakdown enables odontoblasts and progenitor cells to detect and positively respond to the dental tissue

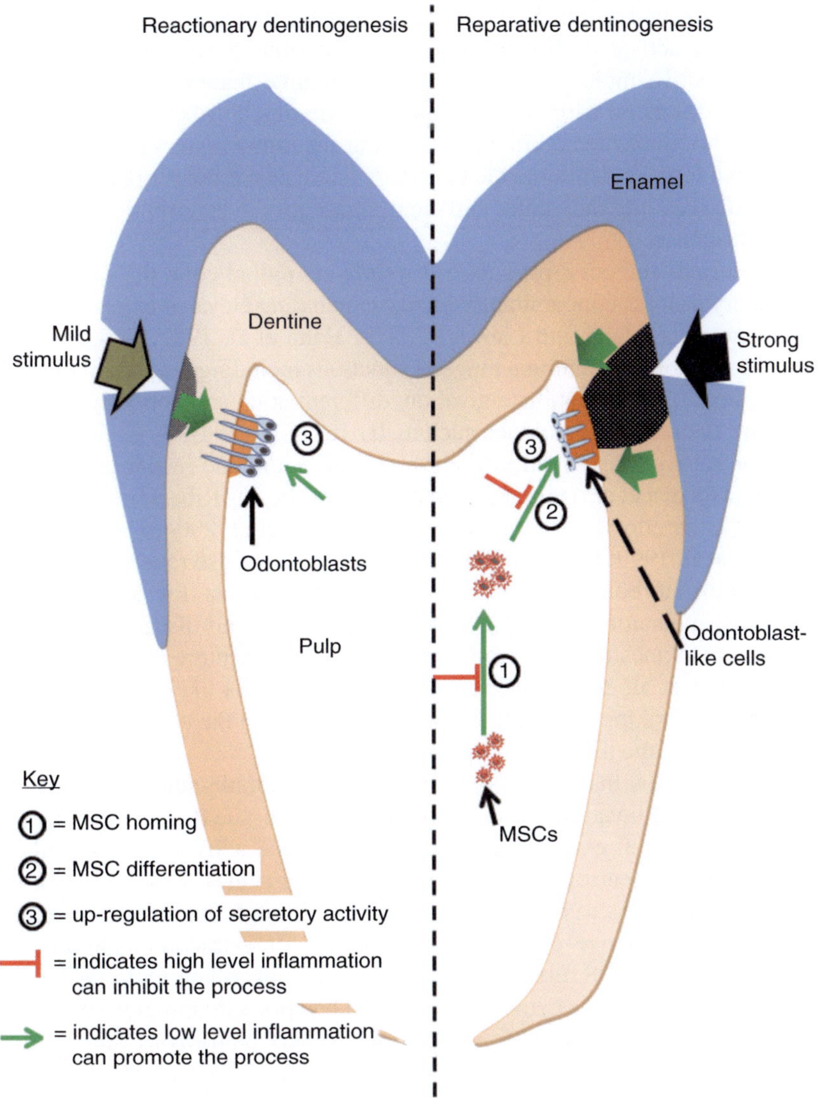

Fig. 6.2 The relationship between inflammation and the tertiary dentinogenic events of reactionary and reparative dentinogenesis. Low-level acute inflammation has the potential to stimulate reactionary dentinogenic events by upregulation of surviving odontoblast's secretory activity. Increased persistent and intense inflammation, such as during a rapidly progressive carious lesion, has the potential to lead to odontoblast death. If the infection is arrested, such as following clinical intervention using restoratives such as calcium hydroxide and MTA, the subsequent low-level resolving inflammation has the potential to signal MSC homing, differentiation and upregulation of their secretory activity. However if high-level inflammation ensues, the relatively high levels of inflammatory mediators may inhibit these MSC tissue repair-associated processes. MSC = mesenchymal stem cell, e.g. dental pulp stem cell (DPSC). Solid green arrows with gradients indicate release of dentine matrix components which signal tertiary dentinogenic events

damage. It is likely that it is the extent of the damage which drives the dentinogenic repair pathway activated. Notably not only do carious bacterial acids release the dentine's bioactive molecules, but certain restorative materials, such as calcium hydroxide and mineral trioxide aggregate, also do this. Furthermore it is now evident that a variety of mediators present during the inflammatory response are also able to signal tertiary dentinogenic events. A fine balance therefore exists between the levels of signalling molecules and their temporality in determining the nature of the tissue response.

As the carious infection progresses towards the pulpal core, the markers of the inflammatory process concomitantly increase including elevated levels of cytokines and immune cells (Hahn and Liewehr 2007b; Hahn et al. 1989; McLachlan et al. 2004). These cytokines exhibit a range of functions including regulation of lymphocyte recruitment, extravasation, activation, differentiation and antibody production. In the pulp, the roles of cytokines such as IL-1α, IL1-β as IL-4, IL-6, IL-8, IL-10 and TNF-α are well described in orchestrating the immune response (McLachlan et al. 2004; Hosoya et al. 1996; Matsuo et al. 1994; Pezelj-Ribaric et al. 2002; Lara et al. 2003; Dinarello 1984; Smith et al. 1980; Silva et al. 2004; Hahn et al. 2000; Barkhordar et al. 1999; Guo et al. 2000). Indeed, we have also reported significantly elevated levels at both the transcript and protein levels for a range of pro-inflammatory mediators, including S100 proteins, in carious diseased pulpal tissue. In addition, cytokines released from the demineralised dentine add to the complex milieu (Cooper et al. 2010; McLachlan et al. 2004). It is likely that not until the levels of these cytokines return to homeostatic ones then the chronic inflammation will persist within the tooth.

The inflammation that occurs within the tooth is double-edged as while it ultimately aims to kill invading bacteria, collateral host tissue damage can occur as a result of immune cell extravasation and antimicrobial activity. In particular it is well described that neutrophils release degradative enzymes, such as matrix metalloproteinases (MMPs), to enable their migration through the soft tissue matrix as well as generate reactive oxygen species (ROS) for extracellular antimicrobial killing. Notably, the ROS released can cause significant collateral tissue damage as well as stimulating further cytokine release via key pro-inflammatory intracellular signalling regulated by the p38 MAPK and NF-κB pathways (Veerayutthwilai et al. 2007; Simon et al. 2010; Fiers et al. 1999; Guha and Mackman 2001; Hagemann and Blank 2001). Notably while these signalling pathways are central to regulating the inflammatory response, they are also known to signal tissue repair events. More recently extracellular traps derived from neutrophils (NETs) have been described as a host antimicrobial mechanism. In this cell death process, termed NETosis, neutrophilic nuclear DNA is extruded via ROS-mediated pathways. The DNA fibres released are decorated with antimicrobial proteins derived from neutrophilic granules which aim to limit the spread of bacteria as well as cause their cell death. Our work in this area (Cooper et al. 2017) has indicated that NET release, while aimed at protecting the host, could have serious deleterious effects on the pulp as it may exacerbate the local inflammatory response as well as induce stem cell death.

It is now becoming apparent that persistent pulpal inflammatory processes impede reparative events, and the accepted paradigm is that pulp healing can only occur after removal of bacteria and significant dampening of the inflammatory process (Bergenholtz 1981; Rutherford and Gu 2000; Baumgardner and Sulfaro 2001). Some of the most significant evidence that infection and inflammation control are necessary to enable healing is derived from classical animal studies. Indeed data has demonstrated that dental tissue healing/repair was apparent only in artificial cavities made in germ-free mice compared with those that were infected and subsequently had inflamed pulps (Inoue and Shimono 1992). Further evidence regarding the effect of inflammation on repair is derived from in vitro studies that demonstrate the biphasic effects of pro-inflammatory mediators. At relatively low levels, these molecules, such as TNF-α and TGF-β and also ROS and LPS, can stimulate repair-associated events in dental cells, while at higher levels, such as during persistent inflammation, they cause cell death. Other work has also shown that stem cell differentiation processes are directly impeded by several pro-inflammatory signalling molecules (Lara et al. 2003; Simon et al. 2010; Smith et al. 2005; He et al. 2005, 2015; Pevsner-Fischer et al. 2007; Chang et al. 2005; Goldberg et al. 2008; Paula-Silva et al. 2009; Wang et al. 2015, 2014; Feng et al. 2013; Lee et al. 2006; Saito et al. 2011).

Further evidence of the link between inflammation and repair is evident from data demonstrating receptor sharing in immune and stem cell populations. The CXC chemokine receptor 4 (CXCR4) is expressed on both cell types (Murdoch 2000; Miller et al. 2008), and along with its ligand, stromal cell-derived factor-1 (SDF-1)/CXCL12, they have been shown to be present within the dentine-pulp complex and are upregulated during dental caries (Jiang et al. 2008a, b). There appears to be a logical explanation for the sharing of this chemotactic receptor by these cell types as infected and damaged tissues need to appropriately modulate the recruitment of both immune and stem cells to injury sites (About and Mitsiadis 2001). Subsequently, the determination as to which of these two cell types gets preferentially recruited appears to be locally regulated. Indeed studies have demonstrated that cytokines modulate the stem cell surface expression of CXCR4 with relatively high levels of pro-inflammatory mediators abrogating CXCR4-expressing stem cell activity at sites where inflammatory cell recruitment predominates (Murdoch 2000).

Differences in the number of steps involved in the two tertiary dentinogenic responses described mean that local tissue inflammation can exert differing effects (Fig. 6.2) (Cooper et al. 2010). Indeed, in reparative dentinogenesis, there is the opportunity for inflammatory modulation at the cell homing, differentiation and secretory stages, whereas during reactionary dentinogenesis, the inflammatory response can lead to upregulation of the odontoblast secretory activity or it may contribute to driving odontoblast death (Fig. 6.3). Potentially it is acute or low levels of these inflammatory signals that are necessary to signal repair responses, while higher chronic levels impede tissue repair and favour signalling of immune cell-related events. This interplay between the inflammatory and reparative responses would appear necessary and pragmatic as protecting the pulp with de novo dentine formation while it is under significant attack from infection, and its own

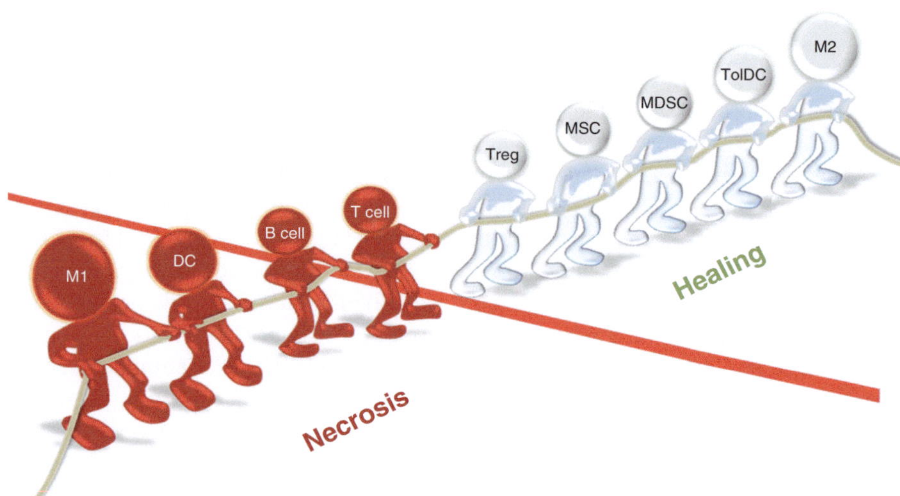

Fig. 6.3 Illustration showing the opposition between immune cells which promote cell and tissue necrosis when inflammation is excessive and those which dampen the immune response and promote healing in the dental pulp tissue (T cell, lymphocyte T helper and T cytotoxic; B cell, B lymphocyte and plasmocytes; DC, dendritic cell; M1, macrophage type 1; Treg, regulatory T cell; MSC, mesenchymal stem cell; MDSC, myeloid-derived suppressor cell; Tol-DC, tolerogenic dendritic cells; M2, macrophage type 2)

inflammatory response, would not be energetically efficient. Combined, the information presented here further support the notion that the modulation of the magnitude as well as temporospatial nature of the inflammatory response is central to determining tissue healing.

6.5 Tissue Inflammation and Healing: Translational Opportunities

Clinical observations following the application of pulp capping agents such as calcium hydroxide and mineral trioxide aggregate (MTA) provide further support for inflammatory events preceding dental tissue repair. These restorative agents are known to enable pulp healing beneath the site of application. Prior to tissue healing in the form of a dentine bridge, pulp tissue inflammatory events are routinely reported (Nair et al. 2008). While calcium hydroxide has been used clinically for over 60 years (Hermann 1930; Schröder 1985; Kardos et al. 1998; Goldberg et al. 2003), its mechanism of action for induction of reparative dentinogenesis still remains unclear. Its beneficial effects have however been attributed to local tissue irritation due to its elevated pH which causes cellular necrosis beneath the site of placement (Kardos et al. 1998; Schröder and Granath 1971; Stanley 2002). Hence, this tissue irritation has been cited as the principal mechanism of action which subsequently leads to the stimulation of an acute sterile inflammatory response

(Brentano et al. 2005; Luheshi et al. 2009; Acosta-Pérez et al. 2008; Magalhães-Santos and Andrade 2005). Furthermore MTA has been shown to stimulate cytokine release, including IL-1α, IL-1β, IL-2, IL-6 and IL-8 expression, from odontoblasts and osteoblasts, and this mild and acute material-induced inflammatory response may also contribute to clinical repair (Huang et al. 2005; Mitchell et al. 1999; Koh et al. 1998). Other studies have reported that the beneficial effects enabled by these restoratives are attributable to their ability to sterilise the site of infection while releasing bioactive components from the dentine (Graham et al. 2006; Tomson et al. 2007). It is therefore likely that several properties of these restoratives are important in generating a locally conducive environment to enable reparative dentinogenesis.

To gain a better understanding of the molecular response of the pulp tissue following carious destruction of enamel and dentine, high-throughput transcriptional profiling using diseased and healthy pulp tissue has been performed. These studies have indicated that the predominant tissue processes detected related to inflammation and there was minimal evidence of repair-associated molecular events (McLachlan et al. 2005). Differential expression of several molecules previously not associated with dental disease were identified, and one particular molecule, adrenomedullin (ADM), provided a candidate modulator for both inflammation and repair. This pleiotropic cytokine has reported antibacterial and immunomodulatory activities, as well as being able to promote angiogenesis and mineralised tissue repair (Zudaire et al. 2006; Montuenga et al. 1997; Ishii et al. 2005; Cornish et al. 1997). Our own studies subsequently demonstrated that ADM can exert similar effects within the dental tissues and that it was archived within the dentine during primary dentinogenesis (Musson et al. 2010). Mining of high-throughput transcriptional data obtained from well-characterised clinical samples has the potential to facilitate our understanding of the link between inflammation and regeneration and identify novel molecular targets for clinical exploitation.

Cell therapy approaches for dental disease are also being considered via the direct action of mesenchymal stem cells (MSCs) or indirectly via their secretome ability to modulate inflammation and promote dental tissue repair. Reported MSC immunomodulatory effects include:

- Inhibition of immune cell proliferation
- Inhibition of cytokine/antibody secretion
- Inhibition of immune cell maturation
- Inhibition of antigen presentation by T cells, B cells, NK cells and DCs (De Miguel et al. 2012; Leprince et al. 2012; Tomic et al. 2011)

Furthermore the direct cell-to-cell contact between stem and immune cells elicits MSC secretion of soluble factors such as TGF-β1 and IDO which have known anti-inflammatory effects. In addition, MSCs in dental pulp express TLR10 (Karim et al. 2016). The role of TLR10 is not well defined, but it appears to act as an inhibitory receptor, with suppressive effects (Oosting et al. 2014). Further work characterising the role of MSCs in inflamed dental tissues and their secreted components may enable development of novel cell therapy approaches.

Therapeutic modulators of inflammation have the potential to be used adjunctively, in particular along with disinfection regimes, to facilitate the healing response and potentially aid restoration longevity. Recent work has reported that dental resin restorative procedures supplemented with antioxidants, such as *N*-acetyl-cysteine (NAC), provide protection to pulpal cells from ROS generated following resin placement. Interestingly, NAC may also limit the activation of the key ROS-activated NF-κB pro-inflammatory pathway (Yamada et al. 2008), and this may minimise tissue inflammation and subsequently create a more conducive environment for healing. Indeed, other work has demonstrated the importance of the modulation of both ROS and RNS to enable repair. It has recently been demonstrated that the anti-inflammatory mechanism of exogenously applied PPARγ in human dental pulp cells was likely due to the removal of both NO and ROS. This application resulted in the suppression of both the NF-κB and extracellular signal-regulated kinase (ERK)1/2 signalling pathways (Kim et al. 2012). There have also been a significant number of studies assessing the anti-inflammatory effects in the pulp of other naturally derived compounds, for example, by pachymic acid, obtained from the mushroom *Formitopsis niagra*. Interestingly, this compound may not only have anti-inflammatory activity but also appears to be able to promote odontoblast differentiation via activation of the HO-1 pathway (Lee et al. 2013b).

Other areas where novel therapeutic anti-inflammatory opportunities exist include the relatively novel and exciting area of microRNA (miRNA) technologies. Recent work has shown the expression of these molecules with immunomodulatory capabilities in the pulp, and hence further work relating to their therapeutic application in the diseased pulp is being explored [(Zhong et al. 2012; Hui et al. 2017); also see Chap. 5]. We and others have been studying the application of low-level light therapy as a means to modulate inflammation and promote tissue repair. While this technology is more widely applied in the treatment of other diseases, there is significant potential for its application in dental disease, therefore further studies are warranted (Milward et al. 2014).

Conclusions

During a progressive carious infection, initially the odontoblasts detect the invading bacteria, and subsequently cells within the pulp core such as resident immune cells, fibroblasts, stem cells and endothelial cells further orchestrate the molecular response. Autocrine and paracrine signalling along with the bacterial acid-mediated release of bioactive molecules from the dentine amplifies the immune reaction which leads to a significant immune cell infiltrate. Until the infection is clinically resolved, the relatively high levels of pro-inflammatory mediators present in the local environment will impede healing events and retention of vital pulp. It is clear that sustained research in this area will result in the development of new diagnostics (see Chap. 2) and therapeutic approaches which will translate into clinical practice and benefit dental patients of the future.

Acknowledgements *Conflict of Interests*: The authors declare that there is no conflict of interests regarding the publication of this paper.

References

About I, Mitsiadis TA (2001) Molecular aspects of tooth pathogenesis and repair: in vivo and in vitro models. Adv Dent Res 15:59–62

Acosta-Pérez G, Maximina Bertha Moreno-Altamirano M, Rodríguez-Luna G, Javier Sánchez-Garcia F (2008) Differential dependence of the ingestion of necrotic cells and TNF-alpha/IL-1beta production by murine macrophages on lipid rafts. Scand J Immunol 68(4):423–429

Arthur JS, Ley SC (2013) Mitogen-activated protein kinases in innate immunity. Nat Rev Immunol 13(9):679–692

Banchereau J, Steinman RM (1998) Dendritic cells and the control of immunity. Nature 392(6673):245–252

Barkhordar RA, Hayashi C, Hussain MZ (1999) Detection of interleukin-6 in human pulp and periapical lesions. Endod Dent Traumatol 15(1):26–27

Baumgardner KR, Sulfaro MA (2001) The anti-inflammatory effects of human recombinant copper-zinc superoxide dismutase on pulp inflammation. J Endod 27(3):190–195

Bergenholtz G (1981) Inflammatory response of the dental pulp to bacterial irritation. J Endod 7(3):100–104

Beutler BA (2009) Microbe sensing, positive feedback loops, and the pathogenesis of inflammatory diseases. Immunol Rev 227(1):248–263

Bjørndal L (2008) The caries process and its effect on the pulp the science is changing and so is our understanding. J Endod 34(7 Suppl):S2–S5

Bjørndal L, Darvann T (1999) A light microscopic study of odontoblastic and non-odontoblastic cells involved in tertiary dentinogenesis in well-defined cavitated carious lesions. Caries Res 33(1):50–60

Bogdan C (2015) Nitric oxide synthase in innate and adaptive immunity: an update. Trends Immunol 36(3):161–178

Brentano F, Schorr O, Gay RE, Gay S, Kyburz D (2005) RNA released from necrotic synovial fluid cells activates rheumatoid arthritis synovial fibroblasts via Toll-like receptor 3. Arthritis Rheum 52(9):2656–2665

Bruno KF, Silva JA, Silva TA, Batista AC, Alencar AH, Estrela C (2010) Characterization of inflammatory cell infiltrate in human dental pulpitis. Int Endod J 43(11):1013–1021

Carrouel F, Staquet M-J, Keller J-F et al (2013) Lipopolysaccharide-binding protein inhibits toll-like receptor 2 activation by lipoteichoic acid in human odontoblast-like cells. J Endod 39(8):1008–1014

Chang J, Zhang C, Tani-Ishii N, Shi S, Wang CY (2005) NF-kappaB activation in human dental pulp stem cells by TNF and LPS. J Dent Res 84(11):994–998

Coleman JW (2001) Nitric oxide in immunity and inflammation. Int Immunopharmacol 1(8):1397–1406

Cooper PR, Takahashi Y, Graham LW, Simon S, Imazato S, Smith AJ (2010) Inflammation-regeneration interplay in the dentine-pulp complex. J Dent 38(9):687–697

Cooper PR, McLachlan JL, Simon S, Graham LW, Smith AJ (2011) Mediators of inflammation and regeneration. Adv Dent Res 23(3):290–295

Cooper PR, Holder MJ, Smith AJ (2014) Inflammation and regeneration in the dentin-pulp complex: a double-edged sword. J Endod 40(4 Suppl):S46–S51

Cooper PR, Chicca IJ, Holder MJ, Milward MR (2017) Inflammation and regeneration in the dentin-pulp complex: net gain or net loss? J Endod 43(9S):S87–S94

Cornish J, Callon KE, Coy DH et al (1997) Adrenomedullin is a potent stimulator of osteoblastic activity *in vitro* and *in vivo*. Am J Physiol 273(6 Pt 1):E1113–E1120

De Miguel MP, Fuentes-Julián S, Blázquez-Martínez A et al (2012) Immunosuppressive properties of mesenchymal stem cells: advances and applications. Curr Mol Med 12(5):574–591

De Wilde V, Van Rompaey N, Hill M et al (2009) Endotoxin-induced myeloid-derived suppressor cells inhibit alloimmune responses via heme oxygenase-1. Am J Transplant 9(9):2034–2047

Di Nardo Di Maio F, Lohinai Z, D'Arcangelo C et al (2004) Nitric oxide synthase in healthy and inflamed human dental pulp. J Dent Res 83:312–316

Dinarello CA (1984) Interleukin-1. Rev Infect Dis 6(1):51–95

Dommisch H, Winter J, Açil Y, Dunsche A, Tiemann M, Jepsen S (2005) Human beta-defensin (hBD-1, -2) expression in dental pulp. Oral Microbiol Immunol 20(3):163–166

Dommisch H, Winter J, Willebrand C, Eberhard J, Jepsen S (2007) Immune regulatory functions of human beta-defensin-2 in odontoblast-like cells. Int Endod J 40(4):300–307

Drujont L, Carretero-Iglesia L, Bouchet-Delbos L et al (2014) Evaluation of the therapeutic potential of bone marrow-derived myeloid suppressor cell (MDSC) adoptive transfer in mouse models of autoimmunity and allograft rejection. PLoS One 9:e100013

Dugast AS, Haudebourg T, Coulon F et al (2008) Myeloid-derived suppressor cells accumulate in kidney allograft tolerance and specifically suppress effector T cell expansion. J Immunol 180(12):7898–7906

Durand SH, Flacher V, Roméas A et al (2006) Lipoteichoic acid increases TLR and functional chemokine expression while reducing dentin formation in in vitro differentiated human odontoblasts. J Immunol 176(5):2880–2887

Eba H, Murasawa Y, Iohara K, Isogai Z, Nakamura H, Nakashima M (2012) The anti-inflammatory effects of matrix metalloproteinase-3 on irreversible pulpitis of mature erupted teeth. PLoS One 7:e52523

Farges J-C, Romeas A, Melin M et al (2003) TGF-beta1 induces accumulation of dendritic cells in the odontoblast layer. J Dent Res 82(8):652–656

Farges J-C, Keller J-F, Carrouel F et al (2009) Odontoblasts in the dental pulp immune response. J Exp Zool Part Mol Dev Evol 312B(5):425–436

Farges J-C, Carrouel F, Keller J-F et al (2011) Cytokine production by human odontoblast-like cells upon Toll-like receptor-2 engagement. Immunobiology 216(4):513–517

Farges J-C, Alliot-Licht B, Baudouin C, Msika P, Bleicher F, Carrouel F (2013) Odontoblast control of dental pulp inflammation triggered by cariogenic bacteria. Front Physiol 4:1–3

Farges JC, Bellanger A, Ducret M et al (2015) Human odontoblast-like cells produce nitric oxide with antibacterial activity upon TLR2 activation. Front Physiol 23(6):185–194

Feng X, Feng G, Xing J et al (2013) TNF-α triggers osteogenic differentiation of human dental pulp stem cells via the NF-κB signalling pathway. Cell Biol Int 37(12):1267–1275

Fiers W, Beyaert R, Declercq W, Vandenabeele P (1999) More than one way to die: apoptosis, necrosis and reactive oxygen damage. Oncogene 18(54):7719–7730

Fitzgerald M, Chiego DJ Jr, Heys DR (1990) Autoradiographic analysis of odontoblast replacement following pulp exposure in primate teeth. Arch Oral Biol 35(9):707–715

Gabrilovich DI, Nagaraj S (2009) Myeloid-derived suppressor cells as regulators of the immune system. Nat Rev Immunol 9(3):162–174

Gaudin A, Renard E, Hill M et al (2015) Phenotypic analysis of immunocompetent cells in healthy human dental pulp. J Endod 41(5):621–627

Goldberg M, Six N, Decup F et al (2003) Bioactive molecules and the future of pulp therapy. Am J Dent 16(1):66–76

Goldberg M, Farges JC, Lacerda-Pinheiro S et al (2008) Inflammatory and immunological aspects of dental pulp repair. Pharmacol Res 58(2):137–147

Graham L, Cooper PR, Cassidy N, Nor JE, Sloan AJ, Smith AJ (2006) The effect of calcium hydroxide on solubilisation of bio-active dentin matrix. Biomaterials 27(14):2865–2873

Guha M, Mackman N (2001) LPS induction of gene expression in human monocytes. Cell Signal 13(2):85–94

Guo X, Niu Z, Xiao M, Yue L, Lu H (2000) Detection of interleukin-8 in exudates from normal and inflamed human dental pulp tissues. Chinese J Dent Res 3(1):63–66

Guzik TJ, Korbut R, Adamek-Guzik T (2003) Nitric oxide and superoxide in inflammation and immune regulation. J Physiol Pharmacol 54(4):469–487

Hagemann C, Blank JL (2001) The ups and downs of MEK kinase interactions. Cell Signal 13(12):863–875

Hahn CL, Liewehr FR (2007a) Innate immune responses of the dental pulp to caries. J Endod 33(6):643–651

Hahn CL, Liewehr FR (2007b) Update on the adaptive immune responses of the dental pulp. J Endod 33:773–781

Hahn CL, Falkler WA Jr, Siegel MA (1989) A study of T and B cells in pulpal pathosis. J Endod 15(1):20–26

Hahn CL, Best AM, Tew JG (2000) Cytokine induced by Streptococcus mutans and pulpal pathogenesis. Infect Immun 68(12):6785–6789

Hamilton IR (2000) Ecological basis for dental caries. In: Kuramitsu HK, Ellen RP (eds) Oral bacterial ecology: the molecular basis. Horizon Scientific Press, Wymondham, pp 219–274

He WX, Niu ZY, Zhao SL, Smith AJ (2005) Smad protein mediated transforming growth factor beta1 induction of apoptosis in the MDPC-23 odontoblast-like cell line. Arch Oral Biol 50(11):929–936

He W, Wang Z, Luo Z et al (2015) LPS promote the odontoblastic differentiation of human dental pulp stem cells via MAPK signaling pathway. J Cell Physiol 230(3):554–561

Hermann BW (1930) Dentinobliteration der Wurzelkanäle nach Behandlung mit calcium. Zahnarztl Rundsch 30:887–899

Heyeraas KJ, Berggreen E (1999) Interstitial fluid pressure in normal and inflamed pulp. Crit Rev Oral Biol Med 10(3):328–336

Hosoya S, Matsushima K, Ohbayashi E, Yamazaki M, Shibata Y, Abiko Y (1996) Stimulation of interleukin-1beta-independent interleukin-6 production in human dental pulp cells by lipopolysaccharide. Biochem Mol Med 59(2):138–143

Huang TH, Yang CC, Ding SJ, Yeng M, Kao CT, Chou MY (2005) Inflammatory cytokines reaction elicited by root-end filling materials. J Biomed Mater Res B Appl Biomater 73(1):123–128

Hui T, Wang C, Chen D, Zheng L, Huang D, Ye L (2017) Epigenetic regulation in dental pulp inflammation. Oral Dis 23(1):22–28

Hunter CA, Jones SA (2015) IL-6 as a keystone cytokine in health and disease. Nat Immunol 16(5):448–457

Inoue T, Shimono M (1992) Repair dentinogenesis following transplantation into normal and germ-free animals. Proc Finn Dent Soc 88(Suppl 1):183–194

Ishii M, Koike C, Igarashi A et al (2005) Molecular markers distinguish bone marrow mesenchymal stem cells from fibroblasts. Biochem Biophys Res Commun 332(1):297–303

Izumi T, Kobayashi I, Okamura K, Sakai H (1995) Immunohistochemical study on the immunocompetent cells of the pulp in human non-carious and carious teeth. Arch Oral Biol 40(7):609–614

Jernvall J, Thesleff I (2000) Reiterative signaling and patterning during mammalian tooth morphogenesis. Mech Dev 92(1):19–29

Jiang HW, Zhang W, Ren BP, Zeng JF, Ling JQ (2006) Expression of toll like receptor 4 in normal human odontoblasts and dental pulp tissue. J Endod 32(8):747–751

Jiang HW, Ling JQ, Gong QM (2008a) The expression of stromal cell-derived factor 1 (SDF-1) in inflamed human dental pulp. J Endod 34(11):1351–1354

Jiang L, Zhu YQ, Du R et al (2008b) The expression and role of stromal cell-derived factor-1alpha-CXCR4 axis in human dental pulp. J Endod 34(8):939–944

Jontell M, Okiji T, Dahlgren U, Bergenholtz G (1998) Immune defense mechanisms of the dental pulp. Crit Rev Oral Biol Med 9(2):179–200

Kaji R, Kiyoshima-Shibata J, Nagaoka M, Nanno M, Shida K (2010) Bacterial teichoic acids reverse predominant IL-12 production induced by certain Lactobacillus strains into predominant IL-10 production via TLR2-dependent ERK activation in macrophages. J Immunol 184(7):3505–3513

Kardos TB, Hunter AR, Hanlin SM, Kirk EE (1998) Odontoblast differentiation: a response to environmental calcium. Endod Dent Traumatol 14(3):105–111

Karim M, El-Sayed F, Klingebiel P, C. E. (2016) Toll-like receptor expression profile of human dental pulp stem/progenitor cells. J Endod 42(3):413–417

Kawai T, Akira S (2010) The role of pattern-recognition receptors in innate immunity: update on Toll-like receptors. Nat Immunol 11(5):373–384

Kawanishi HN, Kawashima N, Suzuki N, Suda H, Takagi M (2004) Effects of an inducible nitric oxide synthase inhibitor on experimentally induced rat pulpitis. Eur J Oral Sci 112(4):332–337

Kawashima N, Nakano-Kawanishi H, Suzuki N, Takagi M, Suda H (2005) Effect of NOS inhibitor on cytokine and COX2 expression in rat pulpitis. J Dent Res 84(8):762–767

Kawashima N, Wongyaofa I, Suzuki N, Kawanishi HN, Suda H (2006) NK and NKT cells in the rat dental pulp tissues. Oral Surg Oral Med Oral Pathol Oral Radiol Endod 102(4):558–563

Keller J-F, Carrouel F, Colomb E et al (2010) Toll-like receptor 2 activation by lipoteichoic acid induces differential production of pro-inflammatory cytokines in human odontoblasts, dental pulp fibroblasts and immature dendritic cells. Immunobiology 215(1):53–59

Keller J-F, Carrouel F, Staquet M-J et al (2011) Expression of NOD2 is increased in inflamed human dental pulps and lipoteichoic acid-stimulated odontoblast-like cells. Innate Immun 17(1):29–34

Kim YS, Min KS, Lee SI, Shin SJ, Shin KS, Kim EC (2010) Effect of proinflammatory cytokines on the expression and regulation of human beta-defensin 2 in human dental pulp cells. J Endod 36(1):64–69

Kim JC, Lee YH, Yu MK et al (2012) Anti-inflammatory mechanism of PPARγ on LPS-induced pulp cells: role of the ROS removal activity. Arch Oral Biol 57(4):392–400

Koh ET, McDonald F, Pitt Ford TR, Torabinejad M (1998) Cellular response to mineral trioxide aggregate. J Endod 24(8):543–547

Korkmaz Y, Lang H, Beikler T et al (2011) Irreversible inflammation is associated with decreased levels of the alpha1-, beta1-, and alpha2-subunits of sGC in human odontoblasts. J Dent Res 90(4):517–522

Kumar H, Kawai T, Akira S (2011) Pathogen recognition by the innate immune system. Int Rev Immunol 30(1):16–34

Lara VS, Figueiredo F, da Silva TA, Cunha FQ (2003) Dentin-induced in vivo inflammatory response and in vitro activation of murine macrophages. J Dent Res 82(6):460–465

Law AS, Baumgardner KR, Meller ST, Gebhart GF (1999) Localization and changes in NADPH-diaphorase reactivity and nitric oxide synthase immunoreactivity in rat pulp following tooth preparation. J Dent Res 78(10):1585–1595

Lee SH, Baek DH (2012) Antibacterial and neutralizing effect of human β-defensins on Enterococcus faecalis and Enterococcus faecalis lipoteichoic acid. J Endod 38(3):351–356

Lee DH, Lim BS, Lee YK, Yang HC (2006) Effects of hydrogen peroxide (H2O2) on alkaline phosphatase activity and matrix mineralization of odontoblast and osteoblast cell lines. Cell Biol Toxicol 22(1):39–46

Lee SI, Min KS, Bae WJ et al (2011) Role of SIRT1 in heat stress- and lipopolysaccharide-induced immune and defense gene expression in human dental pulp cells. J Endod 37(11):1525–1530

Lee CC, Avalos AM, Ploegh HL (2012) Accessory molecules for Toll-like receptors and their function. Nat Rev Immunol 12(3):168–179

Lee JK, Chang SW, Perinpanayagam H et al (2013a) Antibacterial efficacy of a human β-defensin-3 peptide on multispecies biofilms. J Endod 39(12):1625–1629

Lee YH, Lee NH, Bhattarai G et al (2013b) Anti-inflammatory effect of pachymic acid promotes odontoblastic differentiation via HO-1 in dental pulp cells. Oral Dis 19(2):193–199

Leprince JG, Zeitlin BD, Tolar M, Peters OA (2012) Interactions between immune system and mesenchymal stem cells in dental pulp and periapical tissues. Int Endod J 45(8):689–701

Lesot H, Smith AJ, Tziafas D, Bègue-Kirn C, Cassidy N, Ruch J-V (1994) Biologically active molecule and dental tissue repair, a comparative review of reactionary and reparative dentinogenesis with induction of odontoblast differentiation in vitro. Cells Mater 4:199–218

Li MO, Flavell RA (2008) Contextual regulation of inflammation: a duet by transforming growth factor-β and interleukin-10. Immunity 28(4):468–476

Li H, Shi B (2015) Tolerogenic dendritic cells and their applications in transplantation. Cell Mol Immunol 12(1):24–30

Love RM, Jenkinson HF (2002) Invasion of dentinal tubules by oral bacteria. Crit Rev Oral Biol Med 13(2):171–183

Luheshi NM, McColl BW, Brough D (2009) Nuclear retention of IL-1alpha by necrotic cells: a mechanism to dampen sterile inflammation. Eur J Immunol 39(11):2973–2980

MacMicking J, Xie QW, Nathan C (1997) Nitric oxide and macrophage function. Annu Rev Immunol 15:323–350

Magalhães-Santos IF, Andrade SG (2005) Participation of cytokines in the necrotic-inflammatory lesions in the heart and skeletal muscles of Calomys callosus infected with Trypanosoma cruzi. Mem Inst Oswaldo Cruz 100(5):555–561

Magloire H, Joffre A, Bleicher F (1996) An *in vitro* model of human dental pulp repair. J Dent Res 75(12):1971–1978

Mangkornkarn C, Steiner JC, Bohman R, Lindemann RA (1991) Flow cytometric analysis of human dental pulp tissue. J Endod 17(2):49–53

Mansour SC, Pena OM, Hancock REW (2014) Host defense peptides: front-line immunomodulators. Trends Immunol 35(9):443–450

Matsuo T, Ebisu S, Nakanishi T, Yonemura K, Harada Y, Okada H (1994) Interleukin-1 alpha and interleukin-1 beta periapical exudates of infected root canals: correlations with the clinical findings of the involved teeth. J Endod 20(9):432–435

McLachlan JL, Sloan AJ, Smith AJ, Landini G, Cooper PR (2004) S100 and cytokine expression in caries. Infect Immun 72(7):4102–4108

McLachlan JL, Smith AJ, Bujalska IJ, Cooper PR (2005) Gene expression profiling of pulpal tissue reveals the molecular complexity of dental caries. Biochim Biophys Acta 1741(3):271–281

Miller RJ, Banisadr G, Bhattacharyya BJ (2008) CXCR4 signaling in the regulation of stem cell migration and development. J Neuroimmunol 198(1-2):31–38

Milward MR, Holder MJ, Palin WM et al (2014) Dental phototherapy: low level light therapy (LLLT) for the treatment and management of dental and oral diseases. Dent Update 41(9):763–772

Min KS, Kim HI, Chang HS et al (2008) Involvement of mitogen-activated protein kinases and nuclear factor-kappa B activation in nitric oxide-induced interleukin-8 expression in human pulp cells. Oral Surg Oral Med Oral Pathol Oral Radiol Endod 105(5):654–660

Mitchell PJ, Pitt Ford TR, Torabinejad M, McDonald F (1999) Osteoblast biocompatibility of mineral trioxide aggregate. Biomaterials 20(2):167–173

Montuenga LM, Martínez A, Miller MJ, Unsworth EJ, Cuttitta F (1997) Expression of adrenomedullin and its receptor during embryogenesis suggests autocrine or paracrine modes of action. Endocrinology 138(1):440–451

Morelli AE, Thomson AW (2007) Tolerogenic dendritic cells and the quest for transplant tolerance. Nat Rev Immunol 7(8):610–621

Murdoch C (2000) CXCR4: chemokine receptor extraordinaire. Immunol Rev 177:175–184

Musson DS, McLachlan JL, Sloan AJ, Smith AJ, Cooper PR (2010) Adrenomedullin is expressed during rodent dental tissue development and promotes cell growth and mineralization. Biol Cell 102(3):145–157

Nair PN, Duncan HF, Pitt Ford TR, Luder HU (2008) Histological, ultrastructural and quantitative investigations on the response of healthy human pulps to experimental capping with mineral trioxide aggregate: a randomized controlled trial. Int Endod J 41(2):128–150

Nanci A (2003) Dentin-pulp complex. In: Nanci A (ed) Ten cate's oral histology: development structure, and function. Mosby, Saint Louis, MO, pp 192–239

Nathan C (1992) Nitric oxide as a secretory product of mammalian cells. FASEB J 6(12):3051–3064

Nibali L, Fedele S, D'Aiuto F, Donos N (2012) Interleukin-6 in oral diseases: a review. Oral Dis 18(3):236–243

Nussler AK, Billiar TR (1993) Inflammation, immunoregulation, and inducible nitric oxide synthase. J Leukoc Biol 54(2):171–178

Okiji T, Jontell M, Belichenko P, Bergenholtz G, Dahlstrom A (1997) Perivascular dendritic cells of the human dental pulp. Acta Physiol Scand 159(2):163–169

Onoe K, Yanagawa Y, Minami K, Iijima N, Iwabuchi K (2007) Th1 or Th2 balance regulated by interaction between dendritic cells and NKT cells. Immunol Res 38(1-3):319–332

Oosting M, Cheng SC, Bolscher JM et al (2014) Human TLR10 is an anti-inflammatory pattern-recognition receptor. Proc Natl Acad Sci U S A 11(42):E4478–E4484

Paris S, Wolgin M, Kielbassa AM, Pries A, Zakrzewicz A (2009) Gene expression of human beta-defensins in healthy and inflamed human dental pulps. J Endod 35(4):520–523

Paula-Silva FW, Ghosh A, Silva LA, Kapila YL (2009) TNF-alpha promotes an odontoblastic phenotype in dental pulp cells. J Dent Res 88(4):339–344

Pazgier M, Hoover DM, Yang D, Lu W, Lubkowski J (2006) Human beta-defensins. Cell Mol Life Sci 63(11):1294–1313

Pevsner-Fischer M, Morad V, Cohen-Sfady M et al (2007) Toll-like receptors and their ligands control mesenchymal stem cell functions. Blood 109(4):1422–1432

Pezelj-Ribaric S, Anic I, Brekalo I, Miletic I, Hasan M, Simunovic-Soskic M (2002) Detection of tumor necrosis factor alpha in normal and inflamed human dental pulps. Arch Med Res 33(5):482–484

Renard E, Gaudin A, Bienvenu G, Amiaud J, Farges JC, Cuturi MC, Moreau A, Alliot-Licht B (2016) Immune Cells and Molecular Networks in Experimentally Induced Pulpitis. J Dent Res 95(2):196–205

Rutherford RB, Gu K (2000) Treatment of inflamed ferret dental pulps with recombinant bone morphogenetic protein-7. Eur J Oral Sci 108(3):202–206

Saito K, Nakatomi M, Ida-Yonemochi H, Kenmotsu S, Ohshima H (2011) The expression of GM-CSF and osteopontin in immunocompetent cells precedes the odontoblast differentiation following allogenic tooth transplantation in mice. J Histochem Cytochem 59(5):518–529

Saraiva M, O'Garra A (2010) The regulation of IL-10 production by immune cells. Nat Rev Immunol 10(3):170–181

Schröder U (1985) Effects of calcium hydroxide-containing pulp-capping agents on pulp cell migration, proliferation, and differentiation. J Dent Res 64 (Spec No):541–548

Schröder U, Granath LE (1971) Early reaction of intact human teeth to calcium hydroxide following experimental pulpotomy and its significance to the development of hard tissue barrier. Odontol Revy 22(4):379–395

Semple F, Dorin JR (2012) β-Defensins: multifunctional modulators of infection, inflammation and more? J Innate Immun 4(4):337–348

Shiba H, Mouri Y, Komatsuzawa H et al (2003) Macrophage inflammatory protein-3alpha and beta-defensin-2 stimulate dentin sialophosphoprotein gene expression in human pulp cells. Biochem Biophys Res Commun 306(4):867–871

Silva TA, Lara VS, Silva JS, Garlet GP, Butler WT, Cunha FQ (2004) Dentin sialoprotein and phosphoprotein induce neutrophil recruitment: a mechanism dependent on IL-1beta, TNF-beta, and CXC chemokines. Calcif Tissue Int 74(6):532–541

Silva-Mendez LS, Allaker RP, Hardie JM, Benjamin N (1999) Antimicrobial effect of acidified nitrite on cariogenic bacteria. Oral Microbiol Immunol 14(6):391–392

Simon S, Smith AJ, Berdal A, Lumley PJ, Cooper PR (2010) The MAPK pathway is involved in tertiary reactionary dentinogenesis via p38 phosphorylation. J Endod 36(2):256–259

Simon SR, Berdal A, Cooper PR, Lumley PJ, Tomson PL, Smith AJ (2011) Dentin-pulp complex regeneration: from lab to clinic. Adv Dent Res 23(3):340–345

Smith KA, Lachman LB, Oppenheim JJ, Favata MF (1980) The functional relationship of the interleukins. J Exp Med 151(6):1551–1556

Smith AJ, Cassidy N, Perry H, Bègue-Kirn C, Ruch JV, Lesot H (1995) Reactionary dentinogenesis. Int J Dev Biol 39(1):273–280

Smith AJ, Patel M, Graham L, Sloan AJ, Cooper PR (2005) Dentin regeneration: key roles for stem cells and molecular signaling. Oral Biosci Med 2:127–132

Smith AJ, Scheven BA, Takahashi Y, Ferracane JL, Shelton RM, Cooper PR (2012) Dentin as a bioactive extracellular matrix. Arch Oral Biol 57(2):109–121

Song W, Shi Y, Xiao M et al (2009) In vitro bactericidal activity of recombinant human beta-defensin-3 against pathogenic bacterial strains in human tooth root canal. Int J Antimicrob Agents 33(3):237–243

Sørensen OE, Borregaard N, Cole AM (2008) Antimicrobial peptides in innate immune responses. Contrib Microbiol 15:61–77

Stanley H (2002) Calcium hydroxide and vital pulp therapy. In: Hargreaves KM, Goodis HE (eds) Seltzer and Bender's dental pulp. Quintessence, Chicago, IL, pp 309–324

Staquet MJ, Durand SH, Colomb E et al (2008) Different roles of odontoblasts and fibroblasts in immunity. J Dent Res 87(3):256–261

Tanoue T, Umesaki Y, Honda K (2010) Immune responses to gut microbiota-commensals and pathogens. Gut Microbes 1(4):224–233

Tomic S, Djokic J, Vasilijic S et al (2011) Immunomodulatory properties of mesenchymal stem cells derived from dental pulp and dental follicle are susceptible to activation by toll-like receptor agonists. Stem Cells Dev 20(4):695–708

Tomson PL, Grover LM, Lumley PJ, Sloan AJ, Smith AJ, Cooper PR (2007) Dissolution of bioactive dentin matrix components by mineral trioxide aggregate. J Dent 35(8):636–642

Turner MD, Nedjai B, Hurst T, Pennington DJ (2014) Cytokines and chemokines: at the crossroads of cell signalling and inflammatory disease. Biochim Biophys Acta 1843(11):2563–2582

Veerayutthwilai O, Byers MR, Pham TT, Darveau RP, Dale BA (2007) Differential regulation of immune responses by odontoblasts. Oral Microbiol Immunol 22(1):5–13

Viola A, Luster AD (2008) Chemokines and their receptors: drug targets in immunity and inflammation. Annu Rev Pharmacol Toxicol 48:171–197

Wang Y, Yan M, Fan Z, Ma L, Yu Y, Yu J (2014) Mineral trioxide aggregate enhances the odonto/osteogenic capacity of stem cells from inflammatory dental pulps via NF-κB pathway. Oral Dis 20(7):650–658

Wang Z, Ma F, Wang J et al (2015) Extracellular signal-regulated kinase mitogen-activated protein kinase and phosphatidylinositol 3-kinase/Akt signaling are required for lipopolysaccharide-mediated mineralization in murine odontoblast-like cells. J Endod 41(6):871–876

Yamada M, Kojima N, Paranjpe A et al (2008) N-acetyl cysteine (NAC)-assisted detoxification of PMMA resin. J Dent Res 87(4):372–377

Zhong S, Zhang S, Bair E, Nares S, Khan AA (2012) Differential expression of microRNAs in normal and inflamed human pulps. J Endod 38(6):746–752

Zudaire E, Portal-Núñez S, Cuttitta F (2006) The central role of adrenomedullin in host defense. J Leukoc Biol 80(2):237–244

Current and Future Views on Disinfection for Regenerative Strategies

7

Nikita B. Ruparel, Obadah N. Austah, and Anibal Diogenes

7.1   Introduction

Clinicians have routinely applied principles of tissue engineering in dentistry. Reconstruction of craniofacial structures after facial trauma or tumour resections, periodontal regeneration with the goal of regenerating bone in cases of edentulism or periodontal disease and dentine-pulp regeneration after various degrees of tooth infection are some such examples. A prerequisite to tissue engineering is a conducive healing environment, which is devoid of microbial colonisation and inflammation. Several lines of evidence suggest a suboptimal regenerative outcome due to persistent microbial infection. These include studies on bioengineering of skin, bone and dental tissues (Mansbridge 2008; Thomas and Puleo 2011; Yoshinari et al. 1998). Clinical outcomes of periodontal guided tissue regeneration (GTR), for example, show poor regenerative outcomes when an associated bacterial infection persists (Yoshinari et al. 1998; Sander and Karring 1995; Smith MacDonald et al. 1998; Trombelli et al. 1995). Therefore, measures to minimise microbial load by scaling and root planning and use of antimicrobials either locally or systemically are the first steps in creating an environment upon which bone regeneration

N. B. Ruparel (✉) · A. Diogenes
Department of Endodontics, University of Texas Health Science Center at San Antonio, San Antonio, TX, USA
e-mail: ruparel@uthscsa.edu; diogenes@uthscsa.edu

O. N. Austah
Department of Endodontics, University of Texas Health Science Center at San Antonio, San Antonio, TX, USA

Department of Endodontics, Faculty of Dentistry, King Abdulaziz University, Jeddah, Saudi Arabia
e-mail: austah@utexas.edu

© Springer Nature Switzerland AG 2019
H. F. Duncan, P. R. Cooper (eds.), *Clinical Approaches in Endodontic Regeneration*,
https://doi.org/10.1007/978-3-319-96848-3_7

can take place (Yoshinari et al. 2001; Nowzari et al. 1995; Zucchelli et al. 1999). This signifies that the presence of a resistant bacterial colony or a biofilm produces a self-perpetuating inflammatory environment that is detrimental to the process of wound healing. The rationale for the undesirable consequences lies directly with the effect of infection and inflammation on the critical players of regeneration and stem cells. Studies evaluating this phenomenon in oral stem cells have demonstrated that biofilms modulate several key functions of stem cells such as reduced migratory and differentiation capacities as well as altered differentiation fates (Ward et al. 2015; Kato et al. 2014; Morsczeck et al. 2012; Abe et al. 2010). Therefore, both an existing microbial infection and post-therapy infection can dramatically affect the clinical outcome of tissue engineering. This chapter will therefore discuss the role of adequate disinfection in the context of pulp-dentine regeneration.

Vital pulp therapies (VPTs) and regenerative endodontic procedures (REPs) are two commonly used procedures that rely heavily on principles of tissue engineering. The interplay between autologous stem cells, endogenous or exogenous scaffolds and signalling factors that guide regeneration are all players that underlie these treatment modalities. Interestingly, both treatment modalities also aim initially at microbial clearance. While cases treated with VPTs have a relatively low microbial load, the dental pulp of teeth requiring REPs has succumbed to microbial infection secondary to trauma, dental caries or developmental anomalies. REPs have gained significant momentum over the last decade and a half, as these procedures provide the unique opportunity for immature teeth to continue tooth development after pulp necrosis. Therefore, unlike VPTs where maintaining the vitality and health of the uninjured pulp with a biocompatible restorative material is an acceptable goal, in REPs, the goal is far reaching. In REPs, the goals include resolution of disease plus *regeneration*/recapitulation of the lost immunocompetent tissues as well as *generation* of undeveloped tissues such as completion of root development and its associated pulp. Therefore, the role and function of stem cells are far greater in REPs, and every measure must be taken to preserve their function. To this end, the preponderance of the available literature is based on restoring the pulp-dentine complex in the context of REPs used in a clinical setting.

Like all endodontic procedures, the first step in treating immature teeth with pulp necrosis is disinfection. Evidence on the nature of the bacterial flora commonly infecting an immature necrotic tooth is unavailable except for one study. This study (Nagata et al. 2014) identified *Actinomyces naeslundii* as the most prevalent species detected in 66% of root canals, followed by *Porphyromonas endodontalis*, *Parvimonas micra*, *Fusobacterium nucleatum* in 33.34% of root canals, *Porphyromonas gingivalis* and *Prevotella intermedia* in 26.27%, *Tannerella forsythia* in 20% and *Filifactor alocis* and *Treponema denticola* in 13.33%. The prevalence of these organisms is similar to primary infections in mature teeth (Gomes et al. 2007, 2006); however, the microbial contamination in both planktonic and biofilm forms can extend deeper into the inaccessible dentinal tubules in teeth of younger individuals compared to adults (Kakoli et al. 2009). Additionally, the complex anatomical structure of the root canal emphasises the difficulty in eradicating all existing biofilms (Nair et al. 2005). Furthermore, in REPs, the immature teeth present with relatively thin root walls pose limitations to the routinely used debridement protocol such as minimal to no mechanical instrumentation (Kontakiotis et al. 2015). Therefore, the debridement of the infected immature tooth relies greatly on chemical disinfection (Diogenes et al. 2014). Although lowering the threshold of bacteria may be sufficient in healing apical periodontitis in a tooth receiving traditional non-surgical root canal treatment (Siqueira Jr. and Rocas 2008), the presence of a residual biofilm in teeth receiving REPs may pose challenges to the process of regeneration.

Regenerative endodontic procedures can be described in three main steps: disinfection, evoked bleeding and restoration. Prior to 2011, disinfection protocols were employed for thorough debridement of the root canal system (Kontakiotis et al. 2015). However, with the knowledge that evoked bleeding populates the canal systems with increased number of stem cells from the periapical tissues (Lovelace et al. 2011; Chrepa et al. 2015), disinfection agents have been used with caution. Parameters such as disinfectant-induced toxicity to stem cells, function of stem cells as well as their role as dentine conditioners have been previously evaluated (Diogenes et al. 2014). A wide range of irrigants and intracanal medicaments have been used in REPs since 2001 (Fig. 7.1a, b). These data demonstrate that sodium hypochlorite (5.25–6% NaOCl) and full-strength triple antibiotic paste (TAP; 1000 mg/ml) are the most commonly used irrigant and intracanal medicament, respectively. Interestingly, data for every 5-year period from 2001 to 2017 demonstrate substantial changes in trends of various irrigants and medicaments reported for REPs (Fig. 7.2a, b). These changes represent a shift with the increased understanding of the biology of REPs as being stem cell-based therapies. The following subsections will discuss the recent findings and rationale for the observed change in trends.

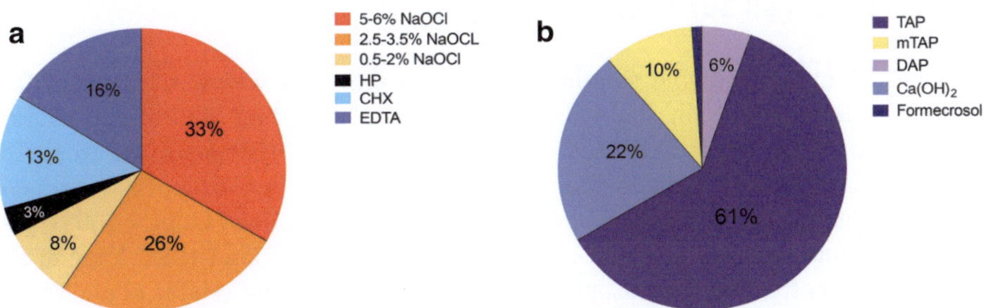

Fig. 7.1 Cumulative representation of various disinfectants used in regenerative endodontic procedures (REPs) from 2001 to 2017. (**a**) Pie chart representation of all the irrigants used in REPs since 2001 (NaOCl, sodium hypochlorite; HP, hydrogen peroxide; CHX, chlorhexidine gluconate; EDTA, ethylenediaminetetraacetic acid). (**b**) Pie chart repräsentation all the intracanal medicaments used in REPs since 2001 (TAP, triple antibiotic paste; DAP, double antibiotic paste; Ca(OH)$_2$, calcium hydroxide)

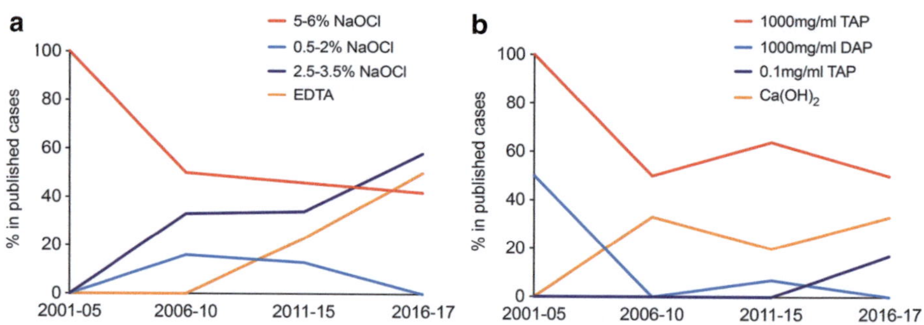

Fig. 7.2 Trends in use of disinfectants in REPs from 2001 to 2017. (**a**) Data representing changes in trends of commonly used irrigating solutions since 2001 (NaOCl, sodium hypochlorite; EDTA, ethylenediaminetetraacetic acid) and (**b**) data representing changes in trends of commonly used intracanal medicaments since 2001 (TAP, triple antibiotic paste; DAP, double antibiotic paste; $Ca(OH)_2$, calcium hydroxide)

7.2 Irrigants as Disinfectants Used in REPs

Irrigation is a critical step used not only in regenerative procedures but also in conventional endodontic therapies. The role of irrigation is manifold; disinfection and removal of disrupted biofilms detoxify bacterial antigens, remove intracanal medicaments and prepare the root surface for receipt of an obturation material (Buck et al. 2001; Oliveira et al. 2012). Therefore, solutions used to irrigate the root canal space (irrigants) are important armamentarium used by clinicians. Since little to no mechanical preparation is advisable, irrigation is the first step in disinfection in REPs. It is therefore imperative to discuss the role of commonly used irrigants on the factors that affect regeneration.

7.2.1 Stem Cell Survival and Attachment

Among the many available solutions, NaOCl is the most widely used agent for chemical debridement in endodontic procedures, including REPs (Fig. 7.1a) (Kontakiotis et al. 2015; Diogenes et al. 2013) and VPTs (Bimstein and Rotstein 2016). It has several desirable characteristics including (1) excellent bactericidal efficacy (Harrison et al. 1990; Vianna et al. 2006; Martinho and Gomes 2008), (2) tissue dissolution capacity (Hand et al. 1978; Harrison and Hand 1981; Yang et al. 1995) and (3) effective haemostatic agent when used topically (Hafez et al. 2002). These are beneficial properties for the disinfection of immature teeth in REPs and VPTs. In VPTs, due to the short duration of application, 5.25–6% NaOCl does not injure the pulp, causing only mild reactions in the most superficial layer of dentine (0.5 mm) (Rosenfeld et al. 1978) with no negative impact on the clinical outcome of these procedures (Akcay et al. 2015). However, unlike in VPTs these concentrations when used for REPs appear to negatively modify the root canal microenvironment reducing stem cell survival and attachment (Ring et al. 2008; Trevino et al. 2011). However, these detrimental effects of NaOCl appear to be concentration dependent. To this end, a study evaluating the effect of various NaOCl concentrations (6%, 3%, 1.5% and 0.5%) on stem cell survival demonstrated that dentine treated with NaOCl decreased stem cell survival in a concentration-dependent manner with 6% showing maximal cell death and 0.5–3% with moderately detrimental effects on the viability of the cells (Martin et al. 2012). These findings are in agreement with other studies demonstrating similar deleterious effects of using full-strength NaOCl (Galler et al. 2011). Additionally, these studies also shed light on the effect of 6% NaOCl on the physical properties of dentine. Dentine treated at this concentration appears to have "clastic" activity resulting in resorption of the dentine surface (Galler et al. 2011). Therefore, the dramatic effect on cell death appears to be the result of an indirect and long-lasting effect of sodium hypochlorite on the physical properties of dentine.

Another frequently used irrigant in endodontic procedures is 17% ethylenedi-aminetetraacetic acid (ETDA). Its role primarily lies within its calcium-chelating properties that allow for removal of the smear layer created on account of mechanical canal preparation. The chelating effect of EDTA also enhances the bactericidal properties of NaOCl due to better penetration of NaOCl into dentinal tubules (Bystrom and Sundqvist 1985). Studies evaluating the cytotoxicity of EDTA show minimal effects on the viability of stem cells (Trevino et al. 2011; Martin et al. 2012; Galler et al. 2015). Moreover, properties of EDTA appear to rescue the detrimental effects of NaOCl (Martin et al. 2012). These effects may be attributed to the unique properties of EDTA in conditioning the dentine surface. Dentine harbours large amounts of proteins beneficial for chemotaxis, attachment, survival and differentiation. Some examples of these include transforming growth factor beta (TGF-β), basic fibroblast growth factor (bFGF), vascular endothelial growth factor (VEGF), bone morphogenetic proteins (BMPs), insulin-like growth factor (IGF-1 and IGF-2), platelet-derived growth factor (PDGF), placenta growth factor (PIGF), hepatocyte growth factor (HGF) and epidermal growth factor (EGF) (Roberts-Clark and Smith 2000; Smith et al. 2012). Dentine conditioning is therefore considered as a critical step in REPs. The cell to cell interaction, cell-extracellular matrix molecule interaction and cell-growth factor interaction, together, provide for an ideal environment for stem cells to thrive and function on. Dentine conditioning therefore relies heavily on agents such as EDTA (Trevino et al. 2011; Martin et al. 2012; Galler et al. 2011, 2015; Smith et al. 2016) that expose the extracellular matrix (for cell adhesion) and promote the release of embedded bioactive molecules (Trevino et al. 2011; Martin et al. 2012; Galler et al. 2011, 2015). This property of EDTA maybe hypothesized for its rescue effects of NaOCl on stem cells. Of note, other irrigants used in clinical cases of REPs include hydrogen peroxide and chlorhexidine gluconate (CHX). CHX has also been used in VPT procedures. Available literature on the effects of these irrigants on regeneration is limited. Two percent CHX appears to be equally detrimental to stem cell survival. Despite the well-documented cytotoxic effects of chlorhexidine (Trevino et al. 2011; Lessa et al. 2010; de Souza et al. 2007), it appears that the reparative capacity of the dental pulp when capped with either calcium hydroxide or a bioceramic material is able to mitigate its cytotoxicity as it has been successfully used in VPT (Tuzuner et al. 2012). Interestingly, these effects are not reversed by 17% EDTA (Trevino et al. 2011). Moreover, CHX has been shown to reduce the thickness of the mineralised bridge induced by MTA (Manochehrifar et al. 2016), and it is important to mention that chlorhexidine does not have the tissue dissolution capability (Okino et al. 2004) or the haemostatic effect of NaOCl. Lastly, the use of chlorhexidine excludes the concomitant use with NaOCl, as a precipitate with strong cytotoxic effect is known to be formed when these two solutions interact (Basrani et al. 2007; Bui et al. 2008). Collectively, these studies suggest that the effects of CHX may also be concentration dependent, and future studies evaluating a permissible dose of CHX, or methodologies to inactivate CHX, may be useful for furthering disinfection while promoting regeneration.

7.2.2 Stem Cell Differentiation

Studies evaluating the differentiation potential of stem cells post irrigation of dentine with various irrigating solutions demonstrate that like the detrimental effects of NaOCl on cell survival, a 6% NaOCl concentration also alters the differentiation potential of mesenchymal stem cells (Martin et al. 2012; Casagrande et al. 2010). This concentration has been shown to result in complete abolishment of odontoblastic differentiation. On the other hand, a 1.5% NaOCl concentration does not alter odontoblastic differentiation of stem cells (Martin et al. 2012). Conversely, dentine conditioned with 17% EDTA favoured odontoblastic differentiation, absence of resorption and the intimate contact of cells, displaying an odontoblast-like phenotype in an ectopic in vivo growth model (Galler et al. 2011). Another study using a tooth slice model evaluating the expression of odontoblastic markers such as matrix extracellular phophoglycoprotein (MEPE), dentin matrix protein-1 (DMP-1) and dentin sialophosphoprotein (DSPP) demonstrated that tooth slices conditioned with 17% EDTA resulted in the significant increase in these markers, while treatment with NaOCl abolished this expression (Casagrande et al. 2010; Galler et al. 2016). Furthermore, similar to findings from survival studies, 17% EDTA also reverses the reduced differentiation potential of stem cells followed by higher concentrations of NaOCl (Martin et al. 2012). The beneficial effects of EDTA are once again attributed to its property of sequestering and resurfacing signalling molecules embedded in the dentin matrix for stem cell differentiation. Collectively, the studies described here support the use of 1.5% NaOCl for its dissolution and disinfecting capabilities followed by 17% EDTA as a final irrigant to promote stem cell survival, attachment and differentiation.

7.3 Intracanal Medicaments as Disinfectants Used in REPs

The second and final step in tooth debridement is placement of an intracanal medicament. This pharmacological intervention is an equally critical step in furthering disinfection prior to the ingress of stem cells into the canal system. Analogous to irrigation studies, considerable efforts have been made for intracanal medicaments to maximise disinfection without hindering the microenvironment required for tissue regeneration (Diogenes et al. 2014).

A combination drug regimen comprising of ciprofloxacin, metronidazole and minocycline has been popular in REPs (Kontakiotis et al. 2015). The triple antibiotic paste (TAP) combination was first studied to evaluate its antibacterial efficacy against endodontic pathogens (Hoshino et al. 1996; Sato et al. 1996, 1993). Since then, REPs have commonly employed this three antibiotic combination owing to the broad-spectrum efficacy of such drugs in a procedure that advocates little to no instrumentation. Several successful clinical cases have been reported demonstrating the applicability of TAP in REPs (Torabinejad et al. 2017). Other commonly used medicaments have been modifications to TAP such as the double antibiotic paste (DAP) with ciprofloxacin and metronidazole, calcium hydroxide ($Ca(OH)_2$) and CHX gel (Torabinejad et al. 2017). As stated throughout this chapter, the purpose of disinfection is twofold: (1) eliminate bacterial aetiology for resolution of pathology and (2) create a microenvironment that is conducive to stem cell function and regeneration. The following subsections will therefore discuss the effect of commonly used medications in REPs and VPT on parameters critical for regeneration.

7.3.1   Stem Cell Survival

Direct contact of stem cells with intracanal medicaments occurs in REPs as well as in VPT. Studies in regenerative endodontics for over half a decade have focused on the effect of various intracanal medicaments on stem cell survival (Diogenes et al. 2014). Therefore, the drug dose in contact with stem cells requires a thorough evaluation on its viability effects. In vitro (Ruparel et al. 2012) as well as ex vivo (Althumairy et al. 2014; Alghilan et al. 2017) studies evaluating the effect of antimicrobials on stem cell survival strongly suggest that the undiluted form (1000 mg/ml) of TAP, DAP, DAP + cefaclor and Augmentin is severely detrimental to stem cell survival. Early recommendations for the use of antibiotic drug concentrations for REPs hail from the notion that the higher the drug dose, the greater the bacteriostatic/bactericidal efficacy. However, it is well known that antibiotic drug dosages must be determined using the minimum inhibitory/bactericidal concentration (MIC or MBC) tests. Although it requires labour-intensive efforts to determine the MIC of a complex polymicrobial biofilm, early work by Hoshino and Sato highlighted that the antibacterial efficacy of TAP does not increase beyond 50–100 µg/ml against clinically acquired planktonic samples from acute and chronically inflamed roots (Hoshino et al. 1996; Sato et al. 1993, 1992). Moreover, with the exception of one study (Latham et al. 2016) that was conducted using a single species biofilm (*Enterococcus faecalis*), recent studies using a multispecies biofilm model have also demonstrated that increasing the dose of antimicrobials beyond 1000 µg/ml (1 mg/ml) does not increase efficacy (Jacobs et al. 2017; Albuquerque et al. 2017) against known endodontic pathogens. Additionally, owing to the inability to remove medicaments entirely from root canal systems (Akman et al. 2015), their residual antibacterial activity has also been evaluated. These studies indicate that antibiotics with low molecular weights such as ciprofloxacin and metronidazole can bind to dentine and therefore retain residual antibacterial effects that last up to 7–14 days after irrigation protocols (Sabrah et al. 2015). Moreover, here again, a 1 mg/ml concentration appeared to be significantly effective in eradicating a single species biofilm (Sabrah et al. 2015). Collectively, there is ample evidence that suggests that TAP/DAP at a 1 mg/ml concentration is optimal for antibacterial properties against endodontic pathogens (Jacobs et al. 2017; Albuquerque et al. 2017; Sabrah et al. 2015; Pankajakshan et al. 2016). Moreover, in vitro as well as ex vivo studies using 1 mg/ml TAP or DAP demonstrate >60% survival of SCAP (Ruparel et al. 2012; Althumairy et al. 2014). Interestingly, the use of $Ca(OH)_2$ has also shown favourable outcomes with stem cell survival at commercially available doses in vitro (Chen et al. 2016) as well as in vivo (Ji et al. 2010). Not surprisingly, clinicians for decades have successfully used $Ca(OH)_2$ formulations with antibacterial and regenerative properties as a pulp capping material in VPT. Overall, the available literature although mostly describing in vitro studies provides some guidelines for the use of medicaments with respect to maintaining stem cell survival.

7.3.2 Stem Cell Attachment

Another critical factor for favourable regeneration is attachment of stem cells to extracellular matrix (ECM). This is an essential property of a surface by which adsorbent proteins facilitate cell attachment, which in turn enables spread, migration and proliferation of cells. This rudimentary property of ECMs is a prerequisite to stem cell differentiation. Cell-to-ECM interactions are primary mediated by membrane expression of attachment proteins called integrins or high-molecular-weight glycoproteins, namely, fibronectin (Frantz et al. 2010). Conceivably, factors that negatively affect this interaction must be minimised in order to reduce loss of stem cell function. Dentine is composed of organic collagenous proteins and inorganic hydroxyapatite (HA) serves as an ECM for stem cells attachment. Furthermore, serum proteins from patients own blood stimulates cell attachment significantly (Sawyer et al. 2005; Kilpadi et al. 2004). Both VPT and REPs involve direct contact of stem cells with such proteins from pulpal blood and periapical blood, respectively. These proteins coat the dentinal surface making HA an already existing ECM for stem cells. Disinfectants such as TAP and $Ca(OH)_2$ have been implicated in modifying HA surface. While TAP at 1000 mg/ml concentration alters dentine surface to significantly reduce its microhardness (Alghilan et al. 2017; Yassen et al. 2015), dentine treated with 1 mg/ml TAP and $Ca(OH)_2$ does not reduce its microhardness or chemical integrity (Yassen et al. 2015; Yilmaz et al. 2016). Furthermore, it is well established that dentine conditioned with $Ca(OH)_2$ has been shown to release bioactive molecules, including chemoattractants (Graham et al. 2006). Dentine-mediated chemotaxis can strongly facilitate cellular migration and attachment (Galler et al. 2016). Supporting evidence for these hypotheses suggests that clinically used TAP at 1000 mg/ml abolishes cell attachment likely due to low survivability as stated before (Yassen et al. 2015). However, lower concentrations at 100 µg/ml have no damaging effects on cell attachment (Yassen et al. 2015). Interestingly, Ca(OH)$_2$ treated dentine surfaces appear to promote cell attachment with increased fibronectin-expressing cells (Kitikuson and Srisuwan 2016). Moreover, cellular morphology of these cells appears to be spindle shaped with long cytoplasmic processes, classical of stem cell phenotype (Kitikuson and Srisuwan 2016). The beneficial effects of Ca(OH)$_2$ are not surprising as previous in vitro work demonstrates increased proliferation of stem cells at 1 mg/ml Ca(OH)$_2$ concentration, potentially due to upregulation of transcription factors such as phosphoERK (Ji et al. 2010). While one study demonstrates high mesenchymal stem cell (MSC) attachment to dentine surface following Ca(OH)$_2$ treatment, another study showed opposing results (Alghilan et al. 2017). Such discrepancies are likely seen due to the different assays being employed for cell attachment. On the other hand, there is consensus that lower concentrations of TAP at 1 mg/ml promote MSC attachment (Alghilan et al. 2017; Kitikuson and Srisuwan 2016). These studies have been critical in framing the currently recommended and still evolving REP protocol.

7.3.3 Stem Cell Differentiation

Dental stem cells represent a unique source of cells that have the multipotency of differentiating into many of the craniofacial tissues. They have been traced to a neural crest origin and have the ability to form mesenchymal tissues such as the bone, cartilage, connective tissue, dental pulp and dentine. These cells can also differentiate into ectodermal derivatives such as neurons and glia. This makes cells of dental neural crest origin a great resource for tooth regeneration. Not surprisingly, therefore, the majority of the existing literature is available on dental pulp stem cells (DPSCs), stem cells from exfoliated deciduous teeth (SHED) and stem cells of apical papilla (SCAP). An ideal outcome for regeneration in REP is *replacement* of lost structures as well as continuation of tooth development, which was arrested due to premature pulp necrosis. Conceivably, cases of immature teeth should be considered a critical size defect (Huang and Garcia-Godoy 2014) which is much larger than one that is encountered in cases of VPT. Moreover, unlike VPT, REP procedures do not have existing pulp architecture to facilitate stem cell differentiation and regeneration. Another equally challenging barrier to stem cell differentiation is chronic bacterial infection and the presence of a plethora of microbial antigens seen with pulp necrosis and REPs. The role of disinfection in stem cell differentiation is therefore critical to outcomes of REPs.

Although lowering the threshold of bacteria via chemomechanical debridement may be sufficient in healing apical periodontitis in a tooth receiving traditional non-surgical root canal treatment (Siqueira Jr. and Rocas 2008), the presence of a biofilm in REPs may pose challenges not yet fully understood. Since the majority of REPs involve little to no mechanical debridement of the canal system (Kontakiotis et al. 2015), it is likely that bacteria are incompletely removed. Indeed, animal studies performed in dogs (Windley 3rd et al. 2005) and ferrets (Verma et al. 2017) showed 30–50% of teeth harboured planktonic as well as biofilm structures on the canal walls post-treatment with 1.25% NaOCl and full-strength TAP at a dose of 1000 mg/ml. Moreover, recently published work demonstrate that incompletely removed bacterial biofilm can shift stem cell differentiation into an osteoblastic phenotype over a dentinogenic phenotype (Vishwanat et al. 2017). Another in vivo animal study demonstrated the direct correlation of presence of bacteria and inflammation with lack of dentine-like tissues on canal walls (Verma et al. 2017). Additionally, histological outcomes of human teeth treated with REPs with necrotic pulps demonstrate non-dentine-like mineralised structures within the canal walls/space (Lin et al. 2014; Martin et al. 2013; Shimizu et al. 2013; Lei et al. 2015; Meschi et al. 2016). These studies suggest lack of optimal stem cell differentiation post-REPs and a strong correlation between the presence of bacterial biofilm and the persistence of microbial antigens that are capable of altering the histological outcomes (Fig. 7.3a, b).

The microbial influence on stem cells can be speculated on two levels: direct and indirect. Direct mechanisms involve the effects of bacterial toxins on stem cell

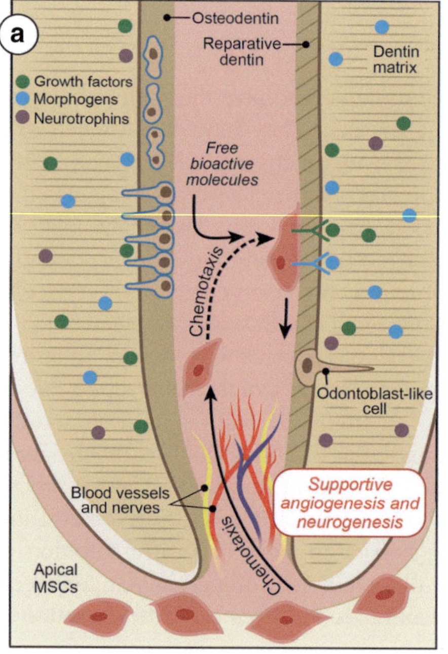

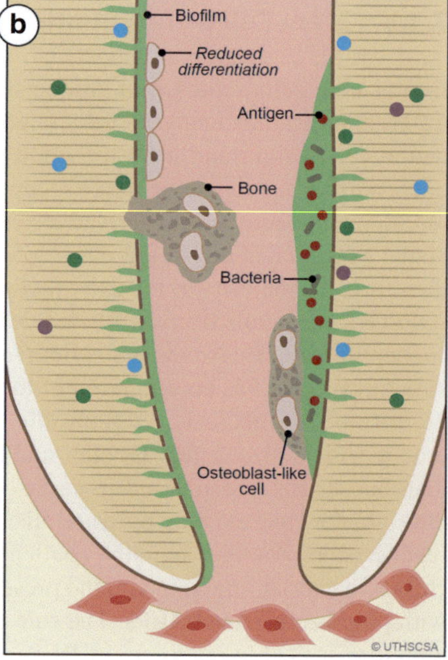

Fig. 7.3 Schematic illustration of tissue engineering after REPs. (**a**) Schematic representation demonstrating ideal histological outcomes post adequate disinfection. Dentine devoid of bacterial colonisation promotes regeneration of dentine-like tissue (osteodentine) lined with newly differentiated odontoblasts-like cells, angiogenesis and neurogenesis. (**b**) Schematic representation demonstrating altered histological outcomes post-inadequate disinfection. Dentine contaminated with either a residual biofilm or residual microbial antigens causes reduced differentiation, altered differentiation in the form of osteoblast-like cells and ectopic tissue formation such as the bone within the intracanal space

differentiation (Ward et al. 2015; Kato et al. 2014; Morsczeck et al. 2012; Abe et al. 2010), while indirect mechanisms involve the effect of bacterial degradation enzymes on signalling molecules required for stem cell differentiation. A study evaluating the direct effects strongly suggests that microbial byproducts can significantly hinder the mineralising phenotype of stem cells (Vishwanat et al. 2017). Indirect mechanisms are equally crucial for investigation as multiple studies demonstrate growth factor release to be a major modulator of stem cell differentiation. Although the ideal cocktail of growth factors required for tooth regeneration is not well known and neither are their specific concentrations, growth factor release from dentine is of utmost importance in regeneration. To this end, studies evaluating the effect of bacterial enzymes on growth factors have demonstrated over 45–60% degradation of growth factors such as platelet-derived growth factor (PDGF), granulocyte macrophage colony-stimulating factor (GM-CSF), transforming growth factor-β (TGF-β) and basic fibroblast growth factor (FGF) (Payne et al. 2002; Slomiany et al. 1996). This effect appears to be a concerted effect of increase in bacterial proteases and bacteria-mediated increase in host matrix metalloproteinases (MMPs) in addition to a decrease in tissue inhibitors of MMPs (Robson 1997; Stadelmann et al. 1998; Chen et al. 1997). Moreover, many of the studied growth factors such as GM-CSF, basic FGF and TGF-β are also molecules that are present in dentine matrix and are crucial for stem cell chemotaxis and migration as well as stem cell differentiation into cells forming mineralised tissues, endothelial cells and connective tissues, respectively. However, the existing literature in the field of dentistry has not evaluated these indirect effects, which represents a significant gap in knowledge.

7.3.3.1 Challenges and Strategies to Improve Disinfection

Clinical examples of failed REPs due to persistent infection and/or lack of significant root development have been reported (Lin et al. 2014; Pinto et al. 2017; Alobaid et al. 2014; Saoud et al. 2014). Moreover, with the exception of one report (Shimizu et al. 2012), the majority of hard tissue histological analyses indicate osteoid- or bone-like and/or cementoid- or cementum-like tissue formation in the regenerated section of REP teeth (Lin et al. 2014; Martin et al. 2013; Shimizu et al. 2013; Lei et al. 2015; Meschi et al. 2016). Thus, dentine formation is not a common outcome. Analyses of preoperative diagnoses of these teeth revealed that all had a diagnosis of pulpal necrosis with either symptomatic apical periodontitis or acute or chronic apical abscess (Fouad and Verma 2014). Moreover, several animal studies have also demonstrated that infected necrotic pulps treated with REP show bone- and cementum-like hard tissue in preference to dentine (Verma et al. 2017; Lei et al. 2015; Zhu et al. 2012, 2013; Torabinejad et al. 2015; Zhang et al. 2014). On the other hand, REPs performed in teeth with vital pulps, in either human (Shimizu et al. 2012; Peng et al. 2017) or animal studies (Kodonas et al. 2012; Iohara et al. 2011; Huang et al. 2010), show promising results. For example, Shimizu and colleagues (Shimizu et al. 2012) and Peng and colleagues (Peng et al. 2017) reported that a REP-treated tooth with a diagnosis of irreversible pulpitis exhibited flattened odontoblast-like cells lining the predentine. Collectively, these studies imply that residual bacteria/biofilm may be detrimental to the ideal fate of stem cells in REPs.

Data on microbial flora commonly infecting immature necrotic teeth is largely unavailable. Findings from a recent study however suggest that the microbial profile of these organisms appears to be similar to that of primary infections in mature teeth (Gomes et al. 2007, 2006). However, the lack of a substantial number of studies precludes the appropriate microbial targeting for disinfection. Antimicrobial efficacy of 16 commonly used antibiotics of known drug classes showed only two antibiotics, namely, Augmentin and tigecycline, having 100% efficacy against all 24 tested endodontic pathogens (Jungermann et al. 2011). Moreover, drugs such as metronidazole used in TAP and clindamycin showed least efficacy (Jungermann et al. 2011). Corroborating findings of this study, another study also revealed high bactericidal efficacy of Augmentin and low bacteriostatic efficacy of metronidazole (Baumgartner and Xia 2003). So far, there are no clinical cases using Augmentin in the literature, and cases with TAP appear to have high success rate; however, in refractory REP cases with persistent infection or lack of root development, drugs such as Augmentin could potentially improve clinical outcomes.

Another strategy to improve disinfection is to increase the residual antimicrobial effects of antibiotics and detoxification of antigens from dentine. To facilitate such mechanisms in the intracanal system, the use of scaffolding matrices is being tested. Photoactivated rose bengal-functionalized chitosan nanoparticles are scaffolds that use light to activate photosensitizers such as rose bengal for detoxification of byproducts including lipopolysaccharide (LPS) (Shrestha et al. 2015). Other strategies include TAP-functionalized polydioxanone (PDS) nanofibers. PDS nanofibers have a unique property of an initial burst release of the drug followed by a sustained action for up to 14 days. In vitro studies using a PDS with 1 mg/ml TAP show excellent antibacterial effects against a dual and multispecies biofilm (Albuquerque et al. 2017; Pankajakshan et al. 2016). These modifications also give body to the diluted form of the drugs, thereby facilitating easy delivery into the canal system.

The technique used to deliver irrigants into root canals also plays an important role in disinfection by providing better distribution, greater evacuation of debris and disruption of microbial biofilms. Sophisticated techniques such as apical negative pressure (EndoVac; KerrEndo, Orange County, CA) irrigation have been advocated for its superior disinfection and safety properties (Desai and Himel 2009; Hockett et al. 2008). However, a study comparing bacterial counts in immature dog teeth after use of EndoVac versus conventional positive-pressure needle irrigation along with TAP failed to demonstrates a significant difference in bacterial reduction between the two irrigation methods (EndoVac group (88.6%) versus conventional irrigation (78.28%)) (Cohenca et al. 2010). However, evaluation of the tissues formed following the regenerative/revascularisation procedures suggested that EndoVac-assisted irrigation promoted better formation of connective tissue, blood vessels and mineralised masses while displaying less inflammatory cells than conventional irrigation group (da Silva et al. 2010). Thus, it appears that adjuvants in irrigation may provide greater benefit than routine positive-pressure needle irrigation.

Although passive ultrasonic or sonic irrigation (Virdee et al. 2018) has not been widely used in regenerative procedures, they have well-documented benefits in the debridement of root canals (Virdee et al. 2018; van der Sluis et al. 2007). This kind of irrigation is particularly suited for REPs due to the lack of mechanical preparation of the dentinal walls. Gentle mechanical disruption of biofilms (circumferential filing with a hand file) and activation of irrigation solutions by sonic (Mancini et al. 2013) or ultrasonic energy may maximise both biofilm disruption and removal. Overall, these approaches appear to have a multifunctional and promising role for enhancement of disinfection.

Conclusions

Appropriate stem cell function is a central tenet in tissue engineering. The field of dentistry routinely applies the concepts of tissue engineering in therapies such as GTR, VPT and REP. With increasing evidence for the role of microorganisms in pulpal inflammation, disinfection becomes a critical modulator of regeneration. Measures to minimise microbial load to maximise stem cell function must be incorporated into regenerative therapies. Owing to the high rate of tooth loss (Garcia-Godoy and Murray 2012) in younger populations due to premature necrosis, therapies such as REPs must be furthered and optimised to minimise a tooth loss epidemic.

Acknowledgements *Disclosure*: The authors deny any conflict of interest related to this work.

References

Abe S, Imaizumi M, Mikami Y, Wada Y, Tsuchiya S, Irie S et al (2010) Oral bacterial extracts facilitate early osteogenic/dentinogenic differentiation in human dental pulp-derived cells. Oral Surg Oral Med Oral Pathol Oral Radiol Endod 109(1):149–154

Akcay M, Sari S, Duruturk L, Gunhan O (2015) Effects of sodium hypoclorite as disinfectant material previous to pulpotomies in primary teeth. Clin Oral Investig 19(4):803–811

Akman M, Akbulut MB, Aydinbelge HA, Belli S (2015) Comparison of different irrigation activation regimens and conventional irrigation techniques for the removal of modified triple antibiotic paste from root canals. J Endod 41(5):720–724

Albuquerque MTP, Nagata J, Bottino MC (2017) Antimicrobial efficacy of triple antibiotic-eluting polymer nanofibers against multispecies biofilm. J Endod 43(9S):S51–SS6

Alghilan MA, Windsor LJ, Palasuk J, Yassen GH (2017) Attachment and proliferation of dental pulp stem cells on dentine treated with different regenerative endodontic protocols. Int Endod J 50(7):667–675

Alobaid AS, Cortes LM, Lo J, Nguyen TT, Albert J, Abu-Melha AS et al (2014) Radiographic and clinical outcomes of the treatment of immature permanent teeth by revascularization or apexification: a pilot retrospective cohort study. J Endod 40(8):1063–1070

Althumairy RI, Teixeira FB, Diogenes A (2014) Effect of dentin conditioning with intracanal medicaments on survival of stem cells of apical papilla. J Endod 40(4):521–525

Basrani BR, Manek S, Sodhi RN, Fillery E, Manzur A (2007) Interaction between sodium hypochlorite and chlorhexidine gluconate. J Endod 33(8):966–969

Baumgartner JC, Xia T (2003) Antibiotic susceptibility of bacteria associated with endodontic abscesses. J Endod 29(1):44–47

Bimstein E, Rotstein I (2016) Cvek pulpotomy - revisited. Dent Traumatol 32(6):438–442

Buck RA, Cai J, Eleazer PD, Staat RH, Hurst HE (2001) Detoxification of endotoxin by endodontic irrigants and calcium hydroxide. J Endod 27(5):325–327

Bui TB, Baumgartner JC, Mitchell JC (2008) Evaluation of the interaction between sodium hypochlorite and chlorhexidine gluconate and its effect on root dentin. J Endod 34(2):181–185

Bystrom A, Sundqvist G (1985) The antibacterial action of sodium hypochlorite and EDTA in 60 cases of endodontic therapy. Int Endod J 18(1):35–40

Casagrande L, Demarco FF, Zhang Z, Araujo FB, Shi S, Nor JE (2010) Dentin-derived BMP-2 and odontoblast differentiation. J Dent Res 89(6):603–608

Chen SM, Ward SI, Olutoye OO, Diegelmann RF, Kelman Cohen I (1997) Ability of chronic wound fluids to degrade peptide growth factors is associated with increased levels of elastase activity and diminished levels of proteinase inhibitors. Wound Repair Regen 5(1):23–32

Chen L, Zheng L, Jiang J, Gui J, Zhang L, Huang Y et al (2016) Calcium hydroxide-induced proliferation, migration, osteogenic differentiation, and mineralization via the mitogen-activated protein kinase pathway in human dental pulp stem cells. J Endod 42(9):1355–1361

Chrepa V, Henry MA, Daniel BJ, Diogenes A (2015) Delivery of apical mesenchymal stem cells into root canals of mature teeth. J Dent Res 94(12):1653–1659

Cohenca N, Heilborn C, Johnson JD, Flores DS, Ito IY, da Silva LA (2010) Apical negative pressure irrigation versus conventional irrigation plus triantibiotic intracanal dressing on root canal disinfection in dog teeth. Oral Surg Oral Med Oral Pathol Oral Radiol Endod 109(1):e42–e46

van der Sluis LW, Versluis M, Wu MK, Wesselink PR (2007) Passive ultrasonic irrigation of the root canal: a review of the literature. Int Endod J 40(6):415–426

Desai P, Himel V (2009) Comparative safety of various intracanal irrigation systems. J Endod 35(4):545–549

Diogenes A, Henry MA, Teixeira FB, Hargreaves KM (2013) An update on clinical regenerative endodontics. Endod Topics 28(1):2–23

Diogenes AR, Ruparel NB, Teixeira FB, Hargreaves KM (2014) Translational science in disinfection for regenerative endodontics. J Endod 40(4 Suppl):S52–S57

Fouad AF, Verma P (2014) Healing after regenerative procedures with and without pulpal infection. J Endod 40(4 Suppl):S58–S64

Frantz C, Stewart KM, Weaver VM (2010) The extracellular matrix at a glance. J Cell Sci 123(Pt 24):4195–4200

Galler KM, D'Souza RN, Federlin M, Cavender AC, Hartgerink JD, Hecker S et al (2011) Dentin conditioning codetermines cell fate in regenerative endodontics. J Endod 37(11):1536–1541

Galler KM, Buchalla W, Hiller KA, Federlin M, Eidt A, Schiefersteiner M et al (2015) Influence of root canal disinfectants on growth factor release from dentin. J Endod 41(3):363–368

Galler KM, Widbiller M, Buchalla W, Eidt A, Hiller KA, Hoffer PC et al (2016) EDTA conditioning of dentine promotes adhesion, migration and differentiation of dental pulp stem cells. Int Endod J 49(6):581–590

Garcia-Godoy F, Murray PE (2012) Recommendations for using regenerative endodontic procedures in permanent immature traumatized teeth. Dent Traumatol 28(1):33–41

Gomes BP, Jacinto RC, Pinheiro ET, Sousa EL, Zaia AA, Ferraz CC et al (2006) Molecular analysis of Filifactor alocis, Tannerella forsythia, and treponema denticola associated with primary endodontic infections and failed endodontic treatment. J Endod 32(10):937–940

Gomes BP, Montagner F, Jacinto RC, Zaia AA, Ferraz CC, Souza-Filho FJ (2007) Polymerase chain reaction of Porphyromonas gingivalis, Treponema denticola, and Tannerella forsythia in primary endodontic infections. J Endod 33(9):1049–1052

Graham L, Cooper PR, Cassidy N, Nor JE, Sloan AJ, Smith AJ (2006) The effect of calcium hydroxide on solubilisation of bio-active dentine matrix components. Biomaterials 27(14): 2865–2873

Hafez AA, Cox CF, Tarim B, Otsuki M, Akimoto N (2002) An in vivo evaluation of hemorrhage control using sodium hypochlorite and direct capping with a one- or two-component adhesive system in exposed nonhuman primate pulps. Quintessence Int 33(4):261–272

Hand RE, Smith ML, Harrison JW (1978) Analysis of the effect of dilution on the necrotic tissue dissolution property of sodium hypochlorite. J Endod 4(2):60–64

Harrison JW, Hand RE (1981) The effect of dilution and organic matter on the anti-bacterial property of 5.25% sodium hypochlorite. J Endod 7(3):128–132

Harrison JW, Wagner GW, Henry CA (1990) Comparison of the antimicrobial effectiveness of regular and fresh scent Clorox. J Endod 16(7):328–330

Hockett JL, Dommisch JK, Johnson JD, Cohenca N (2008) Antimicrobial efficacy of two irrigation techniques in tapered and nontapered canal preparations: an in vitro study. J Endod 34(11):1374–1377

Hoshino E, Kurihara-Ando N, Sato I, Uematsu H, Sato M, Kota K et al (1996) In-vitro antibacterial susceptibility of bacteria taken from infected root dentine to a mixture of ciprofloxacin, metronidazole and minocycline. Int Endod J 29(2):125–130

Huang GT, Garcia-Godoy F (2014) Missing concepts in de novo pulp regeneration. J Dent Res 93(8):717–724

Huang GT, Yamaza T, Shea LD, Djouad F, Kuhn NZ, Tuan RS et al (2010) Stem/progenitor cell-mediated de novo regeneration of dental pulp with newly deposited continuous layer of dentin in an in vivo model. Tissue Eng Part A 16(2):605–615

Iohara K, Imabayashi K, Ishizaka R, Watanabe A, Nabekura J, Ito M et al (2011) Complete pulp regeneration after pulpectomy by transplantation of CD105+ stem cells with stromal cell-derived factor-1. Tissue Eng Part A 17(15-16):1911–1920

Jacobs JC, Troxel A, Ehrlich Y, Spolnik K, Bringas JS, Gregory RL et al (2017) Antibacterial effects of antimicrobials used in regenerative endodontics against biofilm bacteria obtained from mature and immature teeth with necrotic pulps. J Endod 43(4):575–579

Ji YM, Jeon SH, Park JY, Chung JH, Choung YH, Choung PH (2010) Dental stem cell therapy with calcium hydroxide in dental pulp capping. Tissue Eng Part A 16(6):1823–1833

Jungermann GB, Burns K, Nandakumar R, Tolba M, Venezia RA, Fouad AF (2011) Antibiotic resistance in primary and persistent endodontic infections. J Endod 37(10):1337–1344

Kakoli P, Nandakumar R, Romberg E, Arola D, Fouad AF (2009) The effect of age on bacterial penetration of radicular dentin. J Endod 35(1):78–81

Kato H, Taguchi Y, Tominaga K, Umeda M, Tanaka A (2014) Porphyromonas gingivalis LPS inhibits osteoblastic differentiation and promotes pro-inflammatory cytokine production in human periodontal ligament stem cells. Arch Oral Biol 59(2):167–175

Kilpadi KL, Sawyer AA, Prince CW, Chang PL, Bellis SL (2004) Primary human marrow stromal cells and Saos-2 osteosarcoma cells use different mechanisms to adhere to hydroxylapatite. J Biomed Mater Res A 68((2):273–285

Kitikuson P, Srisuwan T (2016) Attachment ability of human apical papilla cells to root dentin surfaces treated with either 3mix or calcium hydroxide. J Endod 42(1):89–94

Kodonas K, Gogos C, Papadimitriou S, Kouzi-Koliakou K, Tziafas D (2012) Experimental formation of dentin-like structure in the root canal implant model using cryopreserved swine dental pulp progenitor cells. J Endod 38(7):913–919

Kontakiotis EG, Filippatos CG, Tzanetakis GN, Agrafioti A (2015) Regenerative endodontic therapy: a data analysis of clinical protocols. J Endod 41(2):146–154

Latham J, Fong H, Jewett A, Johnson JD, Paranjpe A (2016) Disinfection efficacy of current regenerative endodontic protocols in simulated necrotic immature permanent teeth. J Endod 42(8):1218–1225

Lei L, Chen Y, Zhou R, Huang X, Cai Z (2015) Histologic and immunohistochemical findings of a human immature permanent tooth with apical periodontitis after regenerative endodontic treatment. J Endod 41(7):1172–1179

Lessa FC, Aranha AM, Nogueira I, Giro EM, Hebling J, Costa CA (2010) Toxicity of chlorhexidine on odontoblast-like cells. J Appl Oral Sci 18(1):50–58

Lin LM, Shimizu E, Gibbs JL, Loghin S, Ricucci D (2014) Histologic and histobacteriologic observations of failed revascularization/revitalization therapy: a case report. J Endod 40(2):291–295

Lovelace TW, Henry MA, Hargreaves KM, Diogenes A (2011) Evaluation of the delivery of mesenchymal stem cells into the root canal space of necrotic immature teeth after clinical regenerative endodontic procedure. J Endod 37(2):133–138

Mancini M, Cerroni L, Iorio L, Armellin E, Conte G, Cianconi L (2013) Smear layer removal and canal cleanliness using different irrigation systems (EndoActivator, EndoVac, and passive ultrasonic irrigation): field emission scanning electron microscopic evaluation in an in vitro study. J Endod 39(11):1456–1460

Manochehrifar H, Parirokh M, Kakooei S, Oloomi MM, Asgary S, Eghbal MJ et al (2016) The effect of mineral trioxide aggregate mixed with chlorhexidine as direct pulp capping agent in dogs teeth: a histologic study. Iranian Endod J 11(4):320–324

Mansbridge J (2008) Skin tissue engineering. J Biomater Sci Polym Ed 19(8):955–968

Martin DE, Henry MA, Almeida JFA, Teixeira FB, Hargreaves KM, Diogenes AR (2012) Effect of sodium hypochlorite on the odontoblastic phenotype differentiation of SCAP in cultured organotype human roots. J Endod 38(3):e26

Martin G, Ricucci D, Gibbs JL, Lin LM (2013) Histological findings of revascularized/revitalized immature permanent molar with apical periodontitis using platelet-rich plasma. J Endod 39(1):138–144

Martinho FC, Gomes BP (2008) Quantification of endotoxins and cultivable bacteria in root canal infection before and after chemomechanical preparation with 2.5% sodium hypochlorite. J Endod 34(3):268–272

Meschi N, Hilkens P, Lambrichts I, Van den Eynde K, Mavridou A, Strijbos O et al (2016) Regenerative endodontic procedure of an infected immature permanent human tooth: an immunohistological study. Clin Oral Investig 20(4):807–814

Morsczeck CO, Drees J, Gosau M (2012) Lipopolysaccharide from Escherichia coli but not from Porphyromonas gingivalis induce pro-inflammatory cytokines and alkaline phosphatase in dental follicle cells. Arch Oral Biol 57(12):1595–1601

Nagata JY, Soares AJ, Souza-Filho FJ, Zaia AA, Ferraz CC, Almeida JF et al (2014) Microbial evaluation of traumatized teeth treated with triple antibiotic paste or calcium hydroxide with 2% chlorhexidine gel in pulp revascularization. J Endod 40(6):778–783

Nair PN, Henry S, Cano V, Vera J (2005) Microbial status of apical root canal system of human mandibular first molars with primary apical periodontitis after "one-visit" endodontic treatment. Oral Surg Oral Med Oral Pathol Oral Radiol Endod 99(2):231–252

Nowzari H, Matian F, Slots J (1995) Periodontal pathogens on polytetrafluoroethylene membrane for guided tissue regeneration inhibit healing. J Clin Periodontol 22(6):469–474

Okino LA, Siqueira EL, Santos M, Bombana AC, Figueiredo JA (2004) Dissolution of pulp tissue by aqueous solution of chlorhexidine digluconate and chlorhexidine digluconate gel. Int Endod J 37(1):38–41

Oliveira LD, Carvalho CA, Carvalho AS, Alves Jde S, Valera MC, Jorge AO (2012) Efficacy of endodontic treatment for endotoxin reduction in primarily infected root canals and evaluation of cytotoxic effects. J Endod 38(8):1053–1057

Pankajakshan D, Albuquerque MT, Evans JD, Kamocka MM, Gregory RL, Bottino MC (2016) Triple antibiotic polymer nanofibers for intracanal drug delivery: effects on dual species biofilm and cell function. J Endod 42(10):1490–1495

Payne WG, Wright TE, Ko F, Wang X, Robson MC (2002) Bacterial degradation of growth factor. J Appl Res Clin Exp Therap 3(1)

Peng C, Zhao Y, Wang W, Yang Y, Qin M, Ge L (2017) Histologic findings of a human immature revascularized/regenerated tooth with symptomatic irreversible pulpitis. J Endod 43(6):905–909

Pinto N, Harnish A, Cabrera C, Andrade C, Druttman T, Brizuela C (2017) An innovative regenerative endodontic procedure using leukocyte and platelet-rich fibrin associated with apical surgery: a case report. J Endod 43(11):1828–1834

Ring KC, Murray PE, Namerow KN, Kuttler S, Garcia-Godoy F (2008) The comparison of the effect of endodontic irrigation on cell adherence to root canal dentin. J Endod 34(12):1474–1479

Roberts-Clark DJ, Smith AJ (2000) Angiogenic growth factors in human dentine matrix. Arch Oral Biol 45(11):1013–1016

Robson MC (1997) Wound infection. A failure of wound healing caused by an imbalance of bacteria. Surg Clin North Am 77(3):637–650

Rosenfeld EF, James GA, Burch BS (1978) Vital pulp tissue response to sodium hypochlorite. J Endod 4(5):140–146

Ruparel NB, Teixeira FB, Ferraz CC, Diogenes A (2012) Direct effect of intracanal medicaments on survival of stem cells of the apical papilla. J Endod 38(10):1372–1375

Sabrah AH, Yassen GH, Spolnik KJ, Hara AT, Platt JA, Gregory RL (2015) Evaluation of residual antibacterial effect of human radicular dentin treated with triple and double antibiotic pastes. J Endod 41(7):1081–1084

Sander L, Karring T (1995) New attachment and bone formation in periodontal defects following treatment of submerged roots with guided tissue regeneration. J Clin Periodontol 22(4):295–299

Saoud TM, Zaazou A, Nabil A, Moussa S, Lin LM, Gibbs JL (2014) Clinical and radiographic outcomes of traumatized immature permanent necrotic teeth after revascularization/revitalization therapy. J Endod 40(12):1946–1952

Sato T, Hoshino E, Uematsu H, Kota K, Iwaku M, Noda T (1992) Bactericidal efficacy of a mixture of ciprofloxacin, metronidazole, minocycline and rifampicin against bacteria of carious and endodontic lesions of human deciduous teeth in vitro. Microbial Ecol Health Dis 5(4):171–177

Sato T, Hoshino E, Uematsu H, Noda T (1993) In vitro antimicrobial susceptibility to combinations of drugs of bacteria from carious and endodontic lesions of human deciduous teeth. Oral Microbiol Immunol 8(3):172–176

Sato I, Ando-Kurihara N, Kota K, Iwaku M, Hoshino E (1996) Sterilization of infected root-canal dentine by topical application of a mixture of ciprofloxacin, metronidazole and minocycline in situ. Int Endod J 29(2):118–124

Sawyer AA, Hennessy KM, Bellis SL (2005) Regulation of mesenchymal stem cell attachment and spreading on hydroxyapatite by RGD peptides and adsorbed serum proteins. Biomaterials 26(13):1467–1475

Shimizu E, Jong G, Partridge N, Rosenberg PA, Lin LM (2012) Histologic observation of a human immature permanent tooth with irreversible pulpitis after revascularization/regeneration procedure. J Endod 38(9):1293–1297

Shimizu E, Ricucci D, Albert J, Alobaid AS, Gibbs JL, Huang GT et al (2013) Clinical, radiographic, and histological observation of a human immature permanent tooth with chronic apical abscess after revitalization treatment. J Endod 39(8):1078–1083

Shrestha A, Cordova M, Kishen A (2015) Photoactivated polycationic bioactive chitosan nanoparticles inactivate bacterial endotoxins. J Endod 41(5):686–691

da Silva LA, Nelson-Filho P, da Silva RA, Flores DS, Heilborn C, Johnson JD et al (2010) Revascularization and periapical repair after endodontic treatment using apical negative pressure irrigation versus conventional irrigation plus triantibiotic intracanal dressing in dogs' teeth with apical periodontitis. Oral Surg Oral Med Oral Pathol Oral Radiol Endod 109(5):779–787

Siqueira JF Jr, Rocas IN (2008) Clinical implications and microbiology of bacterial persistence after treatment procedures. J Endod 34(11):1291–301.e3

Slomiany BL, Piotrowski L, Slomiany A (1996) Susceptibility of growth factors to degradation by Helicobacter pylori protease: effect of ebrotidine and eucralfate. Biochem Mol Biol Int 40(1):209–215

Smith MacDonald E, Nowzari H, Contreras A, Flynn J, Morrison J, Slots J (1998) Clinical and microbiological evaluation of a bioabsorbable and a nonresorbable barrier membrane in the treatment of periodontal intraosseous lesions. J Periodontol 69(4):445–453

Smith AJ, Smith JG, Shelton RM, Cooper PR (2012) Harnessing the natural regenerative potential of the dental pulp. Dent Clin N Am 56(3):589–601

Smith AJ, Duncan HF, Diogenes A, Simon S, Cooper PR (2016) Exploiting the bioactive properties of the dentin-pulp complex in regenerative endodontics. J Endod 42(1):47–56

de Souza LB, de Aquino SG, de Souza PP, Hebling J, Costa CA (2007) Cytotoxic effects of different concentrations of chlorhexidine. Am J Dent 20(6):400–404

Stadelmann WK, Digenis AG, Tobin GR (1998) Impediments to wound healing. Am J Surg 176(2A Suppl):39S–47S

Thomas MV, Puleo DA (2011) Infection, inflammation, and bone regeneration: a paradoxical relationship. J Dent Res 90(9):1052–1061

Torabinejad M, Milan M, Shabahang S, Wright KR, Faras H (2015) Histologic examination of teeth with necrotic pulps and periapical lesions treated with 2 scaffolds: an animal investigation. J Endod 41(6):846–852

Torabinejad M, Nosrat A, Verma P, Udochukwu O (2017) Regenerative endodontic treatment or mineral trioxide aggregate apical plug in teeth with necrotic pulps and open apices: a systematic review and meta-analysis. J Endod 43(11):1806–1820

Trevino EG, Patwardhan AN, Henry MA, Perry G, Dybdal-Hargreaves N, Hargreaves KM et al (2011) Effect of irrigants on the survival of human stem cells of the apical papilla in a platelet-rich plasma scaffold in human root tips. J Endod 37(8):1109–1115

Trombelli L, Schincaglia GP, Scapoli C, Calura G (1995) Healing response of human buccal gingival recessions treated with expanded polytetrafluoroethylene membranes. A retrospective report. J Periodontol 66(1):14–22

Tuzuner T, Alacam A, Altunbas DA, Gokdogan FG, Gundogdu E (2012) Clinical and radiographic outcomes of direct pulp capping therapy in primary molar teeth following haemostasis with various antiseptics: a randomised controlled trial. Eur J Paediatr Dent 13(4):289–292

Verma P, Nosrat A, Kim JR, Price JB, Wang P, Bair E et al (2017) Effect of residual bacteria on the outcome of pulp regeneration in vivo. J Dent Res 96(1):100–106

Vianna ME, Horz HP, Gomes BP, Conrads G (2006) In vivo evaluation of microbial reduction after chemo-mechanical preparation of human root canals containing necrotic pulp tissue. Int Endod J 39(6):484–492

Virdee SS, Seymour DW, Farnell D, Bhamra G, Bhakta S (2018) Efficacy of irrigant activation techniques in removing intracanal smear layer and debris from mature permanent teeth: a systematic review and meta-analysis. Int Endod J 51:605

Vishwanat L, Duong R, Takimoto K, Phillips L, Espitia CO, Diogenes A et al (2017) Effect of bacterial biofilm on the osteogenic differentiation of stem cells of apical papilla. J Endod 43(6):916–922

Ward CL, Sanchez CJ Jr, Pollot BE, Romano DR, Hardy SK, Becerra SC et al (2015) Soluble factors from biofilms of wound pathogens modulate human bone marrow-derived stromal cell differentiation, migration, angiogenesis, and cytokine secretion. BMC Microbiol 15:75

Windley W 3rd, Teixeira F, Levin L, Sigurdsson A, Trope M (2005) Disinfection of immature teeth with a triple antibiotic paste. J Endod 31(6):439–443

Yang SF, Rivera EM, Baumgardner KR, Walton RE, Stanford C (1995) Anaerobic tissue-dissolving abilities of calcium hydroxide and sodium hypochlorite. J Endod 21(12):613–616

Yassen GH, Eckert GJ, Platt JA (2015) Effect of intracanal medicaments used in endodontic regeneration procedures on microhardness and chemical structure of dentin. Restor Dent Endod 40(2):104–112

Yilmaz S, Dumani A, Yoldas O (2016) The effect of antibiotic pastes on microhardness of dentin. Dent Traumatol 32(1):27–31

Yoshinari N, Tohya T, Mori A, Koide M, Kawase H, Takada T et al (1998) Inflammatory cell population and bacterial contamination of membranes used for guided tissue regenerative procedures. J Periodontol 69(4):460–469

Yoshinari N, Tohya T, Kawase H, Matsuoka M, Nakane M, Kawachi M et al (2001) Effect of repeated local minocycline administration on periodontal healing following guided tissue regeneration. J Periodontol 72(3):284–295

Zhang D-D, Chen X, Bao Z-F, Chen M, Ding Z-J, Zhong M (2014) Histologic comparison between platelet-rich plasma and blood clot in regenerative endodontic treatment: an animal study. J Endod 40(9):1388–1393

Zhu X, Zhang C, Huang GT, Cheung GS, Dissanayaka WL, Zhu W (2012) Transplantation of dental pulp stem cells and platelet-rich plasma for pulp regeneration. J Endod 38(12):1604–1609

Zhu W, Zhu X, Huang GT, Cheung GS, Dissanayaka WL, Zhang C (2013) Regeneration of dental pulp tissue in immature teeth with apical periodontitis using platelet-rich plasma and dental pulp cells. Int Endod J 46(10):962–970

Zucchelli G, Sforza NM, Clauser C, Cesari C, De Sanctis M (1999) Topical and systemic antimicrobial therapy in guided tissue regeneration. J Periodontol 70(3):239–247

Current and Future Views on Cell-Homing-Based Strategies for Regenerative Endodontics

8

Yoshifumi Kobayashi and Emi Shimizu

8.1 Introduction

Once pulpal inflammation or necrosis occurs within the root canal system, the most common strategy to treat the injured dental pulp is its removal and substitution with synthetic materials. However, dental pulp nourishes dentine, serves as a biosensor, contains a dental pulp stem cell population and plays a significant role in tooth viability. Therefore, pulpless teeth become vulnerable to injury, lose the ability to sense environmental change and increase the risk for caries progression, which can lead to tooth loss (Caplan et al. 2005). A healthy pulp is not only important for tooth viability but also for maintaining the capacity to generate tertiary dentine matrix beneath an injury site. Thus, there are increasing needs to develop strategies for dentine-pulp regenerative therapies. This is particularly important for management of immature permanent teeth with incomplete root formation. Pulpal necrosis or chronic apical periodontitis caused by trauma or bacterial infections impedes the mineral deposition process and results in incomplete root development (Luder 2015). Immature permanent teeth with open apexes retain very thin and fragile dentine root walls; subsequently it is difficult to complete root canal obturation in the canal space at the apex (Araújo et al. 2017). Current clinical treatment methods applied for these teeth include apexification or revascularisation.

Apexification is a traditional procedure for an immature permanent tooth with an open apex (Fig 8.1a, b). A calcium hydroxide-based apexification procedure requires at least 6 months to form a calcified apical barrier allowing placement of a root canal filling in the canal. In addition to this disadvantage of the procedure, calcium hydroxide makes the dentine wall fragile, as it reduces the mechanical and physical properties of the dentine. Moreover, calcium hydroxide is less effective in

Y. Kobayashi · E. Shimizu (✉)
Oral Biology Department, Rutgers School of Dental Medicine,
Newark, NJ, USA
e-mail: shimize1@sdm.rutgers.edu

© Springer Nature Switzerland AG 2019
H. F. Duncan, P. R. Cooper (eds.), *Clinical Approaches in Endodontic Regeneration*,
https://doi.org/10.1007/978-3-319-96848-3_8

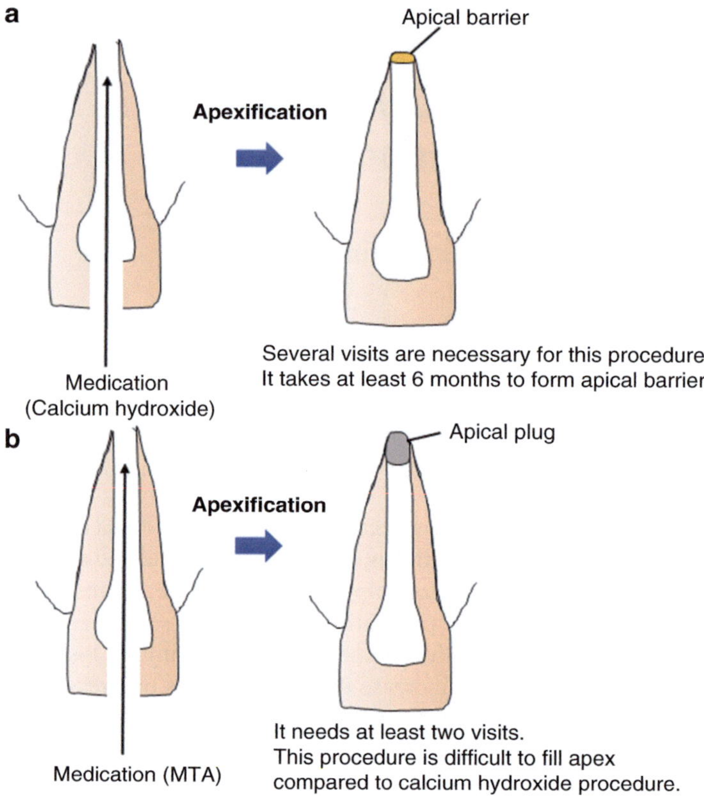

Fig. 8.1 Comparison between apexification procedures with calcium hydroxide and MTA in immature permanent tooth with open apex. In the first clinical visit, an access cavity is prepared with a straight line entry into the root canal. The working length is established within 1 mm of the radiographic apex using a file. The canal space is debrided and instrumented by a root canal file followed by irrigation with normal saline. (**a**) Apexification with calcium hydroxide is performed. After drying of the canal using paper points, calcium hydroxide powder is mixed with normal saline, which is placed into the canal and pushed to the short apex using a plugger or file. (**b**) Apexification with MTA is performed. The canal is dried with paper points, and MTA is placed with pluggers around 5 mm thickness

stimulating root dentine deposition compared with the revascularisation procedure (Jeeruphan et al. 2012). An alternative apexification method is to create an apical barrier with mineral trioxide aggregate (MTA). Although the MTA apexification procedure has a high success rate in comparison with calcium hydroxide treatment, this procedure does not induce extension of root length or root width (Jeeruphan et al. 2012; Alobaid et al. 2014).

Pulp revascularisation/revitalisation procedures in immature pulpless teeth of monkeys and humans have been reported by Nevins and collaborators (Nevins et al. 1976, 1977). In the monkey study, de novo hard tissue and connective tissue formation in the canal space after revitalisation procedure was reported (Nevins et al. 1976) (Fig. 8.2a). In the subsequent human study, a pulp revascularisation procedure induced apical closure and continuous root formation in immature adult teeth (Nevins et al. 1977) (Fig. 8.2b). In 2008, it was histologically shown that reimplanted immature dog teeth can be revascularised from surrounding tissues including blood vessels in the pulp space within 45 days post-procedure (Trope 2008) (Fig. 8.3). In humans, connective tissues including blood vessels, dentine as well as cementum-like tissues were observed filling the root canal space after pulp revascularisation (Shimizu et al. 2012; Peng et al. 2017). These data suggested that this procedure has the potential to regenerate dental pulp tissue including odontoblast-like cells if normal periapical tissues containing Hertwig's epithelial root sheath and the apical papilla are retained in a healthy state.

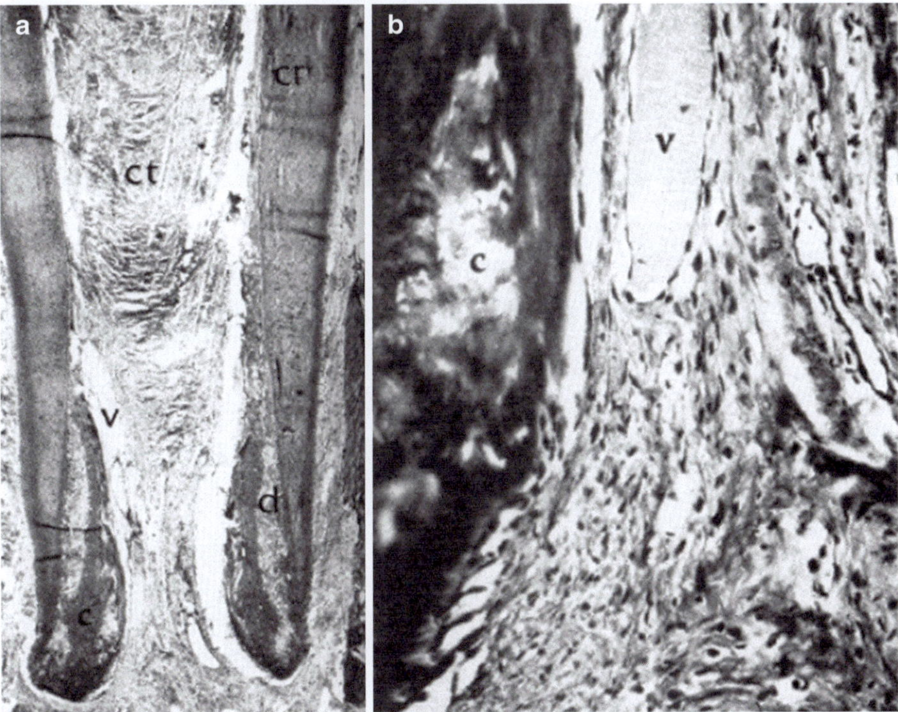

Fig. 8.2 Postoperative observation of pulp revascularisation/vitalisation in monkeys and humans. (**a**) Mandibular central incisor teeth of a rhesus monkey about 2.5 years of age were selected as an experimental model for open apex teeth. Monkey mandibular incisors treated with collagen-calcium phosphate gel showed ingrowth of connective tissue (ct), blood vessel (v) and cement deposition (c) at the apex. d, dentine; cr, cementum repair. (**b**) High magnification of the apical area (**a**). Nevins AJ, Finkelstein F, Borden BG, Laporta R. Revitalization of pulpless open apex teeth in rhesus monkeys, using collagen-calcium phosphate gel. Journal of endodontics. 2, 159–165 (1976). (**c**) Maximally incisors of an 8-year-old boy were damaged due to trauma. Pulpectomy was performed on the incisors. The roots were biomechanically debrided using normal saline as an irrigating solution, and the teeth were filled with a mixture of collagen-calcium phosphate gel. (**d**) The 6 months postoperative radiograph showed continued root formation. Nevins A, Wrobel W, Valachovic R, Finkelstein F. Hard tissue induction into pulpless open-apex teeth using collagen-calcium phosphate gel. Journal of Endodontics. 3, 431–433 (1977)

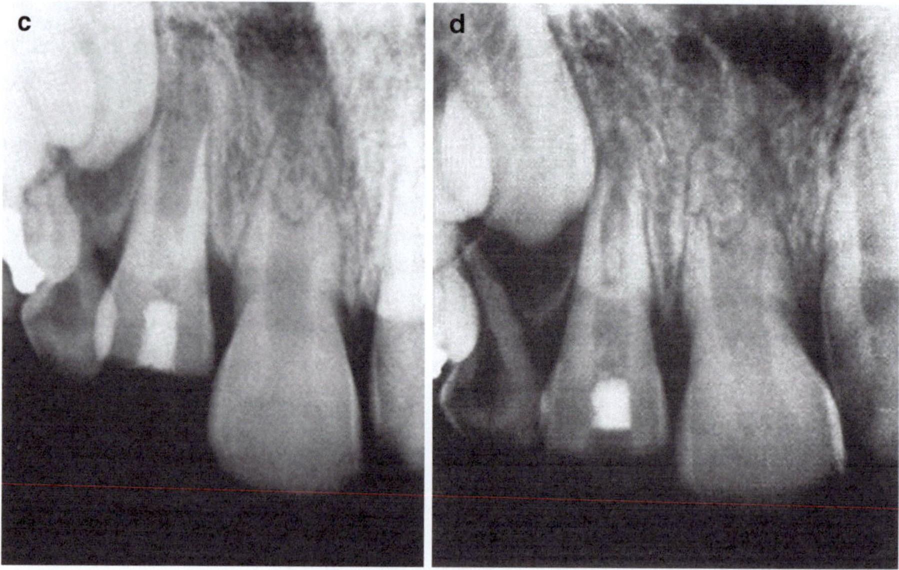

Fig. 8.2 (continued)

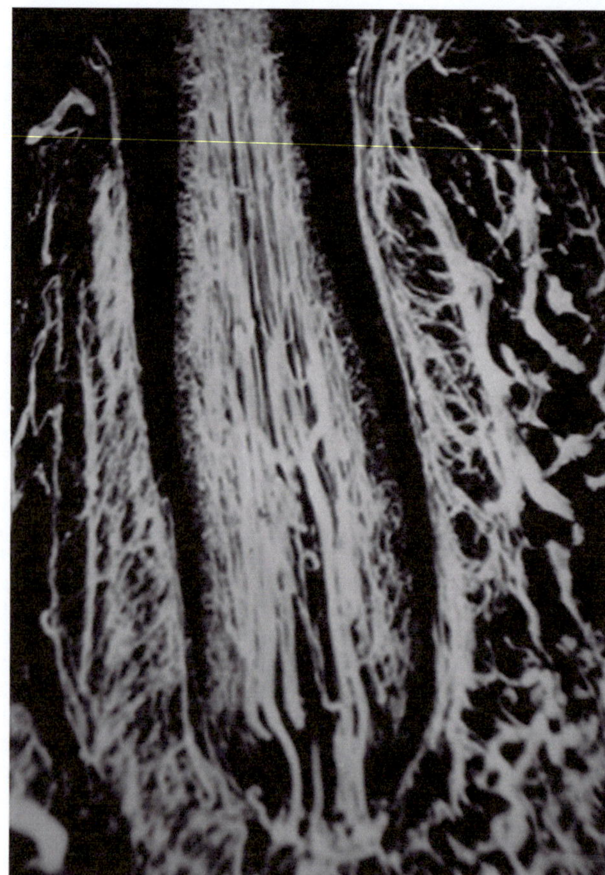

Fig. 8.3 Histological images of revascularisation in immature dog teeth. In extracted dog's teeth, pulpal revascularisation began immediately after reimplantation. Blood vessel formation was completed within approximately 45 days. The apical extension of root structure after healing. Trope M. Regenerative potential of dental pulp. Journal of Endodontics. 34, S13–17 (2008)

Wang et al. have shown the histological outcome of pulp revascularisation for immature dog teeth with apical periodontitis (Wang et al. 2010) (Fig. 8.4). Cementum-like tissue was observed in the dentinal walls in the root canal space, which were thickened by deposition of cementum after the procedure. The root length was increased by the growth of cementum or bone tissues, whereas connective tissue morphology was similar to periodontal ligament including blood vessels in the canal space. Several groups have reported that this characteristic of pulp revascularisation is also observed in human studies (Martin et al. 2013; Shimizu

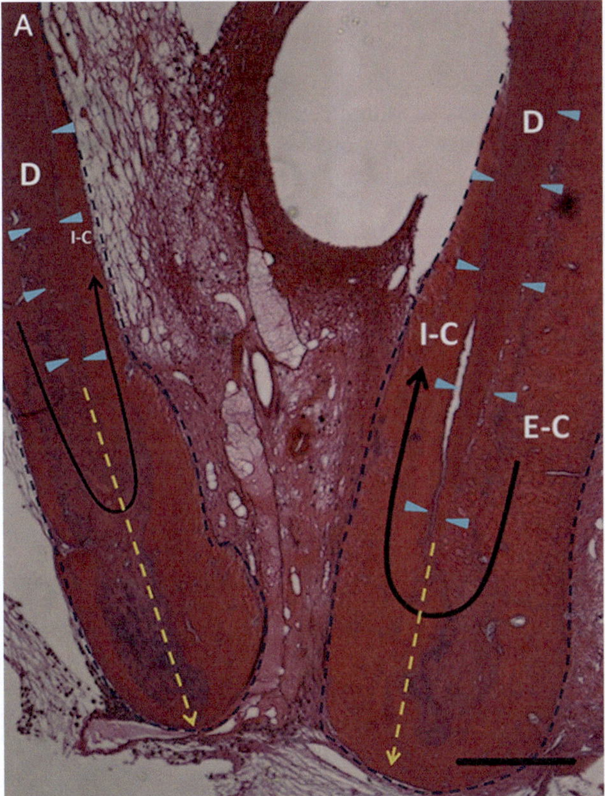

Fig. 8.4 Histological observations after a pulp revascularisation procedure in a dog. Apical periodontitis was induced on a canine from a 6-month-old dog. The canal was irrigated with 1.25% sodium hypochlorite and sterile saline. Bleeding was provoked by a stainless file to fill the canal space. Canal space was filled with soft tissues, and the apex closed by the apposition of cementum and cementum-like tissue. D, dentine. Blue arrowheads indicate the demarcation between dentine and new cementum/cementum-like tissue. Black arrows indicate the continuation of the extracanal cementum (E-C) into intracanal cementum (I-C). Yellow arrows and dashed lines indicate the apical length generated by the cementum. Wang X, Thibodeau B, Trope M, Lin LM, Huang GT. Histologic characterization of regenerated tissues in the canal space after the revitalization/revascularization procedure in immature dog teeth with apical periodontitis. Journal of Endodontics. 36, 56–63 (2010)

et al. 2013; Becerra et al. 2014) (Fig. 8.5). These results indicated that it is difficult to regenerate dental pulp tissues if the apical papilla of immature permanent teeth is already infected or removed. In addition, problematic healing after pulp revascularisation has been reported clinically, including disorganised hard tissue formation in the canal space, limited blood vessel formation in the regenerated connective tissue (periodontal ligament-like tissue) and no-innervation system in the canal. Thus, there is an urgent need to improve current treatment protocols for pulp revascularisation for immature permanent teeth with apical periodontitis.

8.2   Stem Cell Homing

Stem cell-homing is defined as the recruitment of endogenous stem cells by mobilisation factors to an injured site to induce repair or replace the damaged cells or tissues (Andreas et al. 2014). Reported mobilisation factors, which facilitate mobilisation of human bone marrow haematopoietic stem cells from bone marrow, include granulocyte colony-stimulating factor (G-CSF) (Petit et al. 2002) and the closely related granulocyte/macrophage colony-stimulating factor (GM-CSF) (Spitzer et al. 1997), interleukin (IL)-8 (Laterveer et al. 1995), stromal cell-derived factor-1 (SDF-1) (Aiuti et al. 1997; Hattori et al. 2003), Flt-3 ligand (Solanilla et al. 2003), growth factors such as vascular endothelial growth factor (VEGF) (Rafii et al. 2002), angiopoietin-1 (Arai et al. 2004) and macrophage inflammatory protein-2 (Wang et al. 1997).

Fig. 8.5 Histological views of post-pulp revitalisation procedure in human. Twenty-six months after the completion of the revitalisation treatment, the patient presented to a clinic with a horizontal crown fracture at the cervical level of tooth #9. (**a**) Mineralised tissues observed in the apical portion of the root canal (stained with haematoxylin-eosin; original magnification). (**b**) Details of the apical portion in (**a**). An island of soft tissue is present in the calcified tissue apically. The inset shows magnification of the ramification indicated by the lower arrow. Its lumen contains uninflamed connective tissue. (**c**) A high-power view of the apical soft tissue in (**b**). Vital connective tissue with fibroblasts and abundance of collagen fibres. There is an absence of inflammatory cells. (**d**) Magnification of the area indicated by the upper arrow in (**b**). The calcified tissue filling the apical canal is irregular and is demarcated apically by a cementum-like tissue, with some osteoblast-like lacunae. Increased root length is caused by deposition of cementum-like tissue. (**e**) A high-power view of the area of the root canal wall indicated by the left arrow in (**a**). From left to right: area with high concentration of dentinal tubules, area with fewer tubules and calcified tissue with no dentine tubules. (**f**). A high-power view of the area of the root canal wall indicated by the right arrow in (**a**). From right to left: area with high density of dentine tubules, area with relatively few tubules and calcified tissue with no dentine tubules. Shimizu E, Ricucci D, Albert J, Alobaid AS, Gibbs JL, Huang GT, et al. Clinical, radiographic, and histological observation of a human immature permanent tooth with chronic apical abscess after revitalization treatment. Journal of Endodontics. 39: 1078–1083 (2013)

To clinically perform pulp regeneration using a cell-homing strategy is potentially easier than cell-based therapy (cell transplantation) because there is no requirement for exogenous stem cells (Eramo et al. 2018). Pulp regeneration therapy using cell transplantation has several inherent problems, including difficulties in obtaining regulatory approval, stem cell isolation and processing, the relatively high cost associated with storage (cell cryopreservation), the biological risk of immune-rejection, infection and tumorigenesis (Kim et al. 2013).

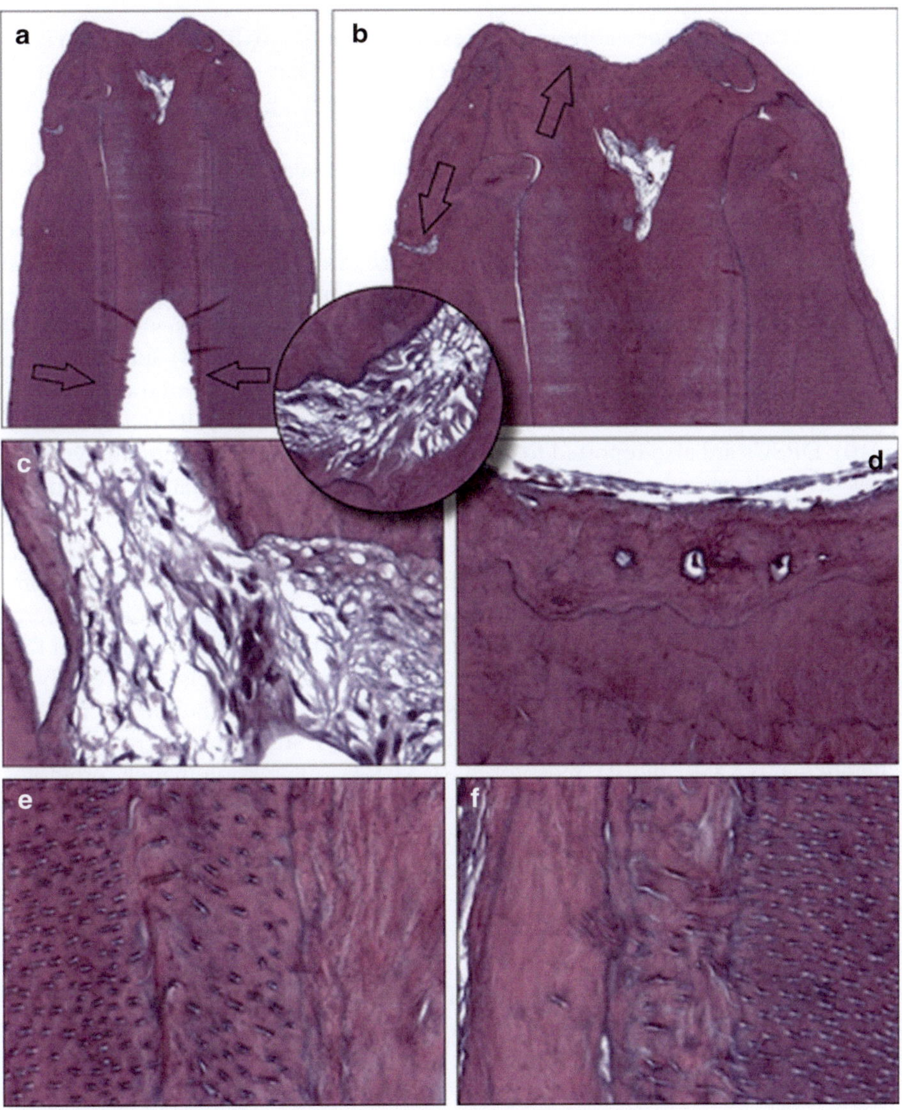

Pulp revascularisation is a cell-homing therapy; however, it is limited to the regeneration or repair of tissues in the pulp space. In addition, this treatment method cannot control the regeneration of specific tissue types in the pulp space. Therefore, the clinical method of pulp revascularisation may need to be modified in the future, for example, with usage of mobilisation factors and precise scaffolds to regulate formation of the vascular system as well as hard tissue in the tooth.

8.3 Dental Stem Cells

Stem cells are self-renewable and possess the potential to differentiate into multiple lineages (Fischbach and Fischbach 2004). They are a key element of regenerative medicine whose aim is to repair or replace cells, tissues or organs as part of therapeutic approaches (Mason and Dunnill 2008). Several stem cell populations have been identified in the dental and oral environment as described below.

Human dental pulp stem cells (DPSCs) have mesenchymal characteristics and are located in the central region of the pulp space (Saito and Oshima 2017). Dental caries or trauma causes inflammation in the dental pulp, which triggers activation of the immune system including the innate and adaptive responses in the dental pulp. Inflammatory cytokines including TNF-α (Ueda et al. 2014) and IFN-γ (He et al. 2017) are released from macrophages, which stimulate cell migration, DPSC proliferation as well as differentiation into odontoblast-like cells (Cooper et al. 2010). DPSCs are also reported to differentiate into osteoblasts, chondrocyte-like cells as well as adipogenic cells under appropriate stimulatory conditions (Gronthos et al. 2000). Even when DPSCs are exposed to inflammatory conditions such as in irreversible *pulpitis*, these cells are able to survive and differentiate down osteogenic/dentinogenic lineages (Alongi et al. 2010). Therefore, DPSCs are a potentially important stem cell source for use in cell-homing therapies. Furthermore, growth factors such as SDF-1 and basic fibroblast growth factor (bFGF) can enhance DPSC migration in 3D collagen gels, whereas bone morphogenic protein-7 (BMP7) induces osteogenic differentiation but not cell migration (Suzuki et al. 2011). Interestingly SDF-1 stimulates its receptor, the chemokine (C-X-C motif) receptor 4 (CXCR4), expression which promotes migration of DPSCs via the GSK3β/β-catenin pathway (Li et al. 2017). Yang et al. have shown that SDF-1 in conjunction with a collagen matrix enhances microvessel formation in DPSCs with involvement of autophagy in vivo (Yang et al. 2015). In addition, stem cell factor (SCF), a haematopoietic chemokine which binds to the c-Kit receptor (CD117), stimulates migration and proliferation of DPSCs in vitro and in vivo (Pan et al. 2013). Interestingly, Gervois et al. have shown that DPSCs indirectly promote cell migration and proliferation of neuronal progenitors, indicating that mobilisation factors produced by DPSCs can recruit progenitors of neural cells and stimulate neuronal maturation and neuritogenesis (Gervois et al. 2017).

8.4 Stem Cells from Human Exfoliated Deciduous Teeth (SHEDs)

SHEDs are multipotent stem cells and are able to differentiate into a variety of cell types including neural cells, adipocytes and odontoblast-like cells. Transplanted SHEDs with hydroxyapatite/tricalcium phosphate (HA/TCP) form hard tissues including bone and dentine-like structures; however, they do not completely regenerate the dentine-pulp complex in contrast to DPSCs in vivo (Miura et al. 2003). SHEDs can promote axon growth, angiogenesis, Schwann cell migration, proliferation and cell survival of neurons as well as differentiation of mature oligodendrocytes, indicating that SHEDs have neuroregenerative activities and potential to be used therapeutically in peripheral nerve and spiral cord injury (Sakai et al. 2012). SHEDs have also relatively high expression of pericyte makers such as NG2, α-smooth muscle actin (α-SMA), PDGF receptor beta (PDGFR β) and CD146. Transplanted SHEDs and human umbilical vein endothelial cells (HUVECs) together form more vessel-like structures compared with SHEDs or HUVECs alone in vivo (Kim et al. 2016). Subsequently, SHEDs can be useful for pulp regeneration, especially, regeneration of nociceptors (A-fibres and C-fibres) as well as blood vessel formation. A disadvantage of tissue regeneration using SHEDs is the difficulty of storing the cells or tissues from exfoliated deciduous teeth until the patient requires them.

8.5 Stem Cells from Apical Papilla (SCAPs)

SCAPs share similar characteristics with DPSCs; however, there are several differences between the cell types. CD24 is present on the surface of SCAPs but not DPSCs (Sonoyama et al. 2006). The apical papilla area contains fewer blood vessels and cellular components than the central pulp. Notably, SCAPs, but not DPSCs, can also be used for root dentine formation (Sonoyama et al. 2008).

SCAPs can be obtained from adult wisdom teeth without adverse health effects, and interestingly, third molar teeth may have the potential to provide high-quality SCAPs for future use. In addition, even when human SCAPs are inflamed, e.g. during apical periodontitis, they retain vitality and stemness and can undergo osteogenic and angiogenic differentiation (Chrepa et al. 2017) (Fig. 8.6).

Chemotactic factors including SDF-1, TGF-β1, PDGF, G-CSF as well as FGF2 can stimulate cell migration of SCAPs, whereas a combination of G-CSF and TGF-β1 can significantly enhance mineralisation responses (Fayazi et al. 2017). Similarly, SDF-1α significantly promotes migration of SCAPs in a 3D collagen gel scaffold (Liu et al. 2015). In addition, transplanted SCAPs in the pulp space of the root form an abundant vascularised pulp-like tissue as well as new dentine-like tissue at the dentinal wall (Huang 2009). Implanted SCAPs in Matrigel conjugated with brain-derived neurotrophic factor (BDNF) and glial cell-derived neurotrophic factor (GDNF) promote axonal outgrowth of trigeminal sensory neurons in vivo (de Almeida et al. 2014), indicating that SCAPs may provide a valuable resource for regeneration of neurites.

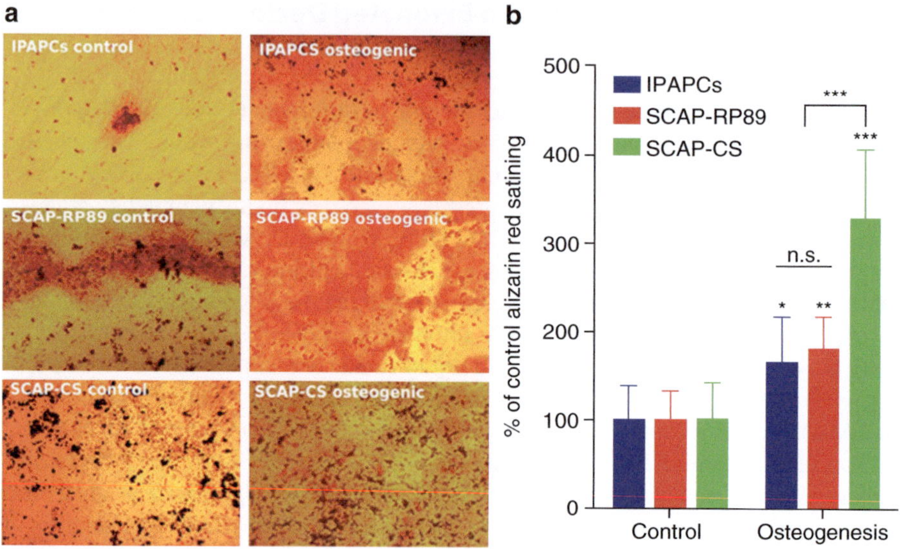

Fig. 8.6 Comparison of osteogenesis in the cell line SCAP CS, SCAP-RP89 and IPAPCs. SCAP CS, inflamed periapical tissue that included part of the apical papilla; SCAP-RP89, normal SCAP; IPAPCs, inflamed periapical progenitor cells. Cells were cultured for 3 weeks in either control or osteogenic medium. (**a**) Alizarin red staining showed the mineralisation potential of all cell lines compared with their respective controls. (**b**) Quantification of osteogenesis confirmed the significantly greater mineralisation of all cell lines compared with their controls (all p values <0.05). SCAP CS exhibited significantly greater mineralisation compared with both SCAP-RP89 and IPAPCs ($p < 0.001$). *$p < 0.05$. **$p < 0.01$. ***$p < 0.001$. n.s: not significant. Chrepa V, Pitcher B, Henry MA, Diogenes A. Survival of the Apical Papilla and Its Resident Stem Cells in a Case of Advanced Pulpal Necrosis and Apical Periodontitis. Journal of Endodontics. 43, 561–567 (2017)

8.6　Human Periodontal Ligament Stem Cells (PDLSCs)

PDLSCs are located between the bone and cementum around the root of the tooth and participate in the formation of the cementum on the root surface as well as bone formation at the bone surface (Isaka et al. 2001). To improve pulp revascularisation strategies, it is necessary to promote an increase in the thickness and length of root dentine wall as well as stimulating an apical closure with cementum. The application of mobilisation factors to PDLCs may contribute to the accomplishment of this. Some mobilisation factors (described below) are known to have specific effects on PDLSCs. Periostin, a ligand for alpha-V/beta-3 and alpha-V/beta-5 integrins, enhances cell migration, proliferation and mineralisation of PDLSCs (Wu et al. 2018). In addition, SDF-1α treatment stimulates perivascular formation by PDLSCs in combination with HUVECs in vitro and in vivo, whereas it cannot induce angiogenesis in PDLSCs or HUVECs (Bae et al. 2017). The combination of parathyroid hormone (PTH) and SDF-1α synergistically stimulates cell proliferation and migration of PDLSCs in vitro, whereas co-therapy increases osteogenic differentiation of

PDLSCs, especially upregulation of osteogenic markers such as type 1 collagen and alkaline phosphatase (Du et al. 2012). In an in vivo study, transplanted hypoxic pretreatments (short term—24 h) of PDLSCs exhibited increased hard tissue deposition (Yu et al. 2016). Other researchers demonstrated that local injection of PDLSCs at an injury site of mental nerve resulted in nerve regeneration, which accomplished a similar level of nerve function obtained after administration of autologous Schwann cells (Li et al. 2013).

Recently, a new class of mobilisation factors, such as enzyme inhibitors, was reported. A ROCK inhibitor, trans-4-[(1R)-aminoethyl]-N-(4-pyridinyl) cyclohexanecarboxamide (Y-27632), has been used for treatment of various cardiovascular diseases such as hypertension, coronary and cerebral vasospasm and pulmonary arterial hypertension (Uehata et al. 1997). Wang et al. reported that Y-27632 enhanced PDLSCs' migration and proliferation, whereas it maintained the stemness of PDLSCs (Wang et al. 2017), indicating that ROCK inhibitors have potential to be used as chemotaxis factors for PDLSCs.

8.7 Human Bone Marrow Stromal Stem Cells (BMSSCs) and Haematopoietic Stem Cells (HSCs)

BMSSCs are capable of differentiation down the mesoderm lineage to osteoblasts, adipocytes and chondrocytes (Abdallah and Kassem 2012). Indeed, BMSSCs may provide the best cell sources for pulp revascularisation therapy. The mobilisation factors described below are known to exert effects on BMSSCs. SCF enhances cell migration, proliferation and osteogenic differentiation of BMSSCs in vivo (Ruangsawasdi et al. 2017). On the other hand, SDF-1α is highly expressed in purified BMSSCs and downregulated during osteogenic differentiation, suggesting that SDF-1 plays a role in the maintenance and survival of immature BMSSCs (Kortesidis et al. 2005). In addition, implantation of BMSSCs pretreated with the key soluble factors, lipocalin-2 and prolactin, significantly increased bone formation in a bone defect compared with the control group (Tsai TL and Lii WJ 2017), suggesting that lipocalin-2 and prolactin enhance repair of a critical-size bone defect in vivo.

Interaction of HSCs and osteoblasts plays an important role in regulation of HSC quiescence in the adult bone marrow niche. The spindle-shaped N-cadherin positive-osteoblasts can adhere to HSCs to maintain HSC quiescence. Calcium and oxygen levels are also associated with N-cadherin-mediated cell adhesion of HSCs (Arai and Suda 2007).

Angiogenesis greatly contributes to HSCs' maintenance and migration from the bone marrow niche. VEGF is a potent angiogenic factor, which stimulates bone marrow-derived endothelial cells. It can also stimulate the recruitment of perivascular cells including CXCR4-positive cells via upregulation of CXCL12 (Tamma and Ribatti 2017; Hattori et al. 2001). Both in vitro and in vivo studies have demonstrated that human recombinant VEGF treatment strongly induced mobilisation of endothelial precursor cells (Asahara et al. 1999).

8.8 Scaffolds

Artificial support systems, called scaffolds, are necessary to assist tissue regeneration with dental stem cells. Specific biochemical materials with specific mechanical and structural properties are used to produce scaffolds. Generating cell-scaffold complexes requires structures capable of maintaining the cell proliferation and differentiation activity (Hosseinkhani et al. 2014). The selection of scaffold materials and appropriate seeding cells is important for the tissue engineering of teeth. In addition, it is necessary to supply sufficient nutrients and oxygen to the transplanted cells, to maintain cell survival and functional activity (Colton 1995). Thus, vascular formation such as neovascularisation should be the first step for tissue regeneration process (Polverini 1995). The scaffold has to retain a specific composition of cells and induce cell interaction and adhesion. In addition, the scaffold needs to be biocompatible, biodegradable, while coordinating tissue formation, and able to provoke minimal risk of inflammation or toxicity (Gathani and Raghavendra 2016).

8.8.1 Natural Scaffolds

There are several types of natural scaffolds:

1. Platelet-rich plasma (PRP)
2. Platelet-rich fibrin (PRF)
3. Collagen
4. Collagen-glycosaminoglycan
5. Chitosan
6. Silk fibroin (SF)
7. Alginate
1. Platelet-rich plasma (PRP) contains a rich source of growth factors and forms a fibrin gel, which is able to stimulate bone and soft tissue healing. Growth factors present in PRP include PDGF, TGF-β, insulin growth factor, VEGF, epidermal growth factor and epithelial cell growth factor.

   The disadvantage of using PRP clinically is the requirement for special equipment (e.g. centrifuge) and reagents for preparing PRP, which increases the cost of the treatment (Jadhav et al. 2012). In order to improve its physical properties, PRP can be formed with collagen to make it more solid and modulate its degradation speed (Rodriguez et al. 2014).
2. Platelet-rich fibrin (PRF) is a fibrin matrix including platelet cytokines and growth factors, which acts as a biodegradable scaffold (Hotwani and Sharma 2014). PRF has been demonstrated to be more efficient clinically compared with PRP (Simonpieri et al. 2012).

   The disadvantage of using PRF is that the volume of product is limited as it is synthesised from autologous blood (Choukroun et al. 2006).

3. Collagen

Collagen is the most abundant fibrous protein in the extracellular matrix. Collagens provide tensile strength, regulate cell adhesion and support chemotaxis and cell migration (Rozario and DeSimone 2010). A combination of SDF-1α and collagen matrix encourages migrating cells from surrounding tissues through the apical foramen and creates vessel formation in the root pulp space (Yang et al. 2015).

A disadvantage of collagen is its rapid degradation, which shrinks the scaffold structure (Vaissiere et al. 2000).

4. Collagen-glycosaminoglycan (CG)

CG has been used within regenerative medicine for dermis, peripheral nerves, bone and cartilage tissue engineering (Caliari et al. 2012; Murphy et al. 2010). The components of CG scaffolds are made by freeze-drying a suspension of collagen and glycosaminoglycans (GAGs), resulting in a highly porous sponge-like material (Caliari et al. 2012). Hyaluronic acid (HA) is one of the GAGs and plays important roles in maintaining morphologic organisation and suppressing pro-inflammatory cytokines from activated macrophages (Shimizu et al. 2003). An in vivo study has shown that more cell-rich reorganising tissues—including dental pulp and blood vessels—were observed in the dentine defect area, when a HA sponge was implanted compared with a collagen sponge (Inuyama et al. 2010).

A disadvantage of HA is its high water solubility, resulting in its rapid degradation by enzymes such as hyaluronidase. HA therefore lacks mechanical integrity in an aqueous environment (Zhang et al. 2016).

5. Chitosan

Chitosan is built up by deacetylation of chitin and is a biocompatible polysaccharide. Chitin is a copolymer composed of N-acetyl-glucosamine and N-glucosamine subunits, which is the primary component of cell walls in fungi and exoskeletons of crustaceans such as crabs or shrimps (Chang et al. 2014). Chitosan is a nontoxic, absorbable and antibacterial product. It can form a gel structure and stimulate osteoblast alkaline phosphatase activity, fibroblast and pulp cell proliferation (Matsunaga et al. 2006).

A disadvantage of chitosan is the difficulty in controlling the size of the hydrogel pores as well as chemical modifications of chitosan (Gathani and Raghavendra 2016).

6. Silk fibroin (SF)

SF is a promising biomechanical material, due to its unique mechanical and biological properties. The mechanical strength, biocompatibility and its slow degradation rate enable its gradual replacement with newly formed tissue indicating that SF might have potential as a material for hard tissue regeneration (Kuboyama et al. 2013). In addition, SF has less immunogenic and inflammatory response, compared with either polylactic-co-glycolic acid (PLGA) or collagens (Meinel et al. 2005).

A disadvantage of SF is its slow degradation, with degradation taking up to 2 years to complete (Cao and Wang 2009).

7. Alginate

Alginate is a natural polysaccharide that offers benefits of biocompatibility and non-toxicity. Its mechanical strength can be improved by increasing the calcium content and cross-linking density. Alginate hydrogel with arginine-glycine-aspartic acid (RGD) stimulates cell adhesion, proliferation and differentiation (Sharma et al. 2014).

A disadvantage of alginate is that it exhibits a low mechanical stiffness.

8.8.2 Synthetic Scaffolds

8.8.2.1 Polymers

Many synthetic polymers such as polylactic acid (PLA), poly-L-lactic acid (PLLA), polyglycolic acid (PGA), PLGA and poly-epsilon-caprolactone (PCL) have been used as scaffold materials for pulp regeneration (Gathani and Raghavendra 2016).

PLA: PLA is an excellent biocompatible and biodegradable polymer and widely used as a medical polymer material. This scaffold can support the adherence of both DPSCs and PDLSCs and reportedly supports enhanced cell proliferation compared with collagen or calcium phosphate scaffolds (Chandrahasa et al. 2011).

PLLA: Karageorgiou et al. have shown that the minimum requirement of pore size for cell migration was around 100 µm, whereas pores larger than 300 µm stimulated new bone and capillaries formation (Karageorgiou and Kaplan 2005). The pore size of PLLA scaffolds is also known to influence cell proliferation and differentiation of DPSCs (Conde et al. 2015).

PGA and PLGA: PGA-PGLA has good biocompatibility as well as advantages for cell growth, without toxicity and inhibitory actions on cells. In addition, a combination of PGA and PLGA can be used to control the degradation rate of the scaffold in tissues in vivo (Singhal et al. 1996).

PCL: This scaffold material is derived from a biodegradable polymer, although it requires an extended period of time for its degradation, indicating that it cannot ideally satisfy the requirement for biomedical application such as for use in bone regeneration (Horst et al. 2012).

The principal disadvantage of the polymers described above is that their degradation time is longer in comparison with most naturally derived scaffolds.

8.8.2.2 Bioceramics

Bioceramics have been used for healing of large bone defects for several years now and include calcium/phosphate materials, bioactive glasses and glass ceramics. Calcium/phosphate scaffolds include β-tricalcium phosphate or hydroxyapatite materials, which have been widely used for bone regeneration. They have biocompatibility, low immunogenicity, osteoconductivity, bone bonding and chemical similarity to mineralised tissues. Conversely, glass ceramics have drawbacks including difficulties in shaping, poor mechanical strength, brittleness and slow degradation rates (Sharma et al. 2014). When used for tissue engineering of dental structures, after the implantation of hydroxyapatite/tricalcium phosphate with PDLSCs/

BMSSCs, PDLSCs develop into PDL-like tissues, while BMSSCs differentiate into bone-like tissues (Wang et al. 2016).

A disadvantage of bioceramics is their slow degradation rates, which restrict their usage as scaffolds for tissue regeneration purposes.

8.8.2.3 Non-rigid/Soft Biomaterials; Synthetic Extracellular Matrix (ECM)

An example of a synthetic ECM is a hydrogel, which presents a three-dimensional (3D) network constructed with hydrophilic homopolymers or copolymers cross-linked to form insoluble polymer matrices. Hydrogels are able to absorb a large amount of water or biological fluids. They demonstrate sol-to-gel conversions and hence can be injected; this property can provide convenience for insertion into narrow and difficult to reach locations, indicating that hydrogels can be applicable to apical areas or narrowed pulpal spaces. Methods employed for forming hydrogels include thermal gelation, ionic interaction, physical cross-linking, photo-polymerisation and chemical cross-linking (Zhao et al. 2015); these processing options also enable hydrogels to relatively easily bind to specific mobilisation factors described earlier in this chapter. These two characteristics of hydrogel, including their invasiveness to narrow space and their high affinity to mobilisation factors, are expected to enable them to contribute significantly to the development of the next generation of biomaterials for biological and biomedical applications, such as self-regulated and site-specific drug delivery systems.

PuraMatrix™ is a self-assembling peptide hydrogel which instantaneously polymerises under normal physiological conditions. DPSC can proliferate and survive in a range of different stiffnesses of this hydrogel. However, reportedly it cannot support odontoblast differentiation without the inclusion of growth factors (Cavalcanti et al. 2013). In contrast, a stiffer gelatin-methacryloyl (GelMA) hydrogel containing RGD domains is known to stimulate cell proliferation and differentiation of both endothelial cells and odontoblast-like cells in vitro (Athirasala et al. 2017).

The principal disadvantage of synthetic ECM-based scaffolds is their low mechanical strength.

8.9 Conclusion and Prospects

8.9.1 Angiogenesis

In vivo experiments targeting angiogenesis in the root canal system have shown that several mobilisation factors such as VEGF and SDF-1α can promote vascular formation (neovascularisation) from DPSCs and PDLSCs, whereas SDF-1α controls the maintenance and survival of immature BMSSCs. SDF-1 also stimulates cell migration of SCAPs, indicating that SDF-1α can be useful for angiogenesis, formation of fibroblasts and odontoblasts from SCAPs in a cell-homing-based regenerative therapy approach. In addition, BDNF and GDNF can enhance neurogenesis from SCAPs, which may be useful for nerve regeneration in situ (Fig. 8.7a).

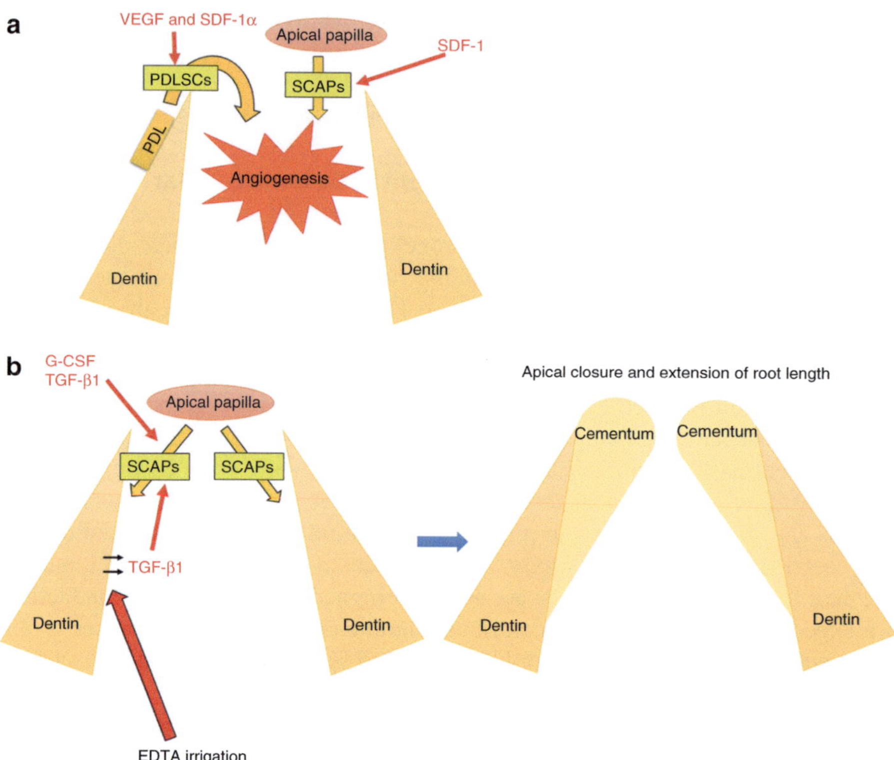

Fig. 8.7 Plausible schemes of cell-homing-based strategies for pulp regeneration in endodontics. (**a**) Angiogenesis in pulp. VEGF and SDF-1α can induce neovascularisation from PDLSCs. SDF-1 also stimulates cell migration of SCAPs, resulting in angiogenesis in the pulp space. (**b**) Apical closure and extension of root length. Combination of G-CSF and TGF-β1 can enhance cementum and bone formation. Irrigating with 17% EDTA can release TGF-β1 from extracellular matrix on dentine wall. After these procedures, the dentine wall at the apex will become thicker, and root length will be extended by deposition of cementum. In addition, the apical foramen will be narrowed

8.9.2 Root Formation

A combination of G-CSF and TGF-β1 can enhance cell mineralisation processes including cementum and bone formation, so that they can be used for root formation and elongation of apical areas in immature adult teeth with open apex. Irrigating with 17% ethylenediaminetetraacetic acid (EDTA) can release TGF-β family members from the extracellular matrix of dentine (Fig. 8.7b). This step should be adopted in cell-homing strategies in dental tissues in the future to aid in thickening of the dentine wall. Improvement of cell-homing strategies may eventually replace current dentine-pulp revascularisation strategies, which cannot reproduce the natural pulp tissue organisation.

Unfortunately, a cell-homing strategies are not likely to be consistently successful under every condition, particularly in adult teeth because differentiation activity of their dental stem cells is substantially reduced compared with stem cells derived from younger patients. Therefore, root canal treatment currently still remains as the standard care for mature teeth in adult or aged patients. On the other hand, cell-based strategies can regenerate dental pulp tissues including blood vessels, nerves as well as odontoblast-like cells using exogenous dental stem cells, independent of the patient's own stem cells. This approach offers the potential for cell-based strategies to be applied for adult patients, whose stem cells may not function optimally.

References

Abdallah BM, Kassem M (2012) New factors controlling the balance between osteoblastogenesis and adipogenesis. Bone 50(2):540–545

Aiuti A, Webb IJ, Bleul C, Springer T, Gutierrez-Ramos JC (1997) The chemokine SDF-1 is a chemoattractant for human CD34+ hematopoietic progenitor cells and provides a new mechanism to explain the mobilization of CD34+ progenitors to peripheral blood. J Exp Med 185(1):111–120

de Almeida JF, Chen P, Henry MA, Diogenes A (2014) Stem cells of the apical papilla regulate trigeminal neurite outgrowth and targeting through a BDNF-dependent mechanism. Tissue Eng Part A 20(23-24):3089–3100

Alobaid AS, Cortes LM, Lo J, Nguyen TT, Albert J, Abu-Melha AS et al (2014) Radiographic and clinical outcomes of the treatment of immature permanent teeth by revascularization or apexification: a pilot retrospective cohort study. J Endod 40(8):1063–1070

Alongi DJ, Yamaza T, Song Y, Fouad AF, Romberg EE, Shi S et al (2010) Stem/progenitor cells from inflamed human dental pulp retain tissue regeneration potential. Regen Med 5(4):617–631

Andreas K, Sittinger M, Ringe J (2014) Toward in situ tissue engineering: chemokine-guided stem cell recruitment. Trends Biotechnol 32(9):483–492

Arai F, Suda T (2007) Maintenance of quiescent hematopoietic stem cells in the osteoblastic niche. Ann N Y Acad Sci 1106:41–53

Arai F, Hirao A, Ohmura M, Sato H, Matsuoka S, Takubo K et al (2004) Tie2/angiopoietin-1 signaling regulates hematopoietic stem cell quiescence in the bone marrow niche. Cell 118(2):149–161

Araújo PS, Silva LB, Neto AS, Almeida de Arruda JA, Álvares PR, Sobral APV et al (2017) Pulp revascularization: a literature review. Open Dent J 10:48–56

Asahara T, Takahashi T, Masuda H, Kalka C, Chen D, Iwaguro H et al (1999) VEGF contributes to postnatal neovascularization by mobilizing bone marrow-derived endothelial progenitor cells. EMBO J 18(14):3964–3972

Athirasala A, Lins F, Tahayeri A, Hinds M, Smith AJ, Sedgley C et al (2017) A novel strategy to engineer pre-vascularized full-length dental pulp-like tissue constructs. Sci Rep 7(1):3323

Bae YK, Kim GH, Lee JC, Seo BM, Joo KM, Lee G et al (2017) The significance of SDF-1alpha-CXCR4 axis in in vivo angiogenic ability of human periodontal ligament stem cells. Mol Cells 40(6):386–392

Becerra P, Ricucci D, Loghin S, Gibbs JL, Lin LM (2014) Histologic study of a human immature permanent premolar with chronic apical abscess after revascularization/revitalization. J Endod 40(1):133–139

Caliari SR, Weisgerber DW, Ramirez MA, Kelkhoff DO, Harley BA (2012) The influence of collagen-glycosaminoglycan scaffold relative density and microstructural anisotropy on tenocyte bioactivity and transcriptomic stability. J Mech Behav Biomed Mater 11:27–40

Cao Y, Wang B (2009) Biodegradation of silk biomaterials. Int J Mol Sci 10(4):1514–1524

Caplan DJ, Cai J, Yin G, White BA (2005) Root canal filled versus non-root canal filled teeth: a retrospective comparison of survival times. J Public Health Dent 65(2):90–96

Cavalcanti BN, Zeitlin BD, Nor JE (2013) A hydrogel scaffold that maintains viability and supports differentiation of dental pulp stem cells. Dent Mater 29(1):97–102

Chandrahasa S, Murray PE, Namerow KN (2011) Proliferation of mature ex vivo human dental pulp using tissue engineering scaffolds. J Endod 37(9):1236–1239

Chang HH, Wang YL, Chiang YC, Chen YL, Chuang YH, Tsai SJ et al (2014) A novel chitosan-gammaPGA polyelectrolyte complex hydrogel promotes early new bone formation in the alveolar socket following tooth extraction. PLoS One 9(3):e92362

Choukroun J, Diss A, Simonpieri A, Girard MO, Schoeffler C, Dohan SL et al (2006) Platelet-rich fibrin (PRF): a second-generation platelet concentrate. Part IV: clinical effects on tissue healing. Oral Surg Oral Med Oral Pathol Oral Radiol Endod 101(3):e56–e60

Chrepa V, Pitcher B, Henry MA, Diogenes A (2017) Survival of the apical papilla and its resident stem cells in a case of advanced pulpal necrosis and apical periodontitis. J Endod 43(4):561–567

Colton CK (1995) Implantable biohybrid artificial organs. Cell Transplant 4(4):415–436

Conde CM, Demarco FF, Casagrande L, Alcazar JC, Nor JE, Tarquinio SB (2015) Influence of poly-L-lactic acid scaffold's pore size on the proliferation and differentiation of dental pulp stem cells. Braz Dent J 26(2):93–98

Cooper PR, Takahashi Y, Graham LW, Simon S, Imazato S, Smith AJ (2010) Inflammation-regeneration interplay in the dentine-pulp complex. J Dent 38(9):687–697

Du L, Yang P, Ge S (2012) Stromal cell-derived factor-1 significantly induces proliferation, migration, and collagen type I expression in a human periodontal ligament stem cell subpopulation. J Periodontol 83(3):379–388

Eramo S, Natali A, Pinna R, Milia E (2018) Dental pulp regeneration via cell homing. Int Endod J 51:405

Fayazi S, Takimoto K, Diogenes A (2017) Comparative evaluation of chemotactic factor effect on migration and differentiation of stem cells of the apical papilla. J Endod 43(8):1288–1293

Fischbach GD, Fischbach RL (2004) Stem cells: science, policy, and ethics. J Clin Invest 114(10):1364–1370

Gathani KM, Raghavendra SS (2016) Scaffolds in regenerative endodontics: a review. Dent Res J 13(5):379–386

Gervois P, Wolfs E, Dillen Y, Hilkens P, Ratajczak J, Driesen RB et al (2017) Paracrine maturation and migration of SH-SY5Y cells by dental pulp stem cells. J Dent Res 96(6):654–662

Gronthos S, Mankani M, Brahim J, Robey PG, Shi S (2000) Postnatal human dental pulp stem cells (DPSCs) in vitro and in vivo. Proc Natl Acad Sci U S A 97(25):13625–13630

Hattori K, Dias S, Heissig B, Hackett NR, Lyden D, Tateno M et al (2001) Vascular endothelial growth factor and angiopoietin-1 stimulate postnatal hematopoiesis by recruitment of vasculogenic and hematopoietic stem cells. J Exp Med 193(9):1005–1014

Hattori K, Heissig B, Rafii S (2003) The regulation of hematopoietic stem cell and progenitor mobilization by chemokine SDF-1. Leuk Lymphoma 44(4):575–582

He X, Jiang W, Luo Z, Qu T, Wang Z, Liu N et al (2017) IFN-γ regulates human dental pulp stem cells behavior via NF-κB and MAPK signaling. Sci Rep 7:40681

Horst OV, Chavez MG, Jheon AH, Desai T, Klein OD (2012) Stem cell and biomaterials research in dental tissue engineering and regeneration. Dent Clin N Am 56(3):495–520

Hosseinkhani M, Mehrabani D, Karimfar MH, Bakhtiyari S, Manafi A, Shirazi R (2014) Tissue engineered scaffolds in regenerative medicine. World J Plastic Surg 3(1):3–7

Hotwani K, Sharma K (2014) Platelet rich fibrin - a novel acumen into regenerative endodontic therapy. Restorat Dentist Endod 39(1):1–6

Huang GT (2009) Pulp and dentin tissue engineering and regeneration: current progress. Regen Med 4(5):697–707

Inuyama Y, Kitamura C, Nishihara T, Morotomi T, Nagayoshi M, Tabata Y et al (2010) Effects of hyaluronic acid sponge as a scaffold on odontoblastic cell line and amputated dental pulp. J Biomed Mater Res B Appl Biomater 92((1):120–128

Isaka J, Ohazama A, Kobayashi M, Nagashima C, Takiguchi T, Kawasaki H et al (2001) Participation of periodontal ligament cells with regeneration of alveolar bone. J Periodontol 72(3):314–323

Jadhav G, Shah N, Logani A (2012) Revascularization with and without platelet-rich plasma in nonvital, immature, anterior teeth: a pilot clinical study. J Endod 38(12):1581–1587

Jeeruphan T, Jantarat J, Yanpiset K, Suwannapan L, Khewsawai P, Hargreaves KM (2012) Mahidol study 1: comparison of radiographic and survival outcomes of immature teeth treated with either regenerative endodontic or apexification methods: a retrospective study. J Endod 38(10):1330–1336

Karageorgiou V, Kaplan D (2005) Porosity of 3D biomaterial scaffolds and osteogenesis. Biomaterials 26(27):5474–5491

Kim SG, Zheng Y, Zhou J, Chen M, Embree MC, Song K et al (2013) Dentin and dental pulp regeneration by the patient's endogenous cells. Endod Topics 28(1):106–117

Kim JH, Kim GH, Kim JW, Pyeon HJ, Lee JC, Lee G et al (2016) In vivo angiogenic capacity of stem cells from human exfoliated deciduous teeth with human umbilical vein endothelial cells. Mol Cells 39(11):790–796

Kortesidis A, Zannettino A, Isenmann S, Shi S, Lapidot T, Gronthos S (2005) Stromal-derived factor-1 promotes the growth, survival, and development of human bone marrow stromal stem cells. Blood 105(10):3793–3801

Kuboyama N, Kiba H, Arai K, Uchida R, Tanimoto Y, Bhawal UK et al (2013) Silk fibroin-based scaffolds for bone regeneration. J Biomed Mater Res B Appl Biomater 101((2):295–302

Laterveer L, Lindley IJ, Hamilton MS, Willemze R, Fibbe WE (1995) Interleukin-8 induces rapid mobilization of hematopoietic stem cells with radioprotective capacity and long-term myelo-lymphoid repopulating ability. Blood 85(8):2269–2275

Li B, Jung HJ, Kim SM, Kim MJ, Jahng JW, Lee JH (2013) Human periodontal ligament stem cells repair mental nerve injury. Neural Regen Res 8(30):2827–2837

Li M, Sun X, Ma L, Jin L, Zhang W, Xiao M et al (2017) SDF-1/CXCR4 axis induces human dental pulp stem cell migration through FAK/PI3K/Akt and GSK3β/β-catenin pathways. Sci Rep 7:40161

Liu JY, Chen X, Yue L, Huang GT, Zou XY (2015) CXC chemokine receptor 4 is expressed paravascularly in apical papilla and coordinates with stromal cell-derived factor-1alpha during transmigration of stem cells from apical papilla. J Endod 41(9):1430–1436

Luder HU (2015) Malformations of the tooth root in humans. Front Physiol 6:307

Martin G, Ricucci D, Gibbs JL, Lin LM (2013) Histological findings of revascularized/revitalized immature permanent molar with apical periodontitis using platelet-rich plasma. J Endod 39(1):138–144

Mason C, Dunnill P (2008) A brief definition of regenerative medicine. Regen Med 3(1):1–5

Matsunaga T, Yanagiguchi K, Yamada S, Ohara N, Ikeda T, Hayashi Y (2006) Chitosan monomer promotes tissue regeneration on dental pulp wounds. J Biomed Mater Res A 76((4):711–720

Meinel L, Hofmann S, Karageorgiou V, Kirker-Head C, McCool J, Gronowicz G et al (2005) The inflammatory responses to silk films in vitro and in vivo. Biomaterials 26(2):147–155

Miura M, Gronthos S, Zhao M, Lu B, Fisher LW, Robey PG et al (2003) SHED: stem cells from human exfoliated deciduous teeth. Proc Natl Acad Sci U S A 100(10):5807–5812

Murphy CM, Haugh MG, O'Brien FJ (2010) The effect of mean pore size on cell attachment, proliferation and migration in collagen-glycosaminoglycan scaffolds for bone tissue engineering. Biomaterials 31(3):461–466

Nevins AJ, Finkelstein F, Borden BG, Laporta R (1976) Revitalization of pulpless open apex teeth in rhesus monkeys, using collagen-calcium phosphate gel. J Endod 2(6):159–165

Nevins A, Wrobel W, Valachovic R, Finkelstein F (1977) Hard tissue induction into pulpless open-apex teeth using collagen-calcium phosphate gel. J Endod 3(11):431–433

Pan S, Dangaria S, Gopinathan G, Yan X, Lu X, Kolokythas A et al (2013) SCF promotes dental pulp progenitor migration, neovascularization, and collagen remodeling - potential applications as a homing factor in dental pulp regeneration. Stem Cell Rev 9(5):655–667

Peng C, Zhao Y, Wang W, Yang Y, Qin M, Ge L (2017) Histologic findings of a human immature revascularized/regenerated tooth with symptomatic irreversible pulpitis. J Endod 43(6):905–909

Petit I, Szyper-Kravitz M, Nagler A, Lahav M, Peled A, Habler L et al (2002) G-CSF induces stem cell mobilization by decreasing bone marrow SDF-1 and up-regulating CXCR4. Nat Immunol 3(7):687–694

Polverini PJ (1995) The pathophysiology of angiogenesis. Crit Rev Oral Biol Med 6(3):230–247

Rafii S, Heissig B, Hattori K (2002) Efficient mobilization and recruitment of marrow-derived endothelial and hematopoietic stem cells by adenoviral vectors expressing angiogenic factors. Gene Ther 9(10):631–641

Rodriguez IA, Growney Kalaf EA, Bowlin GL, Sell SA (2014) Platelet-rich plasma in bone regeneration: engineering the delivery for improved clinical efficacy. Biomed Res Int 2014:392398

Rozario T, DeSimone DW (2010) The extracellular matrix in development and morphogenesis: a dynamic view. Dev Biol 341(1):126–140

Ruangsawasdi N, Zehnder M, Patcas R, Ghayor C, Siegenthaler B, Gjoksi B et al (2017) Effects of stem cell factor on cell homing during functional pulp regeneration in human immature teeth. Tissue Eng Part A 23(3-4):115–123

Saito K, Oshima H (2017) Differentiation capacity and maintenance of dental pulp stem/progenitor cells in the process of pulpal healing following tooth injuries. J Oral Biosci 59(2):63–70

Sakai K, Yamamoto A, Matsubara K, Nakamura S, Naruse M, Yamagata M et al (2012) Human dental pulp-derived stem cells promote locomotor recovery after complete transection of the rat spinal cord by multiple neuro-regenerative mechanisms. J Clin Invest 122(1):80–90

Sharma S, Srivastava D, Grover S, Sharma V (2014) Biomaterials in tooth tissue engineering: a review. J Clin Diagn Res 8(1):309–315

Shimizu M, Yasuda T, Nakagawa T, Yamashita E, Julovi SM, Hiramitsu T et al (2003) Hyaluronan inhibits matrix metalloproteinase-1 production by rheumatoid synovial fibroblasts stimulated by proinflammatory cytokines. J Rheumatol 30(6):1164–1172

Shimizu E, Jong G, Partridge N, Rosenberg PA, Lin LM (2012) Histologic observation of a human immature permanent tooth with irreversible pulpitis after revascularization/regeneration procedure. J Endod 38(9):1293–1297

Shimizu E, Ricucci D, Albert J, Alobaid AS, Gibbs JL, Huang GT et al (2013) Clinical, radiographic, and histological observation of a human immature permanent tooth with chronic apical abscess after revitalization treatment. J Endod 39(8):1078–1083

Simonpieri A, Del Corso M, Vervelle A, Jimbo R, Inchingolo F, Sammartino G et al (2012) Current knowledge and perspectives for the use of platelet-rich plasma (PRP) and platelet-rich fibrin (PRF) in oral and maxillofacial surgery part 2: Bone graft, implant and reconstructive surgery. Curr Pharm Biotechnol 13(7):1231–1256

Singhal AR, Agrawal CM, Athanasiou KA (1996) Salient degradation features of a 50:50 PLA/PGA scaffold for tissue engineering. Tissue Eng 2(3):197–207

Solanilla A, Grosset C, Duchez P, Legembre P, Pitard V, Dupouy M et al (2003) Flt3-ligand induces adhesion of haematopoietic progenitor cells via a very late antigen (VLA)-4- and VLA-5-dependent mechanism. Br J Haematol 120(5):782–786

Sonoyama W, Liu Y, Fang D, Yamaza T, Seo BM, Zhang C et al (2006) Mesenchymal stem cell-mediated functional tooth regeneration in swine. PLoS One 1:e79

Sonoyama W, Liu Y, Yamaza T, Tuan RS, Wang S, Shi S et al (2008) Characterization of the apical papilla and its residing stem cells from human immature permanent teeth: a pilot study. J Endod 34(2):166–171

Spitzer G, Adkins D, Mathews M, Velasquez W, Bowers C, Dunphy F et al (1997) Randomized comparison of G-CSF + GM-CSF vs G-CSF alone for mobilization of peripheral blood stem cells: effects on hematopoietic recovery after high-dose chemotherapy. Bone Marrow Transplant 20(11):921–930

Suzuki T, Lee CH, Chen M, Zhao W, Fu SY, Qi JJ et al (2011) Induced migration of dental pulp stem cells for in vivo pulp regeneration. J Dent Res 90(8):1013–1018

Tamma R, Ribatti D (2017) Bone niches, hematopoietic stem cells, and vessel formation. Int J Mol Sci 18(1):151

Trope M (2008) Regenerative potential of dental pulp. J Endod 34(7 Suppl):S13–S17

Tsai TL, Lii WJ (2017) Identification of bone marrow-derived soluble factors regulating human mesenchymal stem cells for bone regeneration. Stem Cell Reports 8(2):387–400

Ueda M, Fujisawa T, Ono M, Hara ES, Pham HT, Nakajima R et al (2014) A short-term treatment with tumor necrosis factor-alpha enhances stem cell phenotype of human dental pulp cells. Stem Cell Res Ther 5(1):31

Uehata M, Ishizaki T, Satoh H, Ono T, Kawahara T, Morishita T et al (1997) Calcium sensitization of smooth muscle mediated by a Rho-associated protein kinase in hypertension. Nature 389(6654):990–994

Vaissiere G, Chevallay B, Herbage D, Damour O (2000) Comparative analysis of different collagen-based biomaterials as scaffolds for long-term culture of human fibroblasts. Med Biol Eng Comput 38(2):205–210

Wang J, Mukaida N, Zhang Y, Ito T, Nakao S, Matsushima K (1997) Enhanced mobilization of hematopoietic progenitor cells by mouse MIP-2 and granulocyte colony-stimulating factor in mice. J Leukoc Biol 62(4):503–509

Wang X, Thibodeau B, Trope M, Lin LM, Huang GT (2010) Histologic characterization of regenerated tissues in canal space after the revitalization/revascularization procedure of immature dog teeth with apical periodontitis. J Endod 36(1):56–63

Wang ZS, Feng ZH, Wu GF, Bai SZ, Dong Y, Chen FM et al (2016) The use of platelet-rich fibrin combined with periodontal ligament and jaw bone mesenchymal stem cell sheets for periodontal tissue engineering. Sci Rep 6:28126

Wang T, Kang W, Du L, Ge S (2017) Rho-kinase inhibitor Y-27632 facilitates the proliferation, migration and pluripotency of human periodontal ligament stem cells. J Cell Mol Med 21(11):3100–3112

Wu Z, Dai W, Wang P, Zhang X, Tang Y, Liu L et al (2018) Periostin promotes migration, proliferation, and differentiation of human periodontal ligament mesenchymal stem cells. Connect Tissue Res 59:108–119

Yang JW, Zhang YF, Wan CY, Sun ZY, Nie S, Jian SJ et al (2015) Autophagy in SDF-1alpha-mediated DPSC migration and pulp regeneration. Biomaterials 44:11–23

Yu Y, Bi CS, Wu RX, Yin Y, Zhang XY, Lan PH et al (2016) Effects of short-term inflammatory and/or hypoxic pretreatments on periodontal ligament stem cells: in vitro and in vivo studies. Cell Tissue Res 366(2):311–328

Zhang X, Zhou P, Zhao Y, Wang M, Wei S (2016) Peptide-conjugated hyaluronic acid surface for the culture of human induced pluripotent stem cells under defined conditions. Carbohydr Polym 136:1061–1064

Zhao F, Yao D, Guo R, Deng L, Dong A, Zhang J (2015) Composites of polymer hydrogels and nanoparticulate systems for biomedical and pharmaceutical applications. Nanomaterials (Basel, Switzerland) 5(4):2054–2130

Current and Future Views on Pulpal Tissue Engineering

9

Bruno N. Cavalcanti and Jacques E. Nör

9.1 Introduction

The function of stem cells in pulp homoeostasis and response to injury (Gronthos et al. 2000; Miura et al. 2003; Yu et al. 2006; Kawashima 2012) has led the field of endodontics to become more focused on regenerative procedures for treatment of pulp pathosis (Sloan and Smith 2007; Rosa et al. 2012; Hargreaves et al. 2013). Recent studies have suggested the possibility of treating necrotic teeth with cell-based strategies that involve the transplantation of dental pulp stem cells (DPSCs) seeded in enabling scaffolds into the root canal. Several research groups have shown success in promoting *in vivo* regeneration of a connective pulp-like tissue inside the human root canal and/or dentine structures in mouse (Cordeiro et al. 2008; Galler et al. 2012; Rosa et al. 2013) and in canine models (Iohara et al. 2011; Ishizaka et al. 2012). Pilot studies in humans are also beginning to show promising outcomes of stem cell transplantation for treatment of necrotic teeth (Nakashima et al. 2017). As such, the possibility of "making a new pulp" for the treatment of pulp necrosis, particularly for the treatment of immature permanent teeth, is becoming a clinical reality that could transform endodontics.

An important step to achieve this success is the development and testing of scaffolds that enable stem cell survival and differentiation upon transplantation (Cavalcanti et al. 2013; Moore et al. 2015; Kuang et al. 2016). These scaffolds carry the cells that are transplanted inside the root canal and allow for their differentiation into odontoblasts, endothelial cells and other cells that collectively generate a new

B. N. Cavalcanti
Department of Endodontics, College of Dentistry, University of Iowa, Iowa City, IA, USA

J. E. Nör (✉)
Department of Cariology, Restorative Sciences, Endodontics, School of Dentistry, University of Michigan, Ann Arbor, MI, USA
e-mail: jenor@umich.edu

© Springer Nature Switzerland AG 2019
H. F. Duncan, P. R. Cooper (eds.), *Clinical Approaches in Endodontic Regeneration*,
https://doi.org/10.1007/978-3-319-96848-3_9

pulp-like tissue. These findings demonstrate that some of the challenges for clinical translation have already been addressed, including the source of the signalling cues for odontoblastic differentiation. They have demonstrated the role of dentine-derived proteins (e.g. BMP-2) as necessary and sufficient for odontoblastic differentiation of DPSCs (Nakashima and Reddi 2003; Casagrande et al. 2010; Sakai et al. 2010; Yang et al. 2012).

Alongside the research advances in the methods for transplantation of stem cells, other groups have focused on clinical procedures, analysing different aspects of pulp revitalisation by eliciting bleeding inside a necrotic root canal, which may also be considered a form of regenerative endodontics (Banchs and Trope 2004; Andreasen and Bakland 2012; Wigler et al. 2013; Diogenes and Hargreaves 2017). These techniques have increased the impact of pulp regeneration studies, as they have shown an unexplored venue for translation of research to clinical practice by making use of procedures that are clinically accepted today (at least within the USA).

This chapter will discuss advances in the understanding of the biology of DPSCs and will also address ongoing attempts to develop a tissue engineering-based method for dental pulp revitalisation. First, mechanisms of dental pulp development and pulp repair will be discussed as underpinning to understand the pulp tissue regeneration process, that is, the ultimate goal of dental pulp tissue engineering. Clinical and preclinical approaches will be presented in light of critical challenges to the clinical translation of this work. This chapter will also provide a prospectus for the field in attempt to foresee how challenges can be overcome as these therapeutic approaches make their way towards state-of-the-art clinical practice.

9.2   Understanding Dental Pulp Development and Healing

Deep understanding of mechanisms underlying development and healing processes is critical to inform strategies for therapeutic tissue regeneration. Fundamental mechanisms of cell differentiation observed during embryonic development and in response to injury can be co-opted for therapeutic tissue regeneration. Indeed, understanding and mimicking pulp development is considered a rational way to develop a strategy to engineer a new dental pulp. The idea of having cells perfectly aligned and signalling to each other to induce their differentiation and tissue formation reflects what is closer to an "ideal" objective in terms of tissue engineering. It is well known that the development of the tooth starts by the folding of the dental epithelium and formation of a tooth bud, surrounding mesenchymal tissue which will be, in the future, the precursor of the dental pulp and dentine (Balic and Thesleff 2015). The full nature of the interaction between mesenchymal and epithelial cells is difficult to reproduce in whole-tooth tissue engineering (Young et al. 2002; Oshima et al. 2011; Yang et al. 2017a). However, for dental pulp tissue engineering, the most important signalling events for odontoblastic differentiation are initiated by the surrounding dentine, and cell-cell interactions enable differentiation of stem cells into vascular endothelial cells that will provide nutrition and oxygen supply

(Casagrande et al. 2010; Bento et al. 2013; Zhang et al. 2016). From a tissue engineering standpoint, active induction of vasculogenesis is critical for dental pulp regeneration as the root canal offers only one anatomical site for influx of blood vessels, the apical foramen (Casagrande et al. 2011; Rombouts et al. 2017).

Processes regulating the homoeostasis of the pulp tissue and its repair capacity may serve as template for methods aiming at de novo formation of a functional dental pulp that is able of generating new tubular dentine. As such, studies evaluating the healing potential of pulp-capping agents are of interest, since they can assess cell mechanisms, analyse *in vivo* events and answer basic questions about odontoblast differentiation. By critically reviewing the extensive literature in this subject, it becomes immediately clear that cell differentiation towards odontoblasts is not only dependent on stem cells. Indeed, several studies have demonstrated that non-stem dental pulp cell populations exposed to inductive signalling triggered by pulp-capping agents can differentiate into odontoblasts (Min et al. 2009; Paranjpe et al. 2010; Zanini et al. 2012; Schmalz and Smith 2014).

In the initial moments after injury, pulp cells initiate an inflammatory process that is mediated by cytokines and growth factors (Cavalcanti et al. 2011; Rechenberg et al. 2016) and trigger other defence responses as the activation of the complement system (Chmilewsky et al. 2014). These systems are important for recruiting not only inflammatory cells but also for the recruitment and differentiation of progenitor cells in the dental pulp (Goldberg et al. 2008; Xu et al. 2017; Giraud et al. 2017). After this initial contact, biocompatible dental materials may have the potential to stimulate cells, not only by their own action but also due to the potential of dental materials to mobilise calcium and other morphogenic factors from the dentine (Graham et al. 2006; Smith et al. 2012). This cocktail of morphogenic factors can induce cell differentiation and stimulate the production of reparative dentine.

However, little is known about the molecular mechanisms involved in this differentiation. It is expected that new odontoblast-like cells express DSPP, DMP-1 and other genes, which can be used as putative markers of differentiation (Casagrande et al. 2010; Cavalcanti et al. 2013). These genes encode proteins that are directly related to the mineralisation process and are not observed in undifferentiated dental pulp cells. In addition, cells may also express Dlx3 and Dlx5, which are transcription factors involved in dentinogenesis (D'Anto et al. 2006; Zanini et al. 2012). Of course, other markers as alkaline phosphatase activity and mineralised nodule formation are of interest and can be observed both *in vivo* and *in vitro*. However, none of these markers are unique to odontoblastic differentiation as they are also expressed by osteoblasts.

9.3 State of the Art Evidence and Challenges in Pulp Regeneration Studies

Vital pulp therapy (e.g. direct pulp capping, pulpotomy) is a procedure with variable success rates that is considered an alternative for non-surgical root canal treatments for selected cases (Zanini et al. 2017). For instance, the maintenance of a vital pulp tissue in the root canals can be responsible for inducing apexogenesis in immature teeth with open apex. In this context, the use of biomaterials has gained importance as they can induce cell differentiation, promote the mobilisation of biomolecules from the dentine and serve as a mechanical barrier against infection. The limitation of vital pulp therapy relies on the fact that the pulp may be irreversibly inflamed or evolve towards necrosis particularly in the presence of bacteria (Shabahang and Torabinejad 2000).

A major challenge in vital pulp therapy is the diagnosis of the pulp tissue status. Although the identification of pulp necrosis is more straightforward when a periapical lesion is identified, accurately determining differential diagnosis between reversible and irreversible pulpitis can be challenging. Obviously, without accurate diagnosis, the clinician needs to rely on other information to decide if vital pulp therapy is recommended. The direct observation of clinical pulp status (i.e. colour, texture, nature of bleeding), patient's age, status of root formation and response to pulp vitality tests can be performed clinically; however, these show limited correlation with the histological pulp status (Dummer et al. 1980; Bender 2000). The continuous development of improved diagnostic methods constitutes a key step towards the enhanced determination of the potential for pulp tissue repair and indication for pulp regeneration procedures.

The presence of bacterial invasion and pulp necrosis has also led to new approaches that can be used to promote completion of root formation in immature teeth (Fig. 9.1). Recently, the concept of revascularisation has been revisited by the endodontic field, and new insights have been applied in practice with promising success rates (Diogenes and Hargreaves 2017). The use of a blood clot and the induction of the cells present in this blood clot have proven to be feasible ways to promote completion of root formation (Banchs and Trope 2004; Galler 2016).

Dental pulp regeneration is considered to be "biologically based procedures designed to replace damaged structures, including dentine and root structures, as well as cells of the pulp-dentine complex" (Hargreaves et al. 2013). By this definition of pulp regeneration, one must have the replacement of the lost tissue by a new one that exhibits the same histological and functional properties. This differs from the concept of repair, where one may have a different tissue functioning in a similar way as the replaced tissue. This is likely what is observed when the revascularisation method is used. It is important to emphasise that although regeneration is desired, success can also be observed with repair-based procedures. Indeed, from a clinical standpoint, this might be considered a desirable outcome, a clinical success. The clinical use of revascularisation procedures has promoted advances in the understanding of the biology of stem cells by providing clinical data supporting a potential participation of periapical stem cells in the process of pulp repair.

9.4 Cell Transplantation Versus Cell Homing for Dental Pulp Regeneration

Tissue engineering procedures typically involve the use of stem cells, enabling scaffolds and the availability of morphogenic signals to promote the adequate cell differentiation and tissue formation. From this standpoint, most of the research is developing cell-based therapies, i.e. the transplant of autologous DPSCs, the use of

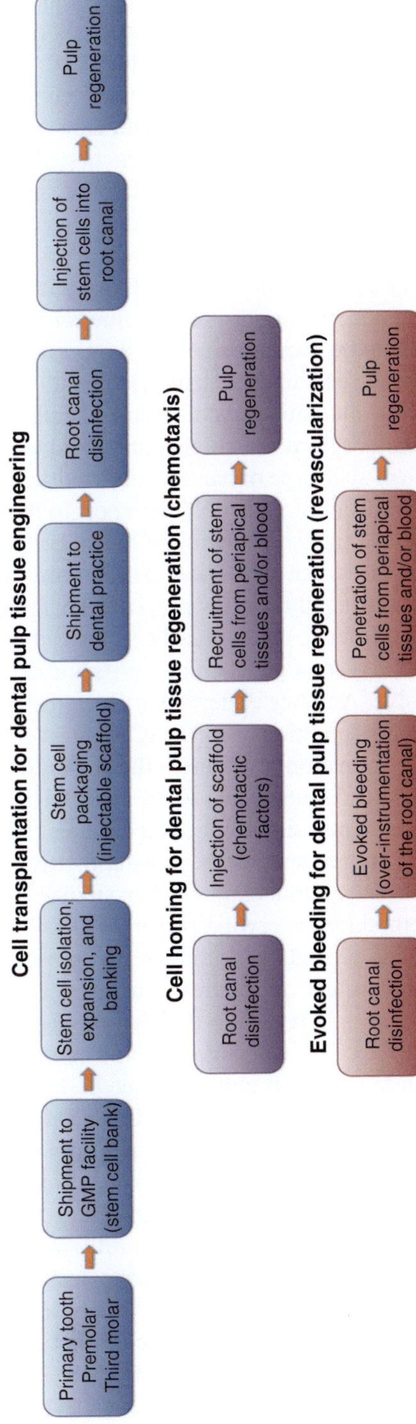

Fig. 9.1 Diagram depicting a panel of strategies for pulp tissue regeneration, i.e. cell transplantation, cell homing and evoked bleeding (revascularisation)

injectable scaffolds and the delivery of the environment signalling molecules either by dentine treatment (Casagrande et al. 2010) or by the incorporation of growth factors in delivery systems for the scaffolds (Kim et al. 2010; Kamocki et al. 2015). The translation of this approach to the clinic required major technical advances, particularly in regard to the use of autologous human cells. Dr. Nakashima's group in Japan has recently published what appears to be the first clinical trial in regenerative endodontics that involves the transplantation of autologous stem cells (Nakashima et al. 2017). This trial can be considered a pilot study with few patients. It suggests feasibility and safety of a stem cell-based approach for pulp regeneration, but still does not fully demonstrate efficacy. Even with these limitations, the initial results are promising and will serve as a baseline for future larger trials.

Several hurdles still need to be overcome before stem cell-based therapies can be used routinely in the clinic. For example, to have viable cells for use in therapeutic regenerative endodontics, one alternative is to use banked cells retrieved from exfoliated primary teeth, premolars or third molars that are extracted for orthodontic reasons. However, the creation of such type of banking demands rigorous quality control in several key steps, tooth collection/extraction, transport to the laboratory, cell culture/expansion process and freezing and thawing of the cells. The clinical trials cited above were able to address the tooth collection/cell handling process by using an infrastructure put in place specifically for this purpose. This may increase the costs of such treatments in the short term, but, as has been seen in dentistry and in other areas of healthcare, this is the type of problem that time and acceptance of the technique may eventually resolve. Another issue that still needs to be addressed is the development of ideal culture conditions for DPSC culture/expansion (Piva et al. 2017). It is known that the elimination of serum in the cell cultures does not alter the cell properties (Ducret et al. 2015; Jung et al. 2016) and that the donor blood can be used as a source for supplement nutrition for the cell cultures (Pisciolaro et al. 2015). However, these studies have not proven that the translation to clinical practice can be achieved under such conditions, demanding further studies to address this point. Also, it is clear that the method for the cryopreservation of DPSCs is a critical factor influencing the success of the procedure. Although cryopreservation appears to be effective in preserving the stem cell properties (Kumar et al. 2015; Hilkens et al. 2016), there is still no consensus in regard to the ideal protocol that should be used for freezing and thawing these cells. This has led some authors to advocate the use of cryopreserved tissues instead of cell cultures (Takebe et al. 2017). And finally, recent evidence on the immunological conditions of DPSCs may have a direct impact on their clinical application. Reportedly, DPSCs are not fully immunologically competent. Indeed, they have exhibited immunosuppressive effects, which may enable the use of DPSCs in allogeneic transplants (Ding et al. 2015; Kwack et al. 2017). However, to our knowledge, this aspect has not been fully tested in humans yet.

One of the areas in development is the use of strategies that do not involve cell transplantation for pulp regeneration. These strategies are based on the use of chemotactic agents to attract periapical mesenchymal stem cells that can promote pulp tissue regeneration (Kim et al. 2010; Suzuki et al. 2011; He et al. 2017). In this case, it is expected that the surrounding tissues, for example, the apical papilla (Liu et al. 2015), circulating blood (Zhang et al. 2015) or the pulp remnants (Galler and Widbiller 2017), would provide the cells required for tissue regeneration. Such an approach can be considered safer in general, as it would not involve *ex vivo* handling of human cells (Galler and Widbiller 2017). Of note, it is important to emphasise that "cell homing" and "cell-free" concepts have been used interchangeably for these types of therapies. In this context, the concept of revascularisation could be classified as a regenerative procedure but does not fulfil the concept of cell-free, since it is clear that the blood clot promoted into the root canal contains cells. This is different from a true cell-free approach where a scaffold devoid of cells will promote the homing towards the root canal.

9.5   Scaffolds for Pulp Tissue Engineering

The second key component of the tissue engineering triad is the use of scaffolds that enable tissue regeneration (Piva et al. 2014). The first research models for pulp tissue engineering, the tooth slice/scaffold model, constitute an approach for proof-of-concept studies, as it promotes close interaction of the implanted cells with the host (e.g. immunodeficient mice), with the dentine, and enables vascularisation of the pulp-like tissue (Cordeiro et al. 2008; Sakai et al. 2011). However, this initial model relies on rigid polymers (e.g. PLLA), which involve the use of a porogen strategy and the use of solvents (Demarco et al. 2010). Although useful for research, it is clear that applications in endodontics would demand the use of injectable scaffolds that can more easily be adapted to the complex anatomy of root canals. The tooth slice/scaffold model was modified to allow for studies of different formulations of scaffolds. These studies demonstrated that DPSCs survive and proliferate in injectable scaffolds within tooth slices of full human roots (Cavalcanti et al. 2013; Rosa et al. 2013). Studies aiming at the development of new scaffolds for dental pulp tissue engineering are focusing on the minimising shrinkage by the use of cross-linking agents (Kwon et al. 2017), enhancing drug delivery and antimicrobial properties (Bottino et al. 2013) and increasing the induction of an angiogenic response that enables fast vascularisation of the pulp-like tissue (Piva et al. 2014). It is worth mentioning that the most advanced clinical study so far uses an atelocollagen gel as scaffold for stem cell transplantation in humans (Nakashima et al. 2017). Recent data also suggest that decellularised human matrices from adjacent tissues are also suitable for this purpose (Zhang et al. 2017). In addition, there is data showing that it is possible to have a scaffold-free approach, by promoting the construction of three-dimensional (3D) structures with DPSCs (Syed-Picard et al. 2014). Nevertheless, all these approaches will have to rely on a clinically feasible method for delivery of care, which includes reasonable costs and a user-friendly technique.

9.6   Morphogenic Signals and Cell Differentiation

And finally, the last component of the tissue engineering triad is the availability of morphogenic signals or "environment" that guides stem cell differentiation (Fig. 9.2). While it has been demonstrated that the dentine provides an ideal source of inducers of odontoblastic differentiation (Smith et al. 1990; Casagrande et al.

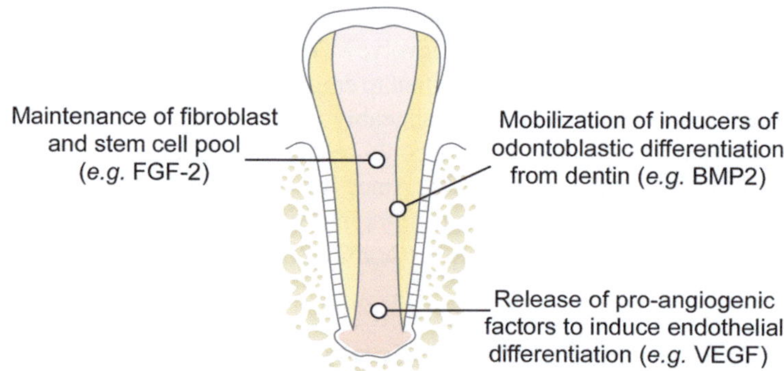

Fig. 9.2 Diagram depicting potential sources of extracellular molecules involved in the promotion of stem cell differentiation and maintenance of phenotypes in regenerated pulp tissues

2010; Liu et al. 2016), it remains unclear what is the best approach to enable optimal release of these morphogenic factors. One possibility is to treat the dentine with a short exposure to ethylenediaminetetraacetic acid (EDTA). Besides being a routine rinsing solution for endodontics, EDTA was shown to mobilise dentine proteins that enable DPSC differentiation into odontoblast-like cells (Casagrande et al. 2010). One possible clinical scenario is to follow the standard root canal instrumentation with a final wash with EDTA immediately before the transplantation of stem cells with an injectable scaffold. While this approach led to promising results in the laboratory (Casagrande et al. 2010; Rosa et al. 2013), it remains to be tested in human patients.

Understanding decisions of cell fate and the nature of specific signalling events is critical to providing an ideal stimulus and to the neo-formed dental pulp-like tissue. An example in dental pulp tissue engineering is that most research has been focused on cell differentiation towards an odontoblastic phenotype, which can be induced by BMP-2 (Nakashima and Reddi 2003; Casagrande et al. 2010; Yang et al. 2012). However, the dental pulp tissue is obviously not comprised only of odontoblasts. Needless to say, it is not desirable that all transplanted stem cells become odontoblast-like cells which would likely lead to full mineralisation of the root canal. Ideally, the newly formed tissue will have odontoblast-like cells lining the dentine tissue, fibroblasts and stem cells in the pulp core, vascular endothelial cells generating blood vessels to provide influx of nutrients and oxygen and neural cells providing for the regulation of cellular function and the recovery of the sensation of protective pain.

The differentiation towards an odontoblastic phenotype is probably one of the most investigated subjects related to pulp tissue engineering, particularly due to the effects of BMP-2 in this process. The literature is rich in examples of studies showing that a number of pathways, including the canonical Smad pathway (Li et al. 2015), the Wnt pathway (Yang et al. 2015), the MAPKinase pathway (Qin et al. 2014) and the Dlx3/Osx pathway (Yang et al. 2017b), are involved in the determination of the odontoblastic fate of stem cells. EDTA-treated dentine serves as a source for inducers of odontoblastic differentiation, including BMP-2 (Casagrande et al. 2010). Moreover, although some intracellular mechanisms are still not clear, studies have shown that dentine-derived BMP-2-induced DPSC differentiation towards odontoblasts is robust and involves upregulated expression of dentine sialophosphoprotein (DSPP) and dentine matrix protein-1 (DMP-1), putative markers of odontoblastic differentiation. A pulp-like tissue requires an odontoblastic layer in close contact with the existing dentine. These cells should serve not only to produce new dentine but also as a barrier to bacteria. Preclinical studies have demonstrated that DPSCs injected into a clean empty tooth slice and transplanted into the subcutaneous immunodeficient mice function as odontoblast-like cells (i.e. generate new tubular dentine as demonstrated by tetracycline staining) and exhibit junctional structures (as demonstrated by transmission electron microscopy) (Cordeiro et al. 2008; Sakai et al. 2010). However, these features of stem cells remain to be demonstrated in humans.

In addition, it is still not clear if DPSCs can respond to extracellular factors and maintain a less differentiated mesenchymal cell phenotype that can be responsible for the fibre and matrix turnover in the core of the pulp connective tissue. Although largely overlooked by researchers, this process can play an important role in maintaining the responsiveness of the neo-formed pulp tissue. Notably, it is known that factors such as FGF-2 may assist in inhibiting the differentiation potential of DPSCs, induce expression of stem cell markers and increase cell proliferation (He et al. 2008; Kim et al. 2014; Gorin et al. 2016). Moreover, the presence of this extracellular matrix "core" in the pulp tissue might be important to promote the supporting structure of fibres in the longer term, as the scaffolds used for cell transplantation are degraded.

Besides requiring odontoblasts and fibroblasts, an engineered pulp requires potent and rapid pro-angiogenic activity due to its particularly challenging anatomical confinement inside the pulp chamber surrounded by rigid walls and with limited access to blood and oxygen influx. It is important to emphasise that the apical tissues are capable of providing pulp blood vessels to occupy, and this can explain, at least in part, successful cases of conservative therapies such as revascularisation. Nonetheless, the current knowledge still lacks information on approaches that consistently induce blood vessel formation throughout the entire root canal and the coronal pulp chamber in necrotic teeth treated with revascularisation approaches. Fortunately, there is mounting evidence supporting the fact that DPSCs can differentiate into endothelial cells when appropriately induced by vascular endothelial growth factor (VEGF) (Sakai et al. 2010). More importantly, studies are showing that these cells cannot only differentiate in endothelial cells but also can organise themselves to promote the formation of blood vessels (Zhang et al. 2016). This happens through the actions of signalling pathways as Wnt and ERK (Bento et al. 2013; Zhang et al. 2016). These studies are providing insights to inform the development of strategies for tissue engineering scaffold involving the controlled delivery of morphogenic factors that can drive rapid vasculogenic response while maintaining a pool of stem cells that are able to differentiate odontoblastically.

9.7   Clinical Hurdles for Dental Pulp Tissue Engineering

Despite substantial scientific developments in the field of dental pulp tissue engineering, many unanswered questions remain, particularly in regard to the optimal clinical protocols. In general, studies that have shown successful pulp engineering using standard procedures for root canal preparation and cleaning, followed by the transplantation of DPSCs seeded in biodegradable scaffolds (Iohara et al. 2011; Ishizaka et al. 2012; Nakashima et al. 2017). As these clinical studies mature with more patients and longer follow-up times, we will have a better understanding for the adequacy of the existing protocol (or need for changes). In addition, there are lingering questions that will have to be addressed by a combination of preclinical and clinical studies, for example, should we shape the root canal? How much dilatation is necessary for injecting cells and scaffolds? Which is the best dentine treatment to allow for cell survival and proliferation? And, which is the best way to disinfect root canals while still maintaining functional dentine-derived morphogenic factors required for pulp regeneration? We propose that questions like these merit further investigation.

The number of endodontic cutting instruments and techniques available in the market is high, and many factors as dentine structure or surface must be considered when preparing a tooth (Peters et al. 2010; Cheron et al. 2011). Extensive information is found on the effects of rotary instruments on the canal walls, but the question raised in this context is "deeper". In general, we shape root canals to remove contaminated dentine and allow for adequate sealing with a plastic material, but is this necessary in a dental pulp tissue engineering procedure? The use of hydrogels as injectable scaffolds for dental pulp tissue engineering has been previously explored when PuraMatrix was tested in preclinical studies (Cavalcanti et al. 2013). As such, it is possible that root canal preparation with minimal shaping could be sufficient. Indeed, self-adjusting files could be an option for root canal preparations of dental pulp regenerative procedures (Peters and Paqué 2011), but this assumption will have to be further evaluated.

If conservative dentine removal approaches are to be used, the integrity of the root canal would be preserved, but concerns regarding disinfection ability may rise. The endodontic literature reports on many examples of approaches for disinfection of root canals for regenerative procedures using antibiotic pastes (Lovelace et al. 2011) or calcium hydroxide (Cehreli et al. 2011). However, it must be kept in mind that the same substance that kills bacteria may also kill stem cells (Martin et al. 2014). In this context, new scaffolds are being developed to allow an efficient and controlled antibiotic release without harming the transplanted cells (Bottino et al. 2013, 2015; Kamocki et al. 2015; Bottino et al. 2017). These materials may constitute an alternative for intracanal dressing before the regenerative procedure. They may also be useful in conjunction with the hydrogel scaffold to disinfect the root canal and promote tissue regeneration at the same time. Notably, the irrigant solution used for root canal treatment may impact the quality and availability of dentine molecules required for cell growth and differentiation. For example, sodium hypochlorite is the most commonly used irrigant in endodontics. However, sodium hypochlorite denatures dentine-derived proteins (e.g. BMP-2) that are required for odontoblastic differentiation (Casagrande et al. 2010; Martin et al. 2014). As an alternative for sodium hypochlorite, one may consider the utilisation of calcium hydroxide, as it has been shown to enable release of active proteins from the dentine substrate (Graham et al. 2006). Another alternative is the use of EDTA, as it also has the property of facilitating release of active dentine-derived proteins that can serve as morphogenic signalling for odontoblastic differentiation (Casagrande et al. 2010).

9.8 Future Perspectives

Regenerative endodontic strategies are becoming a new option in the clinical arsenal that practitioners have at hand for treatment of inflamed or necrotic teeth. They may enable pulp repair/regeneration and perhaps improve the long-term outcome of these teeth. Very recent evidence suggests that dental pulp tissue engineering may be a viable approach for treatment of necrotic teeth (Nakashima et al. 2017). Nevertheless, there are many challenges ahead before dental pulp tissue engineering becomes standard of care for treatment of necrotic teeth. Critical issues include, but are not limited to, the discovery of the ideal method for root canal preparation and disinfection, the ideal stem cell source (e.g. autologous transplant, induction of chemotactic movement of resident stem cells from the periapical region), ideal scaffold for stem cell transplantation, *ex vivo* methods for stem cell handling and the development of approaches that are safe, effective and within reasonable costs.

In conclusion, dental pulp tissue engineering holds much promise as a novel and conservative strategy for the treatment of irreversibly inflamed or necrotic teeth. It is well known that conventional root canal therapy is straightforward, relatively cheap and highly successful in most cases. As such, pulp tissue engineering will likely only be indicated in selected cases where conventional therapy does not allow for excellent prognosis (e.g. treatment of necrotic immature permanent teeth). The challenge for pulp tissue engineering is that it will have to be safe and efficient; it will have to be done within reasonable costs for the patient and lead to improved patient outcomes. We firmly believe that the path to overcome these challenges will require active collaborations among clinicians, pulp biologists and material scientists.

References

Andreasen JO, Bakland LK (2012) Pulp regeneration after non-infected and infected necrosis, what type of tissue do we want? A review. Dent Traumatol 28:13–18

Balic A, Thesleff I (2015) Tissue interactions regulating tooth development and renewal. Curr Top Dev Biol 115:157–186

Banchs F, Trope M (2004) Revascularization of immature permanent teeth with apical periodontitis: new treatment protocol? J Endod 30(4):196–200

Bender IB (2000) Pulpal pain diagnosis: a review. J Endod 26(3):175–179

Bento LW, Zhang Z, Imai A, Nör F, Dong Z, Shi S, Araujo FB, Nör JE (2013) Endothelial differentiation of SHED requires MEK1/ERK signaling. J Dent Res 92(1):51–57

Bottino MC, Kamocki K, Yassen GH, Platt JA, Vail MM, Ehrlich Y, Spolnik KJ, Gregory RL (2013) Bioactive nanofibrous scaffolds for regenerative endodontics. J Dent Res 92:963–969

Bottino MC, Yassen GH, Platt JA, Labban N, Windsor LJ, Spolnik KJ, Bressiani AH (2015) A novel three-dimensional scaffold for regenerative endodontics: materials and biological characterizations. J Tissue Eng Regen Med 9(11):E116–E123

Bottino MC, Pankajakshan D, Nör JE (2017) Advanced scaffolds for dental pulp and periodontal regeneration. Dent Clin N Am 61(4):689–711

Casagrande L, Demarco FF, Zhang Z, Araujo FB, Shi S, Nör JE (2010) Dentin-derived BMP-2 and odontoblast differentiation. J Dent Res 89:603–608

Casagrande L, Cordeiro MM, Nor SA, Nör JE (2011) Dental pulp stem cells in regenerative dentistry. Odontology 99(1):1–7

Cavalcanti BN, Rode Sde M, França CM, Marques MM (2011) Pulp capping materials exert an effect on the secretion of IL-1β and IL-8 by migrating human neutrophils. Braz Oral Res 25(1):13–18

Cavalcanti BN, Zeitlin BD, Nör JE (2013) A hydrogel scaffold that maintains viability and supports differentiation of dental pulp stem cells. Dent Mater 29:97–102

Cehreli ZC, Isbitiren B, Sara S, Erbas G (2011) Regenerative endodontic treatment (revascularization) of immature necrotic molars medicated with calcium hydroxide: a case series. J Endod 37:1327–1330

Cheron RA, Marshall SJ, Goodis HE, Peters OA (2011) Nanomechanical properties of endodontically treated teeth. J Endod 37:1562–1565

Chmilewsky F, Jeanneau C, Laurent P, About I (2014) Pulp fibroblasts synthesize functional complement proteins involved in initiating dentin-pulp regeneration. Am J Pathol 184(7):1991–2000

Cordeiro MM, Dong Z, Kaneko T, Zhang Z, Miyazawa M, Shi S, Smith AJ, Nör JE (2008) Dental pulp tissue engineering with stem cells from exfoliated deciduous teeth. J Endod 34(8): 962–969

D'Anto V, Cantile M, D'Armiento M, Schiavo G, Spagnuolo G, Terracciano L et al (2006) The HOX genes are expressed, in vivo, in human tooth germs: in vitro cAMP exposure of dental pulp cells results in parallel HOX network activation and neuronal differentiation. J Cell Biochem 97(4):836–848

Demarco FF, Casagrande L, Zhang Z, Dong Z, Tarquinio SB, Zeitlin BD, Shi S, Smith AJ, Nör JE (2010) Effects of morphogen and scaffold porogen on the differentiation of dental pulp stem cells. J Endod 36(11):1805–1811

Ding G, Niu J, Liu Y (2015) Dental pulp stem cells suppress the proliferation of lymphocytes via transforming growth factor-β1. Hum Cell 28(2):81–90

Diogenes A, Hargreaves KM (2017) Microbial modulation of stem cells and future directions in regenerative endodontics. J Endod 43(9S):S95–S101

Ducret M, Fabre H, Farges JC, Degoul O, Atzeni G, McGuckin C et al (2015) Production of human dental pulp cells with a medicinal manufacturing approach. J Endod 41(9):1492–1499

Dummer PM, Hicks R, Huws D (1980) Clinical signs and symptoms in pulp disease. Int Endod J 13(1):27–35

Galler KM (2016) Clinical procedures for revitalization: current knowledge and considerations. Int Endod J 49(10):926–936

Galler KM, Widbiller M (2017) Perspectives for cell-homing approaches to engineer dental pulp. J Endod 43(9S):S40–S45

Galler KM, Hartgerink JD, Cavender AC, Schmalz G, D'Souza RN (2012) A customized self-assembling peptide hydrogel for dental pulp tissue engineering. Tissue Eng Part A 18:176–184

Giraud T, Rufas P, Chmilewsky F, Rombouts C, Dejou J, Jeanneau C, About I (2017) Complement activation by pulp capping materials plays a significant role in both inflammatory and pulp stem cells' recruitment. J Endod 43(7):1104–1110

Goldberg M, Farges JC, Lacerda-Pinheiro S, Six N, Jegat N, Decup F, Septier D, Carrouel F, Durand S, Chaussain-Miller C, Denbesten P, Veis A, Poliard A (2008) Inflammatory and immunological aspects of dental pulp repair. Pharmacol Res 58:137–147

Gorin C, Rochefort GY, Bascetin R, Ying H, Lesieur J, Sadoine J et al (2016) Priming dental pulp stem cells with fibroblast growth factor-2 increases angiogenesis of implanted tissue-engineered constructs through hepatocyte growth factor and vascular endothelial growth factor secretion. Stem Cells Transl Med 5(3):392–404

Graham L, Cooper PR, Cassidy N, Nor JE, Sloan AJ, Smith AJ (2006) The effect of calcium hydroxide on solubilisation of bio-active dentine matrix components. Biomaterials 27:2865–2873

Gronthos S, Mankani M, Brahim J, Robey PG, Shi S (2000) Postnatal human dental pulp stem cells (DPSCs) in vitro and in vivo. Proc Natl Acad Sci U S A 97:13625–13630

Hargreaves KM, Diogenes A, Teixeira FB (2013) Treatment options: biological basis of regenerative endodontic procedures. J Endod 39(3 Suppl):S30–S43

He H, Yu J, Liu Y, Lu S, Liu H, Shi J et al (2008) Effects of FGF2 and TGFbeta1 on the differentiation of human dental pulp stem cells in vitro. Cell Biol Int 32(7):827–834

He L, Kim SG, Gong Q, Zhong J, Wang S, Zhou X et al (2017) Regenerative endodontics for adult patients. J Endod 43(9S):S57–S64

Hilkens P, Driesen RB, Wolfs E, Gervois P, Vangansewinkel T, Ratajczak J et al (2016) Cryopreservation and banking of dental stem cells. Adv Exp Med Biol 951:199–235

Iohara K, Imabayashi K, Ishizaka R, Watanabe A, Nabekura J, Ito M, Matsushita K, Nakamura H, Nakashima M (2011) Complete pulp regeneration after pulpectomy by transplantation of CD105+ stem cells with stromal cell-derived factor-1. Tissue Eng Part A 17:1911–1920

Ishizaka R, Iohara K, Murakami M, Fukuta O, Nakashima M (2012) Regeneration of dental pulp following pulpectomy by fractionated stem/progenitor cells from bone marrow and adipose tissue. Biomaterials 33:2109–2118

Jung J, Kim JW, Moon HJ, Hong JY, Hyun JK (2016) Characterization of neurogenic potential of dental pulp stem cells cultured in xeno/serum-free condition: in vitro and in vivo assessment. Stem Cells Int 2016:6921097

Kamocki K, Nör JE, Bottino MC (2015) Dental pulp stem cell responses to novel antibiotic-containing scaffolds for regenerative endodontics. Int Endod J 48(12):1147–1156

Kawashima N (2012) Characterisation of dental pulp stem cells: a new horizon for tissue regeneration? Arch Oral Biol 57:1439–1458

Kim JY, Xin X, Moioli EK, Chung J, Lee CH, Chen M et al (2010) Regeneration of dental-pulp-like tissue by chemotaxis-induced cell homing. Tissue Eng Part A 16(10):3023–3031

Kim J, Park JC, Kim SH, Im GI, Kim BS, Lee JB et al (2014) Treatment of FGF-2 on stem cells from inflamed dental pulp tissue from human deciduous teeth. Oral Dis 20(2):191–204

Kuang R, Zhang Z, Jin X, Hu J, Shi S, Ni L, Ma PX (2016) Nanofibrous spongy microspheres for the delivery of hypoxia-primed human dental pulp stem cells to regenerate vascularized dental pulp. Acta Biomater 33:225–234

Kumar A, Bhattacharyya S, Rattan V (2015) Effect of uncontrolled freezing on biological characteristics of human dental pulp stem cells. Cell Tissue Bank 16(4):513–522

Kwack KH, Lee JM, Park SH, Lee HW (2017) human dental pulp stem cells suppress alloantigen-induced immunity by stimulating t cells to release transforming growth factor beta. J Endod 43(1):100–108

Kwon YS, Kim HJ, Hwang YC, Rosa V, Yu MK, Min KS (2017) Effects of epigallocatechin gallate, an antibacterial cross-linking agent, on proliferation and differentiation of human dental pulp cells cultured in collagen scaffolds. J Endod 43(2):289–296

Li S, Hu J, Zhang G, Qi W, Zhang P, Li P et al (2015) Extracellular Ca2+ promotes odontoblastic differentiation of dental pulp stem cells via BMP2-mediated Smad1/5/8 and Erk1/2 pathways. J Cell Physiol 230(9):2164–2173

Liu JY, Chen X, Yue L, Huang GT, Zou XY (2015) CXC Chemokine receptor 4 is expressed paravascularly in apical papilla and coordinates with stromal cell-derived factor-1α during transmigration of stem cells from apical papilla. J Endod 41(9):1430–1436

Liu G, Xu G, Gao Z, Liu Z, Xu J, Wang J et al (2016) Demineralized dentin matrix induces odontoblastic differentiation of dental pulp stem cells. Cells Tissues Organs 201(1):65–76

Lovelace TW, Henry MA, Hargreaves KM, Diogenes A (2011) Evaluation of the delivery of mesenchymal stem cells into the root canal space of necrotic immature teeth after clinical regenerative endodontic procedure. J Endod 37:133–138

Martin DE, De Almeida JF, Henry MA, Khaing ZZ, Schmidt CE, Teixeira FB, Diogenes A (2014) Concentration-dependent effect of sodium hypochlorite on stem cells of apical papilla survival and differentiation. J Endod 40:51–55

Min KS, Yang SH, Kim EC (2009) The combined effect of mineral trioxide aggregate and enamel matrix derivative on odontoblastic differentiation in human dental pulp cells. J Endod 35:847–851

Miura M, Gronthos S, Zhao M, Lu B, Fisher LW, Robey PG, Shi S (2003) SHED: stem cells from human exfoliated deciduous teeth. Proc Natl Acad Sci U S A 100(10):5807–5812

Moore AN, Perez SC, Hartgerink JD, D'Souza RN, Colombo JS (2015) Ex vivo modeling of multidomain peptide hydrogels with intact dental pulp. J Dent Res 94(12):1773–1781

Nakashima M, Reddi AH (2003) The application of bone morphogenetic proteins to dental tissue engineering. Nat Biotechnol 21:1025–1032

Nakashima M, Iohara K, Murakami M, Nakamura H, Sato Y, Ariji Y, Matsushita K (2017) Pulp regeneration by transplantation of dental pulp stem cells in pulpitis: a pilot clinical study. Stem Cell Res Ther 8(1):61

Oshima M, Mizuno M, Imamura A, Ogawa M, Yasukawa M, Yamazaki H et al (2011) Functional tooth regeneration using a bioengineered tooth unit as a mature organ replacement regenerative therapy. PLoS One 6(7):e21531

Paranjpe A, Zhang H, Johnson JD (2010) Effects of mineral trioxide aggregate on human dental pulp cells after pulp-capping procedures. J Endod 36:1042–1047

Peters OA, Paqué F (2011) Root canal preparation of maxillary molars with the self-adjusting file: a micro-computed tomography study. J Endod 37:53–57

Peters OA, Boessler C, Paqué F (2010) Root canal preparation with a novel nickel-titanium instrument evaluated with micro-computed tomography: canal surface preparation over time. J Endod 36:1068–1072

Pisciolaro RL, Duailibi MT, Novo NF, Juliano Y, Pallos D, Yelick PC et al (2015) Tooth tissue engineering: the importance of blood products as a supplement in tissue culture medium for human pulp dental stem cells. Tissue Eng Part A 21(21-22):2639–2648

Piva E, Silva AF, Nör JE (2014) Functionalized scaffolds to control dental pulp stem cell fate. J Endod 40(4 Suppl):S33–S40

Piva E, Tarlé SA, Nör JE, Zou D, Hatfield E, Guinn T, Eubanks EJ, Kaigler D (2017) Dental pulp tissue regeneration using dental pulp stem cells isolated and expanded in human serum. J Endod 43(4):568–574

Qin W, Liu P, Zhang R, Huang S, Gao X, Song Z et al (2014) JNK MAPK is involved in BMP-2-induced odontoblastic differentiation of human dental pulp cells. Connect Tissue Res 55(3):217–224

Rechenberg DK, Galicia JC, Peters OA (2016) Biological markers for pulpal inflammation: a systematic review. PLoS One 11(11):e0167289

Rombouts C, Giraud T, Jeanneau C, About I (2017) Pulp vascularization during tooth development, regeneration, and therapy. J Dent Res 96(2):137–144

Rosa V, Della Bona A, Cavalcanti BN, Nör JE (2012) Tissue engineering: from research to dental clinics. Dent Mater 28:341–348

Rosa V, Zhang Z, Grande RH, Nör JE (2013) Dental pulp tissue engineering in full-length human root canals. J Dent Res 92:970–975

Sakai VT, Zhang Z, Dong Z, Neiva KG, Machado MA, Shi S, Santos CF, Nör JE (2010) SHED differentiate into functional odontoblasts and endothelium. J Dent Res 89:791–796

Sakai VT, Cordeiro MM, Dong Z, Zhang Z, Zeitlin BD, Nör JE (2011) Tooth slice/scaffold model of dental pulp tissue engineering. Adv Dent Res 23(3):325–332

Schmalz G, Smith AJ (2014) Pulp development, repair, and regeneration: challenges of the transition from traditional dentistry to biologically based therapies. J Endod 40(4 Suppl):S2–S5

Shabahang S, Torabinejad M (2000) Treatment of teeth with open apices using mineral trioxide aggregate. Pract Periodontics Aesthet Dent 12(3):315–320

Sloan AJ, Smith AJ (2007) Stem cells and the dental pulp: potential roles in dentine regeneration and repair. Oral Dis 13:151–157

Smith AJ, Tobias RS, Plant CG, Browne RM, Lesot H, Ruch JV (1990) In vivo morphogenetic activity of dentine matrix proteins. J Biol Buccale 18(2):123–129

Smith JG, Smith AJ, Shelton RM, Cooper PR (2012) Recruitment of dental pulp cells by dentine and pulp extracellular matrix components. Exp Cell Res 318:2397–2406

Suzuki T, Lee CH, Chen M, Zhao W, Fu SY, Qi JJ, Chotkowski G, Eisig SB, Wong A, Mao JJ (2011) Induced migration of dental pulp stem cells for in vivo pulp regeneration. J Dent Res 90(8):1013–1018

Syed-Picard FN, Ray HL Jr, Kumta PN, Sfeir C (2014) Scaffoldless tissue-engineered dental pulp cell constructs for endodontic therapy. J Dent Res 93(3):250–255

Takebe Y, Tatehara S, Fukushima T, Tokuyama-Toda R, Yasuhara R, Mishima K et al (2017) Cryopreservation method for the effective collection of dental pulp stem cells. Tissue Eng Part C Methods 23(5):251–261

Wigler R, Kaufman AY, Lin S, Steinbock N, Hazan-Molina H, Torneck CD (2013) Revascularization: a treatment for permanent teeth with necrotic pulp and incomplete root development. J Endod 39:319–326

Xu JG, Zhu SY, Heng BC, Dissanayaka WL, Zhang CF (2017) TGF-β1-induced differentiation of SHED into functional smooth muscle cells. Stem Cell Res Ther 8(1):10

Yang W, Harris MA, Cui Y, Mishina Y, Harris SE, Gluhak-Heinrich J (2012) Bmp2 is required for odontoblast differentiation and pulp vasculogenesis. J Dent Res 91:58–64

Yang J, Ye L, Hui TQ, Yang DM, Huang DM, Zhou XD, Mao JJ et al (2015) Bone morphogenetic protein 2-induced human dental pulp cell differentiation involves p38 mitogen-activated protein kinase-activated canonical WNT pathway. Int J Oral Sci 7(2):95–102

Yang L, Angelova Volponi A, Pang Y, Sharpe PT (2017a) Mesenchymal cell community effect in whole tooth bioengineering. J Dent Res 96(2):186–191

Yang G, Yuan G, MacDougall M, Zhi C, Chen S (2017b) BMP-2 induced Dspp transcription is mediated by Dlx3/Osx signaling pathway in odontoblasts. Sci Rep 7(1):10775

Young CS, Terada S, Vacanti JP, Honda M, Bartlett JD, Yelick PC (2002) Tissue engineering of complex tooth structures on biodegradable polymer scaffolds. J Dent Res 81(10):695–700

Yu J, Deng Z, Shi J et al (2006) Differentiation of dental pulp stem cells into regular-shaped dentin-pulp complex induced by tooth germ cell conditioned medium. Tissue Eng 12:3097–3105

Zanini M, Sautier JM, Berdal A, Simon S (2012) Biodentine induces immortalized murine pulp cell differentiation into odontoblast-like cells and stimulates biomineralization. J Endod 38:1220–1226

Zanini M, Meyer E, Simon S (2017) Pulp inflammation diagnosis from clinical to inflammatory mediators: a systematic review. J Endod 43(7):1033–1051

Zhang LX, Shen LL, Ge SH, Wang LM, Yu XJ, Xu QC et al (2015) Systemic BMSC homing in the regeneration of pulp-like tissue and the enhancing effect of stromal cell-derived factor-1 on BMSC homing. Int J Clin Exp Pathol 8(9):10261–10271

Zhang Z, Nör F, Oh M, Cucco C, Shi S, Nör JE (2016) Wnt/β-Catenin signaling determines the vasculogenic fate of postnatal mesenchymal stem cells. Stem Cells 34(6):1576–1587

Zhang W, Vazquez B, Oreadi D, Yelick PC (2017) Decellularized tooth bud scaffolds for tooth regeneration. J Dent Res 96(5):516–523

Current Clinical Practice and Future Translation in Regenerative Endodontics

Stéphane Simon

10.1 Introduction

Recent research advances, which demonstrate that the dentine-pulp complex is capable of repairing itself and regenerating mineralised tissue, offer the hope of new odontogenic treatment modalities that can protect the vital pulp, stimulate reactionary dentinogenesis and promote the revascularisation of a necrotic root canal system. The volume of an adult pulp is relatively small (less than 100 μL), so it might be predicted that regeneration of this tissue would be relatively straightforward. Currently, approaches are not, however, translated into clinical practice, as significant obstacles remain which are discussed below.

The dental pulp is a complex and highly specialised connective tissue that is enclosed in a mineralised shell and has a limited blood supply; however, these are only a few of the many obstacles faced by the clinicians and researchers attempting to design new therapeutic strategies for its regeneration. Regenerative endodontics should be considered as two entities. The first is dentine-pulp complex regeneration, which relates to preservation of pulp vitality (pulp capping, partial or complete pulpotomy). The second is dental pulp regeneration which relates to the repopulation and revitalisation of the tissue into an empty but infected root canal space.

S. Simon
Paris Diderot University, Paris, France

Hôpital de Rouen Normandie, Rouen, France

Laboratoire INSERM UMR 1138, Paris, France
e-mail: stephane.simon@univ-paris-diderot.fr

© Springer Nature Switzerland AG 2019
H. F. Duncan, P. R. Cooper (eds.), *Clinical Approaches in Endodontic Regeneration*,
https://doi.org/10.1007/978-3-319-96848-3_10

10.2 Dentine-Pulp Complex Regeneration

During a pulp capping procedure, a biomaterial is placed directly onto the exposed pulp after partial pulp tissue removal which eliminates any necrotic or inflamed areas. The primary aim is to protect the underlying tissue from any external irritants and in particular bacteria, which necessitate that the quality of the filling placement and seal are of the utmost importance. Classically, the seal was thought to be the critical factor that determined the success of the vital pulp procedure. In the 1990s, direct pulp caps and the use of resin-based composite materials appeared to deliver good medium-term clinical results; however, the deterioration of the material resulted in longer-term failures. The breakdown of the material seal with the dentine and subsequent bacterial infiltration prompted either an acute inflammatory response several months after treatment or tissue loss due to pulpal necrosis. These shortcomings have led to a shift in the underlying biological concepts of material development. A complete, biological closure of the wound comprising a long-term seal subsequently came to be seen as essential. To do this, materials with bioactive properties were developed with the explicit goal of inducing dentine bridge formation.

Traditionally, calcium hydroxide has been used as a pulp capping material, either hard setting, non-setting or in combination with resins for ease of manipulation. Application of hard-setting calcium hydroxide materials directly to the pulp stimulates a mineralised tissue barrier to form; however, the barrier is not uniform or bonded to the dentine wall, thereby preventing the formation of a good seal. Furthermore, calcium hydroxide materials dissolve over time, with evidence indicating that after only a matter of months, the capping material dissipates. As a result calcium hydroxide materials are no longer the material of choice for pulp capping indications. There are, however, three properties which are considered essential to these restorative materials (Simon et al. 2009a; Witherspoon 2008):

- The material should create an immediate seal in order to protect the pulp in the first few weeks when the dentine bridge is forming.
- The material should be non-toxic and biocompatible.
- The material should have bioactive properties that stimulate the formation of a mineralised barrier between the pulp and the material itself.

When the pulp is exposed, the odontoblastic palisade is damaged, resulting in the dentine-producing cells being lost. Therefore, to form the mineralised barrier, it is necessary to induce the development of new odontoblast-like cells, which can secrete dentine. As the original odontoblasts are highly differentiated and are post-mitotic, they cannot be replenished easily through mitosis of the cells bordering the wound, as might be the case during cellular repair of other connective tissues. Indeed the only way to rebuild the odontoblastic palisade in the injured area is to reinvoke developmental biological principles within the dental tissue-rebuilding process. To undertake this, progenitor cells (also referred to as 'stem cells') are required. These cells must first be directed to the damaged area through chemotaxis or plithotaxis (Hirata et al. 2014). Once they are in contact with the material, these cells must differentiate into dentine-secreting cells, and subsequently mineralised matrix synthesis must be triggered.

Ideally, the biomaterial used should promote cyto-attraction of progenitor cells and differentiation and stimulate synthesis and mineralisation processes. As these biological mechanisms are only partially understood, it has therefore not yet been possible to develop a truly biologically orientated material. Indeed the results obtained using biomaterials until now have often been discovered by chance. Investigation into how the materials work is currently ongoing, but unfortunately this starts once the dental device has been placed on the market.

With regard to the underlying biology, investigations are ongoing and are delivering results enabling our understanding. Dentine is a partially mineralised tissue whose organic phase consists of chains of collagen-Iα molecules which contain a number of non-collagen matrix proteins. These proteins are initially secreted by the odontoblasts and then encased and protected through the mineralisation process (Smith et al. 2016). The many matrix proteins include a large number of growth factors, especially from the families containing tissue growth factor beta (TGFβ), vascular endothelial growth factor (VEGF) and adrenomedullin (ADM). Any biological or therapeutic process that demineralises dentine will release these proteins and associated growth factors from the matrix. For example, caries-linked demineralisation induces release of these factors. While some of the growth factors may be removed or broken down due to the action of saliva, others will diffuse through the dentinal tubules towards the pulp cells. Another approach for releasing the growth factors in dentine is to use a biomaterial that triggers partial but somewhat controlled demineralisation when the biomaterial comes into contact with dentine. The released proteins subsequently trigger biological processes relating to tissue repair. Many biologically active proteins can be released from dentine using calcium hydroxide (Graham et al. 2006), mineral trioxide aggregate (MTA) (Tomson et al. 2007) or other therapeutic substances that partially demineralise dentine, such as the etching chemicals used during bonding (Ferracane et al. 2010). It is well known that the dentine matrix proteins released promote pulp healing by their stimulation of chemotaxis, angiogenesis (Ricucci et al. 2014) and the differentiation of progenitor cells down the dentinogenic lineage (Liu et al. 2005). Although biologically these effects are important in promoting tissue repair, there are currently no therapeutic solutions available that optimise the use of these proteins' properties.

Odontoblasts are well characterised for their role in the secretion and subsequent regulation of mineralisation of dentine. Genes control the speed of secretion (Simon et al. 2009b), and two distinct phases have been identified: primary and secondary dentinogenesis. If a carious lesion occurs, odontoblasts in the 'quiescent' phase of synthesis can be reactivated to synthesise tertiary dentine, known as reactionary dentine [for more detail, see review (Simon et al. 2009a)]. In addition to this role in synthesis, odontoblasts have two other functions, which include immune competence and mechanosensation. Via Toll-like receptors (TLRs) expressed on their cell surface, odontoblasts can bind bacterial toxins and components to stimulate cellular signalling that is communicated to the underlying connective tissue (Farges et al. 2009). Thus odontoblasts act as a protective barrier for the pulp by 'fending off' aggressors and responding by producing a suitable, intelligible signal for resident and distant immune cell recruitment and activation.

The distinctive structure of odontoblasts, with a cell body and a cytoplasmic extension, has a close resemblance to nerve cells (axon and synapse), and this is only heightened by their intercellular expression of nerve growth factor (NGF). While odontoblasts' involvement in the transmission of nerve impulses during dentine hypersensitivity has been fairly well documented in the literature, their precise role in this response has not yet been elucidated. Baroreceptors, sensors of changes in pressure, may act as an intermediary when they are stimulated by fluid movements in dentinal tubules, while the odontoblasts might also act as nerve cells directly. Regardless of how they are involved, odontoblasts sense this external information and probably act as a buffer during the pressure variations as is described in Brannström's theory, thus transmitting information to the underlying pulp tissue. In view of this topography, a rather semantic trend has recently emerged in which, instead of being called the 'dentine-pulp complex', pulp is referred to as a combination of pulp tissue and an odonto-dentinal complex (Simon et al. 2011).

When odontoblast cells are removed during injury or a therapeutic procedure, an open wound is created leaving an unprotected mass of connective tissue. This wound is closed, protected and stimulated to heal during a pulp capping procedure. The wound is initially closed and protected using a material that is ideally impenetrable to bacteria. For the next step, the chosen capping material should be bioactive in order to stimulate a dentine (or mineralised) bridge to form, which would make a durable, long-term protective barrier against bacteria for the underlying tissue. Notably pulp cells and odontoblasts are sensitive to growth factors and bio-stimulators, which during carious or biomaterial-induced demineralisation are released from the dentine matrix and can diffuse within the dentinal tubules. Growth factors from the TGFβ family signalling are understood to play a key role in dentine-pulp complex repair, and it is understood these molecules can reawaken cells that are in the 'secondary' dentinogenic phase (Simon et al. 2013a). Reactivation can occur via the MAP kinase pathway with the phosphorylation of p38 (Simon et al. 2010).

10.3   Pulp Inflammation and Healing

Pulpitis or 'toothache' is associated with mild to severe pain and has other adverse effects, which leads to the destruction and necrosis of the pulp tissue. Preventing or treating this pain requires removal of the inflamed tissue, and this surgical procedure can be invasive, requiring the removal of the entire pulp (pulpectomy). The adverse effects of inflammation, however, should be balanced with the benefits this systematic pathophysiological step confers in cases of tissue damage. Inflammation is necessary as it marks the first step of tissue convalescence. Clear evidence of this is provided by the fact that immunosuppressed patients, whose inflammatory response is disrupted, experience complications in the healing process or do not heal at all (Shanmugam et al. 2012). Host inflammation is arguably beneficial in two ways, by cleaning and disinfecting the wound area and by secreting a variety of substances and molecules that facilitate the healing and regeneration process.

In a clinical setting, pulpal inflammation is commonly classified as either 'reversible' or 'irreversible' pulpitis. This idea of reversibility originates from the fact that, in some cases, the process is controlled and it can be halted and then guided to aid in healing. In other cases, where the inflammation is too advanced to be controlled, the only viable option is to completely remove the inflamed tissue in order to preserve the unaffected tissue. The concept of 'irreversible' pulpitis thus merely refers to a certain clinical or therapeutic situation associated with relatively basic diagnostic elements (type of pain, persistence, etc.). In no way do these 'clinical clues' provide any actual information on the state of inflammation of the tissue. This lack of correlation has been demonstrated for many years (Dummer et al. 1980) and has been confirmed in other studies since (Ricucci et al. 2014).

Many studies have assessed the markers of pulp inflammation and their potential use in diagnosis or treatment. Both quantitative (number of inflamed cells) and qualitative variations have been demonstrated and directly correlated with the depth of the carious lesion, the pulp's proximity to the lesion and inflammatory state of the pulp (Fig. 10.1). Certain biological markers could potentially be used to identify inflammatory standards that must not be exceeded if the pulp is to be saved. Although these markers are known to exist, more specific information remains elusive. Studies are also required to develop reliable diagnostic tools that are robust and reproducible. Until these markers and diagnostic tools are commercially available,

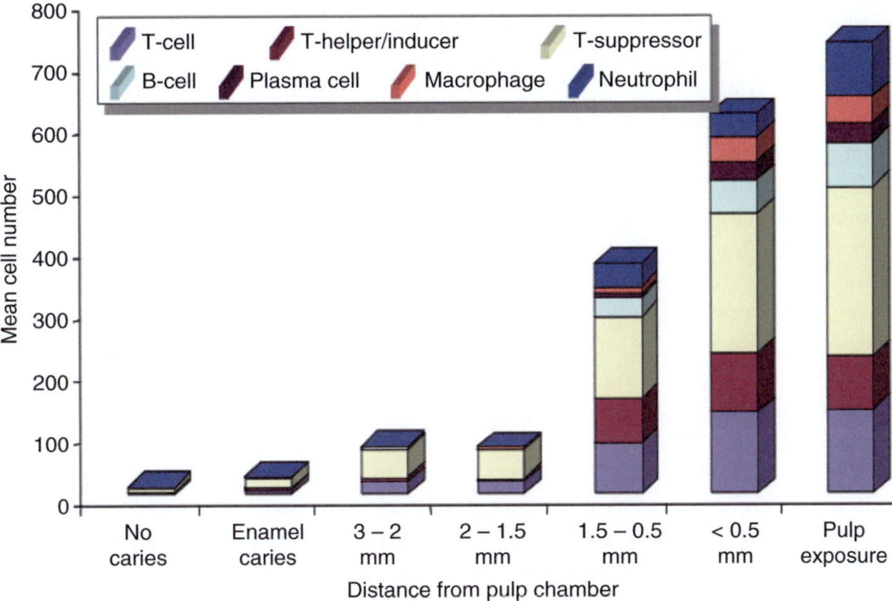

Fig. 10.1 Quantitation of inflammatory cells associated with increasing depth of the carious lesion (from Cooper et al. (2011))

practitioners must continue with rather basic tools, such as dental anamnesis to define the patient's pain as well as thermal and electrical tests whose reliability remains suboptimal. Other options include controlling haemostasis at the time of pulp exposure and/or partial pulpectomy. Inflammation is associated with hypervascularisation, which means that the damaged tissue can be identified clinically (though this might not always be relevant). This hypervascularisation can be identified by the bleeding that arises when vascular connective tissue is cut. In practice, the lesion can be packed with a damp cotton wool ball placed directly on the tissue with pressure applied for 1–2 min. This is sufficient time to achieve haemostasis under physiological conditions. If bleeding persists, it may be assumed that some of the pulp tissue is still inflamed and partial removal is necessary until healthy tissue is exposed.

To conclude it is clear that the tools for identifying and testing for the presence of inflamed tissue in exposed pulp are both arbitrary and inadequate. Still, no other methods are currently available to improve diagnostics in situ, which renders it impossible to list all of the formal indications for a pulp cap. Additional research is therefore necessary to identify new diagnostic markers, develop suitable, accurate diagnostic tools and improve long-term results. This is critical as controlling inflammation remains central to the success of pulp capping therapies.

10.4 Pulp Capping and Biomaterials

MTA, commercially marketed as ProRoot MTA® (Dentsply Maillefer), and other products have gradually become the vital pulp treatment material of choice over recent years. Packaged as a powder to be mixed with water, the substance is placed onto a glass tray and applied directly to the pulp using a dedicated instrument such as the MAP System® (PDSA, Vevey, Switzerland) or other carrier. As with an Amalgam Carrier, the material is loaded into the tip and then ejected from the syringe by the Teflon piston. The material is not packed in but instead lightly tapped into contact with the pulp and the dentine wall using thick paper or a cotton pellet (Fig. 10.2). The manufacturer's instructions stipulate that the material should set before placing the final coronal restoration; however, as the material takes over 4 h to set, this is not readily possible, and placing the final restoration immediately is necessary. Care must be taken during this procedure to avoid washing away the recently placed restoration. Note, if the preparation protocol stipulates spraying dental tissue with water, it is recommended to complete this step first before applying the MTA (Fig. 10.3).

The beneficial biological properties of this material have been shown in the literature in vitro and in vivo as well as in clinical trials which compare it with other biomaterials (Hilton et al. 2013). The enhanced histological quality of the dentine bridges formed using this material compared with calcium hydroxide has previously been demonstrated (Nair et al. 2007). A commonly reported disadvantage of this material however relates to its handling difficulties. Several manufacturers have tried developing galenic forms that are easier to use, both in terms of preparation

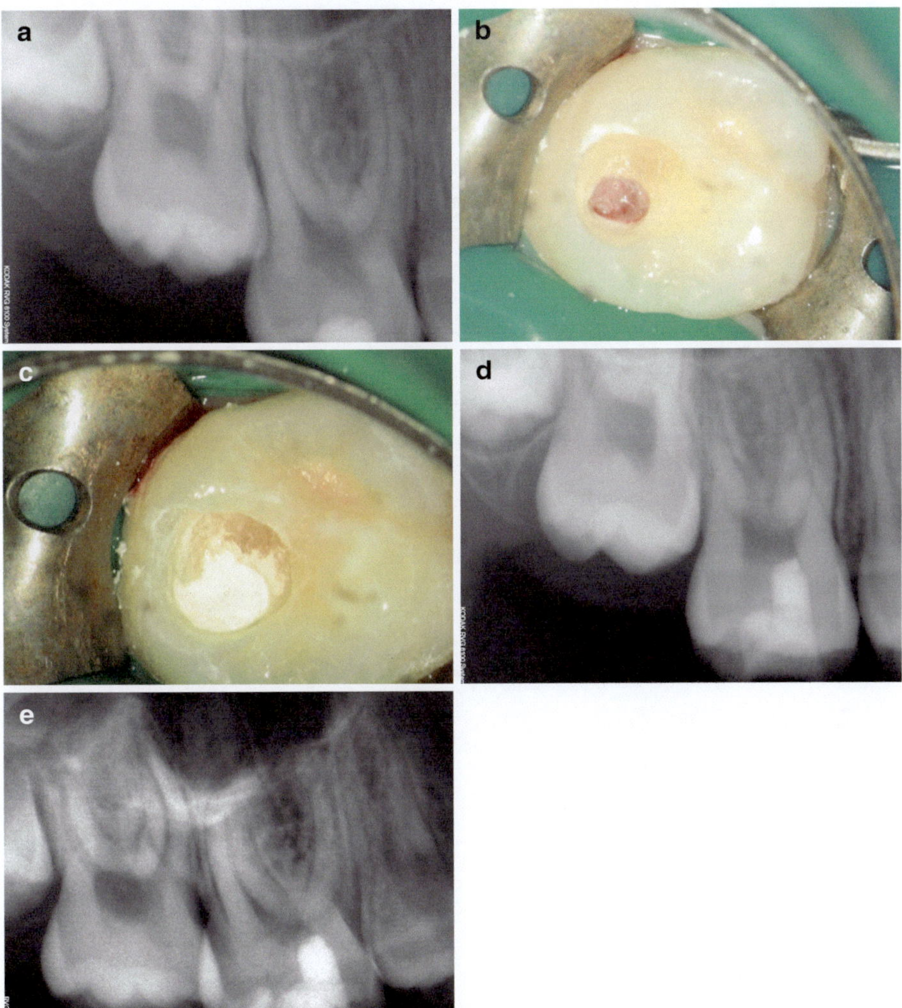

Fig. 10.2 Pulp capping procedure on the first upper molar of a 9-year-old child. After carious tissue excavation, dental pulp was exposed up to 2 mm in diameter. Pulp capping was completed with ProRoot MTA (Dentsply Sirona). (**a**) Preoperative radiograph, (**b**) pulp exposure and haemostasis control, (**c**) material placement, (**d**) postoperative radiographs and (**e**) 1-year radiographic review. Note the presence of the mineralised bridge in direct contact with the applied material

and application. While ergonomically these substances are promising, there has not been a study to date that demonstrates that the results achieved are the same as those of the non-modified form. Such studies are essential if the modified material is to be considered eligible for pulp capping.

More recently, a tricalcium silicate-based material (Biodentine®, Septodont, France) has appeared on the market. Initially developed as a dentine substitute for coronal fillings, the positive effects it was shown to have on biological tissues led to

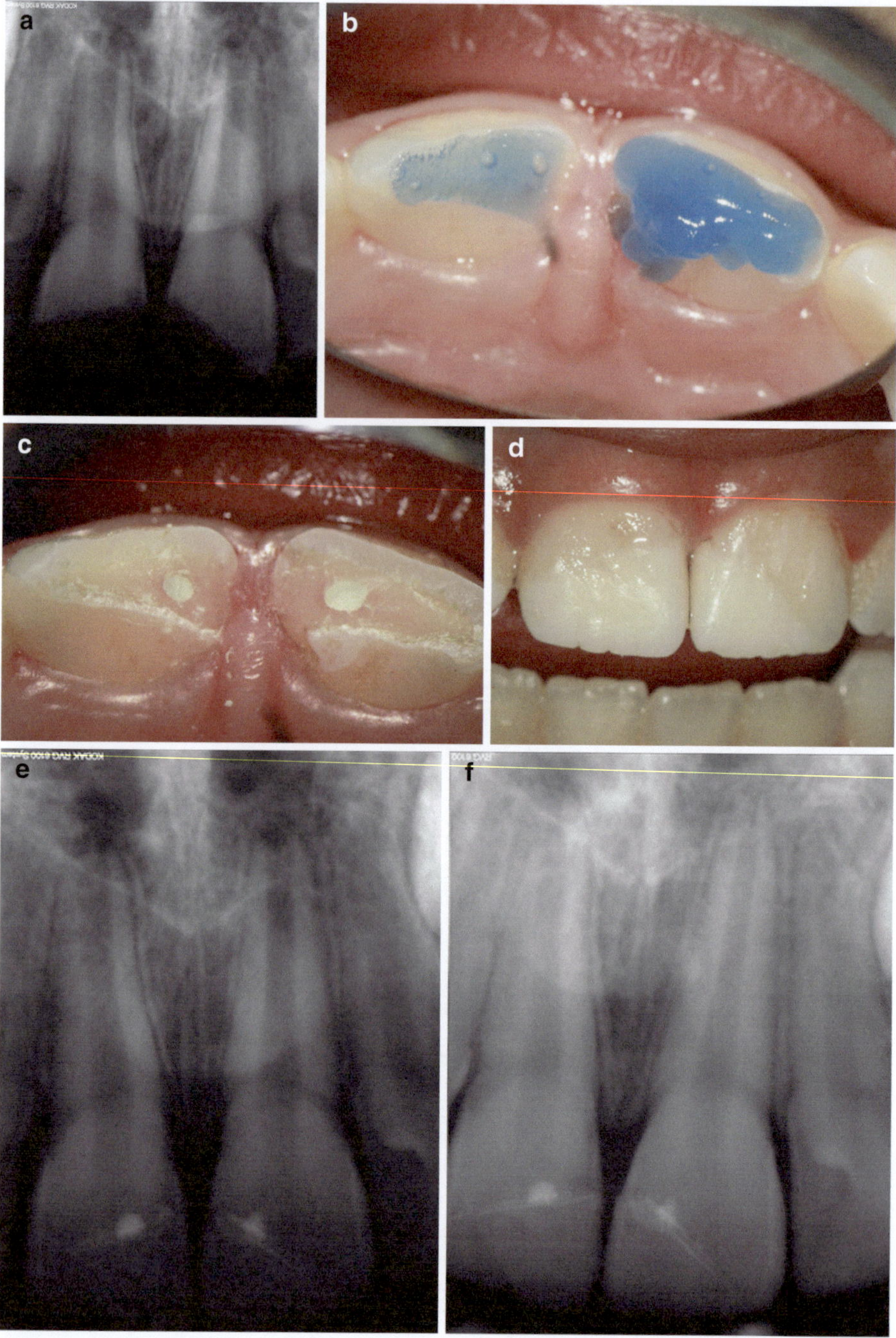

Fig. 10.3 Pulp capping of an immature tooth with direct coronal restoration. (**a**) Preoperative radiographs. (**b**) Hard tissue etching with phosphoric acid. (**c**) Pulp capping material (Pro-Root MTA (Dentsply Sirona)) is directly applied on the pulp tissue. (**d**) Fractured fragments of the traumatised teeth were replaced and bonded at the same session. (**e**) Postoperative radiograph. (**f**) One-year review radiograph. The tooth responds positively and normally to sensitive tests. Note that apexogenesis and root canal lengthening occurred due to the maintenance of pulp vitality

an extension of its indications to include pulp capping. One of its notable qualities is its effect on the initiation of mineralisation (Laurent et al. 2012) and on cellular differentiation (Zanini et al. 2012). These results provide excellent grounds for optimism for its long-term clinical potential. While positive biological interaction of these materials with pulp cells has been shown, the materials also have the ability to induce dentin matrix protein release upon contact. This has been demonstrated for both calcium hydroxide (Graham et al. 2006) and MTA (Tomson et al. 2007), but not Biodentine® as of yet. The materials described above are of particular interest as they combine a direct biological effect on the pulp with an indirect effect by causing a gradual, delayed release of growth factors, including some with anti-inflammatory activities. Given these results, it may therefore be worthwhile in the future to not only apply the material to the exposed pulp but to extend the application area to include the adjacent dentine walls where preparation of the cavity has made the dentine thinner. Subsequently, the material in contact with the dentine could liberate the matrix components, which could diffuse through the dentinal tubules and thereby promote the healing process within the pulp. There is particular potential for Biodentine® to aid in this regard as it is marketed as a bulk-fill restorative material designed to fill the entire cavity, unlike MTA. Indeed, Biodentine® could be used as a bulk-filling material to enable the undertaking of the pulp capping and coronal filling procedures in the same step. Notably, however, the mechanical behaviour of the material necessitates an additional procedure in which it is coated with a bonded composite which both makes the restoration more aesthetically pleasing and stops the substitution material from 'dissolving' in the oral fluids.

10.5 Application of Pulp Capping and 'Bio-products' to Stimulate Regeneration

The dentine extracellular matrix (ECM) contains a variety of molecules involved in the regulation of dentinogenesis. Attempts have been made to use ECM proteins (expressed in recombinant bacteria) to stimulate pulp regeneration. For example, Rutherford and co-workers (Rutherford et al. 1993, 1994) implanted bone morphogenetic protein-7 (BMP-7, also known as OP-1) into the pulp of monkeys using agarose beads as carriers. Osteodentine was formed, which completely filled the root canal space. The authors obtained better results with the application of bone sialoprotein (BSP), which induced formation of a more solid, homogenous dentinal bridge that occluded the pulp exposure. The biological effects of several other dental tissue-derived molecules have also been examined, including dentonin, an acid synthetic peptide derived from matrix extracellular phosphoglycoprotien (MEPE), and A + 4 and A − 4, two splice products of the amelogenin gene. Each molecule induced regeneration of a superficial pulp (Goldberg et al. 2009).

In the tissues surrounding the agarose beads used as carriers, pulp cells were recruited and showed differentiation towards an osteo-/odontogenic lineage. Furthermore, the cells were mitotically active, as evidenced by their staining with antibodies to proliferating cell nuclear antigen (PCNA). Indeed pulp cells migrated and underwent early differentiation, forming a ring around and adjacent to the surface of the agarose beads. Furthermore while they initially expressed mesenchymal markers, they subsequently became osteopontin and dentine-sialoprotein positive, both markers indicative of cell differentiation and necessary for the formation of a reparative dentine matrix. This cascade of differentiation events leads to the formation of ortho- or osteodentine. Such biological analyses have helped elucidate the processes occurring during pulp capping and tissue regeneration; however, before the direct clinical application of biomolecules, more studies are required to confirm the advantages and safety of such bio-products versus the mineral cements currently available.

10.6   New Developments

Considerable improvement in the development of biomaterials during the last 10 years has helped reawaken interest in techniques to preserve pulp vitality. Alongside these developments, our understanding of pulp biology continues to progress, which makes it possible to explain the reason for certain clinical failures. It must be noted that the weakness of these minimally invasive procedures remains the assessment of the state of inflammation of the pulp in need of treatment. In a clinical situation, it remains impossible to predict how much pulp tissue needs to be removed to eliminate the risk of leaving any inflamed tissue. Recently it has been proposed that a relatively large swathe of tissue should be removed so as to ensure that all of the inflamed tissue is eliminated; however, this should be undertaken without resulting in a complete pulpectomy of the tooth. Traditionally, coronal pulpotomies were restricted to primary teeth or immature teeth with open apices; however, in the future pulp chamber pulpectomies might come to be seen as an endodontic therapeutic alternative to pulpectomies and root canal treatment for cases with irreversible pulpitis (Fig. 10.4). In this procedure, all of the pulp from the pulp chamber is removed, and the radicular stumps are capped via the same procedure described earlier. Preliminary studies have shown promise (Simon et al. 2013b), but these must be supplemented with more formal studies before it can be deemed a generally viable procedure.

10.7   Revascularisation, Revitalisation and Pulp Regeneration

The therapeutic strategies discussed above are aimed at limiting tissue degeneration and maintaining the vitality of the remainder of the pulp. Importantly, if there is severe pulp damage, severe inflammation or necrosis, then it is probable that preservation of the pulp will not be possible. In such cases, the clinician must perform a pulpectomy, disinfect the entire canal and place a root canal filling to prevent reinfection by bacteria. While current root canal therapeutic approaches do provide reliable outcomes, a better approach for endodontic treatment in the future might be to stimulate de novo synthesis of pulp or connective tissue inside the root canal system in situ. However, regeneration of pulpal tissue within an empty canal has technical hurdles that remain need to be overcome. For example, questions remain

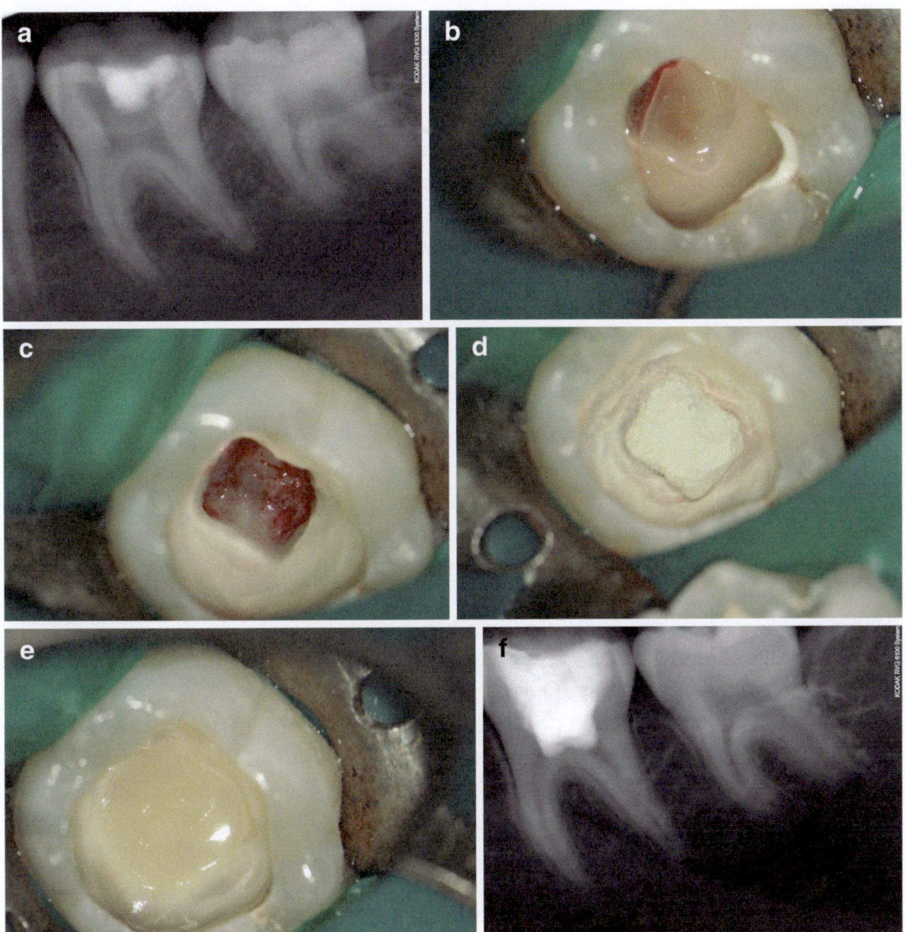

Fig. 10.4 Endodontic treatment of a first lower molar by pulp chamber pulpotomy. (**a**) Preoperative radiograph. (**b**) Occlusal view after removal of caries. The pulp is largely exposed and bleeding is difficult to control. (**c**) Removal of the dental pulp from the entire pulp chamber and haemostasis control of the pulp at the entrance of the root canals. (**d**) Placement of the bioactive material in direct contact with the pulp chamber floor and the pulp at the entrance of the root canals. (**e**) Coronal restoration ongoing with glass ionomer and resin-based composite. (**f**) One-year postoperative review radiograph. Tooth is asymptomatic, and no periapical signs of inflammation are evident. This can be considered as a clinical success

concerning the optimal type of scaffold to be used, the source and recruitment of stem cells and the exact cocktail of signalling molecules required for tissue development, maturation and neovascularisation.

The first successful attempts at root canal revascularisation were made in the 1960s, with the principal aim being to regenerate dental pulp tissue de novo (Ostby 1961). One of the biggest limitations of this early approach was that viable cells could only be obtained by inducing bleeding into the root canal space, which resulted in these cells being derived from the circulation, cementum, periodontal ligament or alveolar bone—that is, they were not of pulpal origin. It was not until 2001 that the goal of root canal revascularisation gained renewed interest (Iwaya et al. 2001). A relatively recent proposal was to use stem cells from the apical papilla (SCAP), obtained by disorganising the apical papilla tissue with an endodontic file and allowing the SCAP to be carried into the empty canal space by the blood flow forming the blood clot.

Despite a significant number of published case studies, little is known about the exact cellular processes involved in this therapeutic approach. Most case studies show examples of revascularisation of the pulp space where there was a pre-existing lesion of endodontic origin. Several of these publications demonstrate completion of apexogenesis, which previously ceased because of pulp necrosis, as well as increased dentinal thickness of the root end and reduced volume of the root canal space. These observations tend to support regeneration of a dental pulp-like tissue inside the root canal, with peripheral cells showing dentinogenic capability. However, this treatment is not always predictable, as some case reports described teeth which subsequently need to be extracted following treatment.

The first histological observations of regenerated tissue using the revascularisation technique inside a tooth were obtained in a dog model (Thibodeau et al. 2007). Within the root canal space, dentinal walls covered with a layer of cementum were evident accompanied by a neo-ligament and an osteoid structure. More recently, histological analysis of teeth treated by simple revascularisation (Shimizu et al. 2013) or by filling with platelet-rich plasma (Martin et al. 2013) showed a mineralised layer deposited on the radicular walls. This newly formed tissue appeared to be of periodontal tissue rather than pulpal origin and therefore was not formed by dentinogenesis. Instead, the recruited progenitor cells likely migrated from the apical papilla or from the surrounding periradicular tissues and differentiated into periodontal tissue-like cells. Perhaps, radiographic analysis in these studies may have incorrectly inferred that the mineralised tissue was dentine rather than cementum, as shown by recent histological analysis. If this histological evidence is supported in the future, then apexogenesis becomes difficult to assess when formed by revascularisation. As an alternative, apical closure (apexification) with periodontal structure can be induced by MTA as described in the literature (Nosrat et al. 2013; Simon et al. 2007). This treatment is really root canal treatment, but not a regenerative procedure per se.

Whether or not this treatment modality can be considered efficacious depends on the therapeutic objective. If it is to induce healing of the periapical tissue, stimulate bone regeneration and relieve the patient of signs or symptoms, then it could be termed a success. However, if the objective is to regenerate new pulp tissue, then this treatment would be considered a failure. In other words, although it might be a clinical success, the result would not have been achieved via the intended biological mechanism and could not be termed regenerative endodontics.

The objectives of endodontic treatment of an infected tooth are (1) to disinfect the root canal system and (2) to prevent reinfection over time. Both these objectives should lead to favourable bone healing and regeneration of the periradicular tissues. Filling the root canal space with a biological tissue avoids many of the disadvantages of using a synthetic material, such as potential loss of seal and toxicity. Furthermore, treatment using biological tissue has the important advantage of keeping the root canal immunocompetent to protect it against further reinfection (Fig. 10.5).

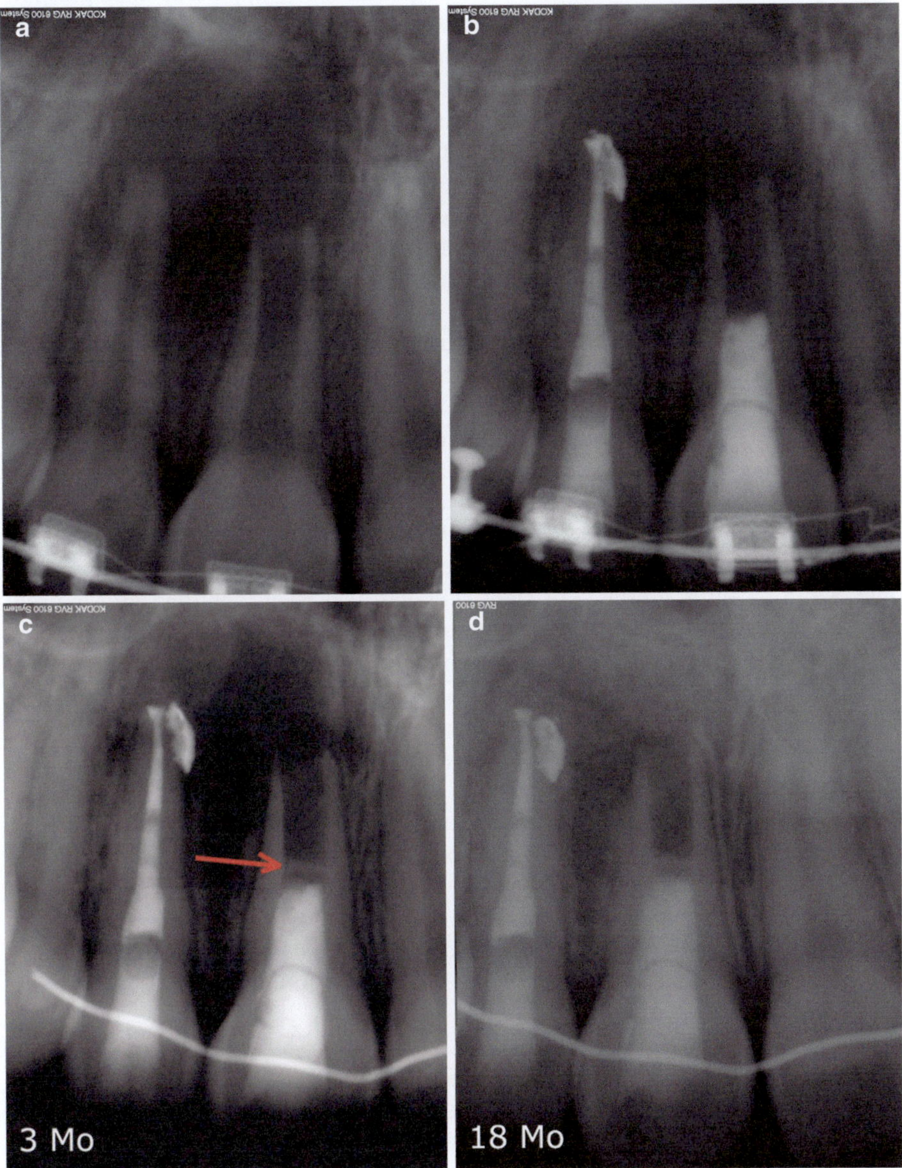

Fig. 10.5 (**a**) Preoperative radiograph of tooth #11 and #12 demonstrating a large periapical radiolucency in a 15-year-old teenager. Both teeth were unresponsive to sensitivity tests. (**b**) Tooth #12 has been root canal treated and #11 with revitalisation procedure. (**c**) At 3 months postoperatively. The size of the radiolucency decreased, and a mineralised barrier was clearly visible. (**d**) 18-month recall—bone healing is complete

Revitalisation is a technique which aims to fill the pulp space with a vital tissue. This replacement tissue is different from what was initially present in the canal and will not transform into dentine. Among the 132 cases published to date, only one showed the presence of dental pulp inside the treated canal—a true palisade of odontoblasts and well-organised dental pulp tissue. An important distinguishing feature of this latter case was that the tooth experienced pulpitis, not necrosis. Thus, the odontoblastic layer was generally intact, and the treatment consisted of disorganising the remaining pulp tissue without destroying it. Although the dentine-odontoblastic complex is highly specialised and difficult to regenerate, resident cells still present were able to regenerate the pulp tissue and preserve it. By definition, 'regeneration' requires that the pulp tissue reforms in the vacant root canal space and subsequently for it to perform normal homeostatic function. If this definition is accepted, then none of our present therapeutic strategies can be said to be regenerative as they do not fulfil these requirements. Instead, the treatments should be regarded as reparative modalities only.

While these considerations are obviously important, they remain as scientific problems in need of solutions. Clinically, however, these therapeutic strategies have their place even though clear indications and contraindications have not yet been determined for them. Beyond the semantics of definitions, many questions remain about how a vital tissue can form in a vacant biological space. The presence of stem cells in a revascularised canal has been clearly demonstrated (Lovelace et al. 2011). The most plausible hypothesis to explain this is that recruitment of SCAP is critical to the formation of this new tissue; however, the origin of these cells remains debatable. More recently, presence of stem cells has also been identified into the root canal of mature teeth after equivalent treatment of revitalisation. By extrapolation the presence of the apical papilla seems not to be absolutely necessary for the revitalisation process. Further investigations are ongoing in an attempt to identify the role of stem cell niches involved in the healing process (Chrepa et al. 2015).

At this point these assumptions suggest that the clinical indications of revascularisation treatment should be confined to immature teeth; however, if progenitor cells could be recruited from a niche other than the apical papilla, then the indications of treatment could be extended to mature teeth. If progenitor cell niches lie inside periradicular tissues, then their recruitment into the root canal space should in theory be achievable. This may explain why the newly formed tissue is closer to periodontal as opposed to pulpal tissue-like. If proven successful, then treatment of mature teeth using this method may be possible in the future.

10.8 Revitalisation Protocol (ESE Guideline Recommendation) (Galler et al. 2016)

Session 1:

– Tooth cleaning, anaesthesia, field isolation, disinfection of work field (e.g. iso-betadine).
– Preparation of access cavity.

- Remove loose or necrotic pulp tissue using suitable endodontic instruments.
- Avoid mechanical instrumentation of the root canal walls.
- Irrigate with 1.5–3% sodium hypochlorite (20 mL, 5 min), use of side-vented needle, placement 2 mm above vital tissue.
- Bleeding or exudate (control with paper points) may require extended irrigation.
- Irrigate with 0.9% saline (5 mL) to minimise cytotoxic effects of sodium hypochlorite on vital tissues.
- Dry with paper points.
- Irrigate with 20 mL of 17% EDTA.
- Insert a non-discolouring calcium hydroxide product homogenously into the root canal.
- Place coronal seal directly onto intracanal dressing with a minimum thickness according to the used restoration material.

Session 2 (2–4 weeks later):

- If signs of inflammation have not subsided, replace calcium hydroxide. Administration of systemic antibiotics may be considered at this stage.
- Cleaning, anaesthesia, field isolation, disinfection of work field.
- Remove temporary seal.
- Irrigate with 17% EDTA (20 mL, 5 min), use of side-vented needle, placement 2 mm above vital tissue.
- Irrigate with 0.9% saline (5 mL) to reduce adverse effects of irrigants to target cells.
- Remove access liquid with paper points.
- Induce bleeding by mechanical irritation of periapical tissue and rotational movement of an apically prebent file (e.g. Hedström ISO 40).
- Allow the canal to fill with blood until 2 mm below the gingival margin, and wait for blood clot formation for 15 min.
- Cut a collagen matrix to a diameter larger than the coronal part of the root canal and a height of 2–3 mm, place on top of the blood clot, allow the matrix to soak with liquid and avoid formation of a hollow space.
- Place calcium-silicate-based cement (e.g. MTA) over the collagen matrix in a thin homogeneous layer of about 2 mm. Should be placed below the cement-enamel junction.
- Apply a flowable light-curable glass ionomer or calcium hydroxide cement.
- Refresh the cavity walls with a diamond bur or grit blast with aluminium oxide.
- Seal with adhesive restoration.

Follow-up appointments should be performed after 3, 6, 12 and 18 and 24 months, after that annually for up to 5 years. Clinical diagnostic tests should be performed according to the flow chart.

10.9　Regeneration, Repair and Remodelling: Concluding Remarks

Bone undergoes constant remodelling, with turnover rates of less than a few months. Therefore, newly secreted bone tissue will merge with older tissue such that the bone becomes a combination of old and new tissue. Remodelling can also lead to partial or complete destruction of regenerated tissue in cases where the tissue is not biologically compatible with its microenvironment (Leucht et al. 2008).

In contrast with bone, remodelling of dentine does not occur, and newly formed tissue is not replaced. Histologically, tertiary dentine can appear similar to secondary dentine; however, it is not truly the same nor does it exhibit tubular continuity with the pre-existing dentine. The dentine-pulp interface may be considered a dentine-odontoblastic complex, because dentine is uniquely penetrated by odontoblast processes which extend to and intermingle with the odontoblastic palisade beneath, forming a cohesive layer. This layer acts like a membrane, separating itself from the pulp underneath by the acellular zone of Weil. Breakage of this odontoblastic membrane by caries, trauma or iatrogenic damage exposes the pulp tissue, leaving it vulnerable to further degradation.

Determination of the origin of tissue laid down by the processes of repair/regeneration generally relies on identification of cellular markers (usually proteins) sequestrated by the cells that produced the tissue. Based on the presence of such markers as well as the cellular behaviour (especially biomineralisation) and structure of the new tissue, conclusions can be drawn about the origin of these dental tissue secretions. Nonetheless, because the newly secreted tissues often lack specific molecular markers, the implicated cells are given the suffix '-like' (e.g. odontoblast-like). By using this approach, it is possible to distinguish between normal tissue and altered tissue, suggesting that the latter is formed from reparative rather than regenerative processes. In the field of tooth biology, it is conventional to consider the mineralised tissue secreted by dental cells to be dentine; however, very few experiments have sought to characterise the type of mineral produced during the synthesis of tertiary dentine. It was recently demonstrated by X-ray analysis that the crystal structure of the reparative dentine formed after pulp capping was close to that of orthodentine but differed in terms of protein levels (Simon et al. 2008). However, so little is known about the precise nature of mineralised tissue that the formal differences that may exist between dentine and bone have not been properly elucidated. Such knowledge would allow us to describe the precise nature and composition of secreted tissue and identify the healing process as truly regenerative or reparative.

References

Chrepa V, Henry MA, Daniel BJ, Diogenes A (2015) Delivery of apical mesenchymal stem cells into root canals of mature teeth. J Dent Res 94:1653

Cooper PR, McLachlan JL, Simon S, Graham LW, Smith AJ (2011) Mediators of inflammation and regeneration. Adv Dent Res 23:290–295

Dummer PM, Hicks R, Huws D (1980) Clinical signs and symptoms in pulp disease. Int Endod J 13(1):27–35

Farges JC, Keller JF, Carrouel F, Durand SH, Romeas A, Bleicher F et al (2009) Odontoblasts in the dental pulp immune response. J Exp Zool B Mol Dev Evol 312B(5):425–436

Ferracane JL, Cooper PR, Smith AJ (2010) Can interaction of materials with the dentin-pulp complex contribute to dentin regeneration? Odontology 98(1):2–14

Galler KM, Krastl G, Simon S, Van Gorp G, Meschi N, Vahedi B, Lambrechts P (2016) European Society of Endodontology position statement: revitalization procedures. Int Endod J. 49(8):717–723. https://doi.org/10.1111/iej.12629 Epub 2016 Apr 23

Goldberg M, Six N, Chaussain C, DenBesten P, Veis A, Poliard A (2009) Dentin extracellular matrix molecules implanted into exposed pulps generate reparative dentin: a novel strategy in regenerative dentistry. J Dent Res 88:396–399

Graham L, Cooper PR, Cassidy N, Nor JE, Sloan AJ, Smith AJ (2006) The effect of calcium hydroxide on solubilisation of bio-active dentine matrix components. Biomaterials 27(14): 2865–2873

Hilton TJ, Ferracane JL, Mancl L (2013) Comparison of CaOH with MTA for direct pulp capping: a PBRN randomized clinical trial. J Dent Res 92(7 Suppl):16S–22S

Hirata A, Dimitrova-Nakov S, Djole S-X, Ardila H, Baudry A, Kellermann O et al (2014) Plithotaxis, a collective cell migration, regulates the sliding of proliferating pulp cells located in the apical niche. Connect Tissue Res 55(Suppl 1):68–72

Iwaya SI, Ikawa M, Kubota M (2001) Revascularization of an immature permanent tooth with apical periodontitis and sinus tract. Dent Traumatol 17(4):185–187

Laurent P, Camps J, About I (2012) Biodentine(TM) induces TGF-β1 release from human pulp cells and early dental pulp mineralization. Int Endod J 45:439

Leucht P, Kim J-B, Amasha R, James AW, Girod S, Helms JA (2008) Embryonic origin and Hox status determine progenitor cell fate during adult bone regeneration. Development 135(17):2845–2854

Liu J, Jin T, Ritchie H, Smith A, Clarkson B (2005) In vitro differentiation and mineralization of human dental pulp cells induced by dentin extract. In Vitro Cell Dev Biol Anim 41(7): 232

Lovelace TW, Henry MA, Hargreaves KM, Diogenes A (2011) Evaluation of the delivery of mesenchymal stem cells into the root canal space of necrotic immature teeth after clinical regenerative endodontic procedure. J Endod 37(2):133–138

Martin G, Ricucci D, Gibbs JL, Lin LM (2013) Histological findings of revascularized/revitalized immature permanent molar with apical periodontitis using platelet-rich plasma. J Endod 39:138–144

Nair PN, Duncan HF, Pitt Ford TR, Luder HU (2007) Histological, ultrastructural and quantitative investigations on the response of healthy human pulps to experimental capping with mineral trioxide aggregate: a randomized controlled trial. Int Endod J 41(2):128–150

Nosrat A, Li KL, Vir K, Hicks ML, Fouad AF (2013) Is pulp regeneration necessary for root maturation? J Endod 39(10):1291–1295

Ostby BN (1961) The role of the blood clot in endodontic therapy. An experimental histologic study. Acta Odontol Scand 19:324–353

Ricucci D, Loghin S, Siqueira JF (2014) Correlation between clinical and histologic pulp diagnoses. J Endod 40:1932–1939

Rutherford RB, Wahle J, Tucker M, Rueger D, Charette M (1993) Induction of reparative dentine formation in monkeys by recombinant human osteogenic protein-1. Arch Oral Biol 38(7):571–576

Rutherford RB, Spångberg L, Tucker M, Rueger D, Charette M (1994) The time-course of the induction of reparative dentine formation in monkeys by recombinant human osteogenic protein-1. Arch Oral Biol 39(10):833–838

Shanmugam V, Schilling A, Germinario A, Met M, Kim P, Steinberg J et al (2012) Prevalence of immune disease in patients with wounds presenting to a tertiary wound healing center. Int Wound J 9(4):403–411

Shimizu E, Ricucci D, Albert J, Alobaid AS, Gibbs JL, Huang GT-J et al (2013) Clinical, radiographic, and histological observation of a human immature permanent tooth with chronic apical abscess after revitalization treatment. J Endod 39:1078–1083

Simon S, Rilliard F, Berdal A, Machtou P (2007) The use of mineral trioxide aggregate in one-visit apexification treatment: a prospective study. Int Endod J 40(3):186–197

Simon S, Cooper P, Smith A, Picard B, Naulin Ifi C, Berdal A (2008) Evaluation of a new laboratory model for pulp healing: preliminary study. Int Endod J 41(9):781

Simon S, Cooper PR, Lumley PJ, Berdal A, Tomson PL, Smith AJ (2009a) Understanding pulp biology for routine clinical practice. Endod Pract Today 3(3):171–184

Simon SR, Smith AJ, Lumley PJ, Berdal A, Smith G, Finney S et al (2009b) Molecular characterisation of young and mature odontoblasts. Bone 45(4):693–703

Simon S, Smith AJ, Berdal A, Lumley PJ, Cooper PR (2010) The MAP kinase pathway is involved in odontoblast stimulation via p38 phosphorylation. J Endod 36(2):256–259

Simon SRJ, Berdal A, Cooper PR, Lumley PJ, Tomson PL, Smith AJ (2011) Dentin-pulp complex regeneration: from lab to clinic. Adv Dent Res 23(3):340–345

Simon SR, Smith AJ, Lumley PJ, Cooper PR, Berdal A (2013a) The pulp healing process : from generation to regeneration. Larjava H, editor. Endod Topics 26:41–56

Simon S, Perard M, Zanini M, Smith AJ, Charpentier E, Djole SX et al (2013b) Should pulp chamber pulpotomy be seen as a permanent treatment? Some preliminary thoughts. Int Endod J 46(1):79–87

Smith AJ, Duncan HF, Diogenes A, Simon S, Cooper PR (2016) Exploiting the bioactive properties of the dentin-pulp complex in regenerative endodontics. J Endod 42(1):47–56

Thibodeau B, Teixeira F, Yamauchi M, Caplan DJ, Trope M (2007) Pulp revascularization of immature dog teeth with apical periodontitis. J Endod 33(6):680–689

Tomson PL, Grover LM, Lumley PJ, Sloan AJ, Smith AJ, Cooper PR (2007) Dissolution of bioactive dentine matrix components by mineral trioxide aggregate. J Dent 35(8):636–642

Witherspoon DE (2008) Vital pulp therapy with new materials: new directions and treatment perspectives--permanent teeth. J Endod 34(7 Suppl):S25–S28

Zanini M, Sautier JM, Berdal A, Simon S (2012) Biodentine induces immortalized murine pulp cell differentiation into odontoblast-like cells and stimulates biomineralization. J Endod 38(9):1220–1226

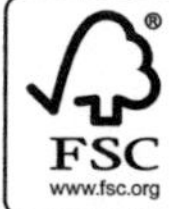